Health Care Politics

Health Care Politics

**Ideological and
Interest Group
Barriers to Reform**

Robert R. Alford

**The University of Chicago
Press** Chicago and London

ROBERT ALFORD is professor of sociology at the University of California at Santa Cruz and director of a new interdisciplinary graduate program. He is the author of various publications in the fields of sociology and political science.

The University of Chicago Press, Chicago 60637
The University of Chicago Press, Ltd., London

Library of Congress Cataloging in Publication Data

Alford, Robert R
  Health care politics.

  Bibliography: p.
  1. Medical care—United States. 2. Medical care—New York (City). 3. Medical policy—United States. I. Title. [DNLM: 1. Community health services—New York City. 2. Politics—New York City. WA546 AN7 A3h]
RA395.A3A59   362.1′0973   74-75611
ISBN   0-226-01379-0 (cloth)
ISBN   0-226-01380-4 (paper)

To Ann Wallace,
without whom this and many
other projects would never
have been finished.

Contents

Acknowledgments

This monograph was prepared under a grant to the Center for Policy Research, New York City, from the National Center for Health Research and Development, National Institute of Mental Health, Department of Health, Education, and Welfare. I am indebted to the Center for Policy Research for providing research facilities and particularly for making it possible for Ann Wallace to serve as my research associate during 1970-71.

A remarkable number of friends and colleagues have commented on various drafts of chapters 5 and 6, including Howard Aldrich, Astrida Butners, Jay Demerath, Nancy DiTomaso, David Elesh, Amitai Etzioni, Norman Fainstein, Roger Friedland, Richard C. Hill, Joel and Lily Hoffman, Ira Katznelson, Mark Kesselman, Judith Ladinsky, Edward Lehman, Sandra Lichty, David Mechanic, Murray Milner, Samuel Norich, Charles Perrow, Marc Renaud, Milton I. Roemer, and Edward T. Silva. Since I have sometimes neglected their severe criticisms, they can all dissent in good conscience.

I have accumulated a large number of intellectual debts in the course of undertaking this research in what is for me a new field—combining a problem of interorganizational theory with a substantive problem in medical sociology. Although I bring to this problem some background in political sociology, I hope my concern with power, conflict, and the stratification of interest groups adds rather than detracts from the analysis.

The hypothesis which most influenced this study is Murray Edelman's suggestion, set forth in two books—*The Symbolic Uses of Politics* (Urbana: University of Illinois Press, 1964) and *Politics as Symbolic Action: Mass Arousal and Quiescence* (Chicago: Markham Publishing

Company, 1971)—that politics serves simultaneously to provide tangible benefits to various elites and symbolic benefits to mass publics, quieting potential unrest, deflecting potential demands, and blurring the true allocation of rewards.

The research reported on in this book is entirely qualitative in character, since preliminary investigation of the available quantitative data on hospitals and clinics in New York City indicated that they were not appropriate for my purposes. Some of the reasons for this approach are given in my article "Problems of Data and Measurement in Interorganizational Studies of Hospitals and Clinics," appearing in the December 1974 issue of the *Administrative Science Quarterly*.

Earlier versions of the basic argument have been published in *Politics and Society* (Winter 1972) and in *The Social Welfare Forum* (1971).

Introduction

Health care in the United States is allegedly in a state of crisis. High and rising costs, inadequate numbers of medical and paramedical personnel, a higher infant mortality rate in 1969 than in thirteen other countries, a lower life expectancy in 1965 for males than in seventeen other countries, and poor emergency room and ambulatory care are among the diverse facts or allegations which have justified a wide variety of proposed reforms. And yet the numbers of health personnel, the proportion of the gross national product spent on health care, and the sheer quantity of services rendered have grown considerably faster than the economy as a whole.[1]

If health care is in "crisis" now, then it was in crisis ten, twenty, and forty years ago as well. Several qualified observers have commented on the similarity between the 1932 analysis by the Committee on the Costs of Medical Care[2] and reports issued thirty-five or more years later. Dr. Sumner N. Rosen, an economist on the staff of the Institute of Public Administration in New York City, has said that the "catalogue of problems drawn up almost forty years ago strongly resembles the latest list—inadequate services, insufficient funds, understaffed hospitals. Virtually nothing has changed."[3] Economist Eli Ginzberg, summarizing the results of his study of New York City, concludes, "While changes have occurred in response to emergencies, opportunities, and alternatives in the market place, the outstanding finding is the inertia of the system as a whole."[4]

"Crises" are usually creations of specific interest groups seeking to make political capital out of a situation that has existed for many years and will continue to exist after the "crisis" has disappeared from public view. The New York City hospitals, as well as prisons, schools, welfare system, and police corruption, are cases in point. The mass media cooperate in attempts to discredit political leaders because crises —whatever their reality or character—are news. That prisoners are beaten, that poor patients are "dumped" from voluntary to municipal hospitals, or that policemen take bribes are not news *unless* some notable or political leader announces that it is occurring and calls for an investigation and legislative or executive action to correct it.

However, health care in New York City is not in any more (or any less) of a "crisis" than it has been for many years. My hypothesis is that advertisements of crisis serve as political weapons in the hands of interest groups, inside and outside of government, which divert resources and services from one program to another, one social group or class to another. Sayre and Kaufman, citing a 1957 condemnation of conditions in Bellevue Hospital by a number of administrators of that institution, note that "the impending crisis is also used as a public relations method. . . . This is not to say these problems are not real or that the crises are deliberately invented or manufactured. In every case the facts tend to bear out the anxieties of the agencies. Nevertheless, the agency heads or their subordinates employ these situations to arouse public opinion."[5]

The quantity and quality of medical care given in New York City may actually be better than that available in most other areas of the country. More specialists are available, there is more public pressure for medical care, and medical professionals and planners are constantly pressing for state and federal funds for facilities and staff. The controversies over the New York hospitals may actually be part of the process of political and social battles which produce relatively good medical care and do not indicate a low level of care.

This does not mean that medical care in New York City is good or distributed equally in the population by any absolute standard, or even by comparison with the best offered nationally or internationally. But it should not be inferred, from the revelations of crisis and inadequate care, that New York City's medical care is objectively worse than any other city's.

Classic sociological theories provide grounds for suspecting that at stake in the present system are powerful and strategically located interests which effectively resist change. Discovering via a new study or investigation that the same "defects" exist does not create any levers for change. In fact, one would further suspect that the commissioning of more studies or investigations is evidence that the standard or classic response to a "crisis" is being followed. Rather than a program of systematic change being advocated, another study of the situation is called for. Thus, the studies themselves become part of the system to be understood, as part of the barriers to significant structural change. After describing different theories of reform and alternate ways of studying health care politics, I shall argue in chapter 1 that the principal barriers to health care reform lie in the powers of strategically structured interests and that this view of the politics of health care provides a broader explanation than one which focuses on specific innovations or pieces of legislation such as Medicare.

This theoretical perspective is used to focus upon the more specific problem of the links of hospitals and clinics with overarching funding, regulating, and planning agencies, both governmental and private. One selected "output" is analyzed in chapter 2: the reports of a series of commissions of investigation of New York City's hospitals between 1950 and 1970. These commissions included in their membership representatives of many agencies, both public and private, and were explicitly directing their analyses and recommendations at state and federal agencies. Their reports are important empirical materials in our specification of the attempts to create effective interorganizational coalitions within the city vis-a-vis external sources of funding and control. The next step—not taken in this study—would be to assess the actual consequences of such investigations upon subsequent state and federal government activity and upon the actual performance of New York City hospitals and clinics.

A second "output" is analyzed in chapter 3: the efforts to create neighborhood family care centers in New York City by means of a variety of state and federal as well as private and city sources of funds. The primary data used were the files of the Health and Hospital Planning Council of Southern New York dealing with this program, which was an important instance of complex interorganizational relations in which an effective coalition at the local level required sponsorship at higher levels. Again, given limited time and resources, the story told in chapter 3 is limited both historically and empirically.

Chapter 4 presents some evidence for the argument that the observations of New York City hospitals, the commissions of investigation, and the attempts to coordinate health care are not atypical of other cities, other policy areas, and higher levels of government. Even though New York City may exhibit a higher concentration of "crises" of all kinds, the typical processes and their causes seen there are also found elsewhere.

Chapters 5 and 6 are theoretical essays on the political economy of health care which generalize far beyond the empirical materials presented in the first four chapters but attempt to place their findings within the context of some hypotheses about the barriers to change which the matrix of conflicting structural interests creates within health institutions.[6]

Chapter 7 considers the consequences for health research, and chapter 8 summarizes the argument and presents some conclusions about the character of "pluralism" in health care and the possibility of different types of reform.

To conclude, the present book is an attempt to add only two major substantive points to the array of analyses and critiques of health care in the United States. First, responses to periodic "crises" take the form of symbolically reassuring investigations, whose reports call for new administrative devices to "coordinate" and "integrate" the health care delivery system and thus heal the deep-seated disease of fragmentation. Second, the call for coordination and integration, and the reactive defense of pluralism and diversity in the market, are part of a battle—sometimes manifest, sometimes latent—of deeply embedded structural interests for control of key health care resources and institutions.

My general theoretical perspective is that health care institutions, whether described as "fragmented" or as "pluralistic," must be understood in terms of a continuing struggle between major structural interests operating within the context of a market society—"professional monopolists" controlling the major health resources, "corporate rationalizers" challenging their power, and the community population seeking better health care via the actions of equal-health advocates.

1 Health Care Reform and Structural Interests

Although health care in the United States is generally described as fragmented, unresponsive, uncoordinated, costly, and inefficient, diagnoses of the causes and possible reforms differ considerably. Two of the major reform points of view complement each other almost precisely, each pointing to the other as the cause and itself as the solution.

1. Types and Significance of Reform

One point of view—that of "market reformers"—blames bureaucratic interference and cumbersomeness for the defects of the system and calls for the restoration of market competition and pluralism in health care institutions. The other point of view—that of "bureacratic reformers"—blames market competition for the defects of the system and calls for increased administrative regulation and government financing and control of health care.

Both are pointing to real aspects of the system. The market reformers validly point to the elaborate and overlapping medical and health care bureaucracies, both private and public, and properly ridicule the absence of real health care planning. The bureaucratic reformers validly point to the unresponsiveness to health needs of market-oriented hospitals and doctors and properly suggest that a system oriented to profit cannot meet those needs. Each emphasizes reforms appropriate to the functions and institutions it considers crucial.

Market reformers would expand the diversity of facilities available, the number of physicians, the competition between health facilities, and the quantity and quality of private insurance. Their assumptions are that the public sector should underwrite medical bills for the poor and that patients should be free to choose among various health care providers. The community population is regarded as consumers of health care, like other commodities, and is assumed to be able to evaluate the quality of service received. Market pressures will thus drive out the incompetent, excessively high-priced or duplicated service and the inaccessible physician, clinic, or hospital. The market reformers wish to preserve the control of the individual physician over his practice, over the hospital, and over his fees, and they simply wish to open up the medical schools in order to meet the demand for doctors, to give patients more choice among doctors, clinics, and hospitals, and to make that choice a real one by providing public subsidies for medical bills.

These assumptions are questioned by the bureaucratic reformers. They stress the importance of the hospital as the key location and organizer of health services and wish to put individual doctors under the control of hospital medical boards and administrators. The bureaucratic reformers are principally concerned with coordinating fragmented services, instituting planning, and extending public funding. Their assumption is that the technology of modern health care requires a complex and coordinated division of labor between ambulatory and in-hospital care, primary practitioners and specialists, and personalized care and advanced chemical and electronic treatment. The community population is regarded as an external constituency of the health providers to be organized to represent, if necessary, its interests in maintaining the equilibrium of the system.

These contrasting modes of reform are partly illustrated by recent articles by Harry Schwartz of the *New York Times* and Dr. Milton I. Roemer of UCLA, who represent the market and bureaucratic reform views respectively.[1] Both recognize the rocketing costs, criticize duplicated facilities, and call for such reforms as health insurance. But they differ sharply both in their image of the health system and in their proposals for reform.

According to Schwartz,

these needed and useful improvements can be made within the context of a continued pluralistic system. Different people have different tastes and different needs. Those who want to use prepaid groups should be permitted to do so; those who want to go to a physician and pay him each time should be free to do so, too. The result may not seem to be as neat on an organization chart as a uniform national system, and it may have seeming inefficiencies and duplications. But the right of choice for doctors and patients alike is worth such costs —at least in a really humane society. (p. 55)

Schwartz argues that the pluralistic market system in the U.S. not only "provides choices for both physicians and patients," but also "gives [the physician] an economic interest in satisfying the patient" and provides "reassurance and psychological support" to the patient because of the "intimate, long-term, and humane" contact between physician and patient. He argues that to "nationalize and bureaucratize" the American health system like that in Britain will reduce the amount of choice, reduce the incentives to please the patient, and thus depersonalize treatment.

This position is essentially a defense of the present system or an advocacy of further extension of the market principle. Critics of this position argue that the choices allegedly provided by the plurality of health care providers are not real for most people, that the economic incentives to physicians result in much over-doctoring, over hospitalization, and over-operating, and that the alleged intimate and humane quality of most doctor-patient relationships is a myth.

Thus, Dr. Roemer, in sharp contrast to Schwartz, asserts that, indeed, "our spectrum of health services in America has conventionally been described as 'pluralistic.' More accurate would be to describe it as an irrational jungle in which countless vested interests compete for both the private and the public dollar, causing not only distorted allocations of health resources in relation to human needs but all sorts of waste and inefficiency along the way" (p. 36).

The image of the ideal health system presented by Dr. Roemer is worth summarizing because it appears in many reports and studies aimed as coordinating health facilities and services. Integrating the system is advocated simultaneously with differentiating its components into a rational division of labor. The ideal system provides primary health centers for every neighborhood, close to people's homes, staffed by general practitioners and medical assistants, to provide basic diagnoses and preventive services. "Each person served by this health center would be attached to a particular doctor and his team of colleagues" (p. 34). "For each four or five such health centers . . . there should be a district hospital" with 120 to 150 beds to handle relatively common conditions: maternity cases, trauma, less complex surgery. For the service areas of about ten district hospitals, there would be a regional hospital with about 500 beds serving even "more complex medical or surgical problems" and engaged actively in medical research. "At the highest echelon, serving the population coming under three to five regional hospitals (that is, from 1½ million to 2½ million people), should be a university medical center" providing basic medical training and treating all types of cases as part of their research and teaching objectives.

According to Dr. Roemer, "Ideally health care should be a public service like schools or roads, paid for from general tax revenues." All professional personnel would be salaried, with salaries varying "according to qualifications, skills and responsibilities." The quality of medical care would be assured by a "framework of authority and responsibility, backed up by continuous education. Surveillance and reasonable professional controls would also be provided, with rewards and penalties as necessary." In charge of the system would be a hierarchy of officials, beginning with the district hospital director who would serve as a "public health director" in the "broadest social sense," being responsible for seeing to it that "the whole health service operates effectively. . . . He would be responsible for coordination of the several parts of the system, through proper use of records, statistics and information exchange. . . . [He] would be responsible to a health official above him" (p. 36).

Another plan for bureaucratic reform envisions automated multiphasic screening of patients upon first contact in order to use scarce medical manpower efficiently, and an integrated system of health maintenance organizations, clinics, and specialized hospitals. The greater supervision and checking of medical decisions in the hospital context is seen as far outweighing the possible loss of personal contact.[2]

Contrasting images both of present institutions and of the viability of reform are seen in Schwartz' and Roemer's analogy of health to education. Dr. Roemer cites the public school system as an "achievement" of the American political system which did not require a revolution, along with a sharply graduated income tax and an extensive social security program. These achievements constitute grounds for his optimism that a reorganized health system can be achieved without a fundamental modification of American political and economic institutions. Harry Schwartz, on the other hand, cites the public school system as a "debacle" and says that "in every community, public school education is free to the recipients; yet, everywhere—or almost everywhere—there is bitter complaint of the failure of this system to teach effectively or to satisfy the psychological needs of our young people" (p. 55).

Reacting against the strategy of bureaucratic reform on the grounds that it has been tried and failed, some social scientists have turned to market reform. Sociologist Roland Warren asserts that for a hundred years the standard assumption has been that central planning and avoidance of duplication of services is the best way of providing health and welfare ("human") services.[3] But this strategy has met with little success. "A century of coordinative effort in the social service field since the inception of the Charities Organization Movement has resulted in a much vaster patchquilt, with ever greater need for coordination and ever greater efforts in that direction, with agencies set up to coordinate which then in turn have to be coordinated" (p. 116). Warren asserts that "virtually none ... of the four conditions deemed necessary for adequate planning of human services ... is met in most inter-agency planning ventures" (p. 117) (those four conditions are: [1] centralized decision making; [2] avoidance of duplication of services; [3] techniques of calculation of distribution of resources efficiently; and [4] devices for insuring conformity of service-providing agencies to the general plan). As a solution, Warren calls for extension of the market principle of competition to as many human services as possible, assuming that "domain overlap" (p. 115) (which he does not want to call duplication of services) will increase efficiency and responsiveness *if* a substantial part of the income of an agency is produced by demand from consumers. Thus his recommended principle of inter-agency coordination is to "encourage competitiveness among service agencies wherever feasible" (p. 123). Wherever feasible, he would put the necessary money in the hands of the consumer to buy his services.

The assumptions for the market strategy are clear: that (1) consumers have the required information to allow them to choose between provider agencies; (2) agencies will in fact arise in response to the demands which are presently unfulfilled more readily than they do now; and (3) an "elite" centralized planning apparatus is less likely to know what people want than people do themselves. Warren calls his system "interactional field planning" (p. 126) and would leave to central planning agencies the decision as to where this strategy would work.

As is clear from the mixed version presented by Dr. Warren, the two contrasting diagnoses, images of the future, and proposals for reform of health care which I have called "market" and "bureaucratic" reform are only partially ideologies which are accepted or rejected mainly because of one's moral and political values. They are also analyses of the structure of health care which rest upon different empirical assumptions about the nature and power of the health profession, the nature of medical technology, the role of the hospital, and the role of the patient (or the "community") as passively receiving or actively demanding a greater quality and quantity of health care.

However, neither type of reformer sees the interdependence of the defects they identify. I will argue that the proliferation of bureaucratic agencies which fail to plan or coordinate health care intrinsically sustains the unresponsiveness of the separate market-oriented units. Bureaucratic agencies, market-oriented physicians, clinics, and hospitals can all be more adequately understood from yet a third point of view on reform, which I shall label the "structural interest" perspective. Powerful interests benefit from the health care system precisely as it is—with its ineffective layers of bureaucratic "planning" and "administration" and its uncoordinated separate organizational and professional components responding to demands by the sick for care. These interests do not have to exert "power" to influence particular "decisions," except to block proposals for change.

The proposals for change emanating from the market and bureaucratic reformers do not challenge any of the institutional roots from which the power of structural interests derives. None of the decisions called for by the market reformers (to dismantle government agencies attempting to supervise and plan and to allow the free play of the market to operate) or the decisions called for by the bureaucratic reformers (to set up still more or reorganized government agencies to interfere with the market process) will challenge the effective institutionalized and legal control of the system as a whole by the dominant structural interests which benefit from its continuance in its present form.

Because each of the types of analyses which lead to the different recipes for reform is incomplete and represents an exaggeration of the importance and independence of professional work, on the one hand, and corporate organization, on the other, there is a strong ideological component in the policy recommendations of each group. This ideological component leads to a neglect of the discrepancy between the claims of each interest group about its performance and role in the health system and its actual role.

The overwhelming fact about the various reforms of the health system that have been implemented or proposed—more money, more subsidy of insurance, more manpower, more demonstration projects, more clinics—is that they are absorbed into a system which is enormously resistant to change. The reforms which are suggested are sponsored by different elements in the health system and favor one or another element, but they do not seriously damage any interests. This pluralistic balancing of costs and benefits successfully defends the funding, powers, and resources of the producing institutions against any basic structural change.

This book does not pretend to have the "solution" to the organization of health care, and in fact the author resists as inappropriate those criticisms which ask "But what would *you* do?" One of the most general thrusts of my argument is that a myriad of recipes for health reform have been tried and found wanting and that serious and sustained theoretical, historical, and empirical analyses of the origins, development, and consequences of the functioning of health care institutions and personnel are necessary. Without these analyses, social movements which strike out at the clearly inhumane and inadequate health care available to millions of Americans will almost inevitably be trapped in still another set of chimerical demands. Perhaps the best recent example is the volume *The American Health Empire*, written by the group of New York activists in the Health Policy Advisory Committee, which stresses "community control" as the solution.[4]

Professor Roemer accepts almost all of the diagnosis presented by Health PAC. As he says, "there can be no doubt of the corrupting influence of profit-making in American health service. The unnecessary surgery, the waste and inefficiencies of private solo practice, the profiteering of the drug industry, the entrepreneurialism of substandard nursing homes and proprietary hospitals—these and other problems are real. A reliable and documented book on profits in health care is needed, especially in this period when the federal administration of the United States is moving to *enhance* the proprietary sector of medicine."[5] But, Roemer argues, *The American Health Empire* is not that book, mainly because it contains "virtually no historical perspective on the long social struggles in back of the development of medical care for the poor or social insurance for the aged."

The underlying issue is really the role of knowledge in contributing to social change. As Roemer points out in his review, some twelve comprehensive and complete critiques of health care in the United States were written between 1927 and 1970. Unlike the authors quoted at the very beginning of the Introduction to this book, Roemer argues that

each of these books has made a contribution to public understanding, pulling aside the mask of secrecy which shielded the healing arts from public scrutiny and accountability for too many decades. Generally these books have resulted from painstaking study of the problems of medical care, they have exposed the enormous inequities caused by the private entrepreneurial market in which American medicine is immersed, and they have offered constructive solutions for improving the system. Many of the recommendations of these critics have been acted upon—improved public health services, increased outputs of health personnel, expanded health insurance, extension of hospitals into rural areas, more care for the aged and the poor. The substantial progress in America's health over the last 40 years can be traced, in good part, to the aroused demands of people—demands dependent on knowledge and awareness to which these books have significantly contributed. (p. 119)

There is probably no contradiction between this optimistic view of what has been achieved in the provision of health care to Americans in the last half century and the pessimistic view of others. Dr. Roemer is measuring very real improvements against what existed before, taking into account the barriers to change, and he is paying tribute to the devoted and detailed analyses of two generations of critics. Drs. Rosen and Ginzberg, cited in the Introduction, are comparing what has been achieved against what might or what could be accomplished, given our national resources of wealth, manpower, and technology.

The expansion of health insurance and the extension of federal funds to cover health costs for the poor and the elderly can be regarded as real and important, and yet one can still argue that health *institutions* have not changed and that the barriers to change vitiate those reforms. The dilemma of reform intensifying the elements of "crisis" is seen most sharply in Medicaid, the federal legislation enacted in 1965 which extended health payments for the poor via matching grants to funds provided by the states. According to Rosemary Stevens, Medicaid, while undeniably improving the quantity of care provided, "quickly threatened a crisis in state budgetary arrangements," since costs were nearly twice what had been predicted. "The problems besetting Medicaid were epitomized in New York City, where the costs of welfare and Medicaid payments doubled between 1965 and 1969 and where one million people are on welfare and another 900,000 of welfare and Medicaid payments doubled between 1965 and 1969 and where one million people are on welfare and another 900,000 deemed medically indigent. The changes in Medicaid forced additional people into the city's already overwhelmed hospital system, developing still further the chronic understaffing and underfinancing [of] facilities." The result has been that "... a slow-burning sense of crisis has been engendered, born not of social revolution but of administrative chaos. The combined effect of one piece of legislation after another, poured into an unconnected health service system, has been to produce increasing dysfunction in the way the system works."[6]

A double point is found here. New York City specifically, as Stevens says, exhibits a concentrated dose of the conditions leading to health "crises," but its situation is *not* unique. More generally, reforms such as Medicaid have certain short-term benefits, but do not constitute significant institutional change, since the additional funding they provide simply feeds into increased costs and soon leads to cutbacks of services and payments.

2. Alternative Views of the Study of Health Care

There is widespread recognition among medical sociologists that interest-group politics are central to the resistance of health institutions to change. According to medical sociologist David Mechanic, "medical care involves a variety of interest groups that tend to view priorities from their own particular perspectives and interests, and it is enormously difficult to achieve a consensus. Groups are usually reluctant to yield rights and privileges that they have already exercised, and will resist significant restructuring unless it appears that there is something in it for them."[7]

Despite this recognition, there are remarkably few studies which take interest groups in health as their major subject. Frequently the conflicts between interest groups are mentioned but then are either glossed over or resolved by sheer assertion. Another medical sociologist, Odin W. Anderson, cites an example from a Swedish medical journal which argued both that a hospital could be run more like a business, rationalized and planned, and simultaneously that this "does not mean that the humanitarian, the so-called personal care, cannot be taken into account." Anderson adds that "this view appears as an inherent conflict everywhere." He also quotes what he calls a "bland statement" produced by one of the national commissions whose reports he evaluates: "The responsible participation and involvement of all sectors of the community, coordination of efforts, and development of cooperative working arrangements are fundamental to effective action-planning." As Anderson says, such statements do not recognize the politics of health care.[8] Unfortunately, they are all too typical, as we shall see, of analyses of health care hoping to produce change via consensus.

Older sociological studies of "health and sickness" frequently bear little or no trace of concern with the larger society and its impact on the resources made available for medical care. One example is a 1960 volume of collected studies, representing some of the leading medical sociologists of the time. Three sections are almost entirely social-psychological: "The Recognition of Need for Health Care," "The Patient's Point of View," and "Psychosocial Processes in Illness." The fourth, "The Organization of Hospitals," contains six articles, but all of them refer to processes internal to hospitals. None deals with the larger social environment.[9] More recently, there has been an increase of concern with the "interorganizational" relationships of hospitals—their links, interdependence and reliance on external resources.[10] But there has been no full theoretical revision which treats the health system as a whole in more than a rhetorical sense. The term "health delivery system," now bandied about, may be more a part of the ideological repertoire of an interest group than a term used for analytic purposes.

The conventional view of "public policy," "decision making," "pluralist competition," "party organization," "leadership," the "role of the mayor," and all of the other topics beloved of political science sharply separates the public, governmental sector of decision making and policy from the private, corporate sector. This distinction makes it possible to ignore many knotty theoretical and policy problems. A good example relevant to the present study is the classic study by political scientists Wallace S. Sayre and Herbert Kaufman, *Governing New York City: Politics in the Metropolis*.[11] This book provides a good starting point for my review of the various studies, commission reports, planning investigations, and surveys which have been done in the twenty years from 1950 to 1970 and of the attempt to create "neighborhood family care centers." This study was the most comprehensive survey of the politics of New York City done up to that time, and its view of the health system and health politics in New York provides a background setting for this study.

Unfortunately—and this is exactly my point—the book does not deal with the "health system." It does not deal with *any* problem of function or service which any institution in the city provides to the population, whether it is in the area of education, transportation, or police or fire protection—among those services already "public" in character—or with the production and distribution of those goods and services still defined as "private" by their ownership and control. The book deals only with "politics" in the narrow sense—the struggle for control of appointments, recruitment, the battles between city agencies, the attempts to influence the mayor, who gets nominated by the parties, and so forth.

Strange as it may seem, there are relatively few studies of the politics of health care policy. As recently as 1966 Herbert Kaufman could review major treatises in public health and conclude that none contained "more than a passing reference to politics." Even more startling was his conclusion after reviewing major textbooks on local, state, and national government in the United States that there were "virtually no references to the politics of public programs."[12] While this lack has been remedied to some extent in the intervening years, systematic analyses are still few.

The recent book by political scientist Theodore Marmor, *The Politics of Medicare*, epitomizes a pluralist focus on the political strategies within and outside Congress which influenced the timing and outcome of the Medicare bill of 1965. Marmor argues convincingly that the 1964 Johnson landslide made possible an extension of the bill past what most legislative strategists thought possible and that earlier attempts were doomed mainly because of the sheer absence of votes in Congress.[13] Interest groups are dealt with only in the narrow context of the extent and kind of their participation in the effort to pass or defeat Medicare. Marmor notes that the disputes over national health insurance in the 1970's essentially pit the same issues and contestants against each other (pp. 90-93), but the reasons for the persistence of dominant structural interests are not juxtaposed to the reasons certain changes are politically possible at times.

Two other examples of approaches different from mine—both chosen because their titles are essentially the same as that of this book—also illustrate the way the definition of the theoretical problem influences the choice of appropriate concepts and methods.

In *The Politics of Health Care: Nine Case Studies of Innovative Planning in New York City*, Herbert Harvey Hyman, a health planner at Hunter College and former director of the Model Cities Program for the Human Resources Administration in New York City, concluded the final essay in a way which seemed to contradict the optimism of the book's subtitle. Summarizing the results of nine case studies (ghetto medicine, Medicaid, family planning, abortion, rat eradication, the Health and Hospitals Corporation, ambulatory health care, Regional Medical Programs, and Comprehensive Health Planning), he concluded that "regardless of the nature of the programs, support or service, they were mostly underfinanced and thus hardly able to meet the overwhelming needs for health services in the New York City community."[14] Only two programs—abortion and family planning—met their original objectives to a significant degree. "All other programs had major financial limitations, organizational inhibiting constraints, or poor commitment as factors that prevented their achievement.... None of these programs have had any real impact on these already existing basic health services" (p. 195).

Hyman found the reason for this situation in the nature of our society.
"The nature of our political society with its pluralistic self-interest groups, operating to protect their varied interests or to expand them when opportunities arise, encourages only incremental or marginal changes. The delicate balance that must be constantly maintained between what is and what is needed, or ought to be, precludes dramatic departures from the known, safe and accepted methods.... Established health forces are not idle with respect to the attempted innovations" (pp. 197–98).

Unfortunately, Hyman's methodology of the study, by focusing upon the specifics of the events surrounding the introduction of each of the "innovations," ignored the powerful forces battling to maintain or change the existing structure of health care. The analytic difficulty is that each case was treated as a discrete program, with separate evaluations of its own sequence of events, participants, decisions, definition of problems, objectives, and consequences. Also, as is the case with much health planning, the focus was not (as the editor himself said) upon "program or planning product as such," but rather with "people and their actions and how those actions change the objectives they seek to implement" (p. 7). "Innovation" is thus defined as the process of *initiating* some program and of *attempting* to carry it through. Whether or not the program changed anything didn't matter.

The result of this way of looking at innovations is that consequences are separated from the process or events and that the interrelations of events with each other are lost. More fundamentally, the institutions which control and shape the allocation of resources within health care cannot be analyzed in any systematic way, but only appear within the "cracks" of the analysis, so to speak. Thus, Hyman's book contains many scattered references to the "established health forces," but nowhere were they described and analyzed in any coherent way. The author of the chapter on comprehensive health care planning asserted, for example, that "the delivery of health care in New York City is primarily in the hands of the private sector. The voluntary hospitals and medical schools control the flow of manpower and funds into the city" (p. 161). However, the overall structure and argument of the book, which isolated nine different local and federal programs for separate treatment, did not allow the reader to come to grips with the implications of that description of the underlying structure of power.

Another recent article, entitled "The Politics of Health," exemplifies the analytic difficulties of the so-called systems approach to health politics.[15] Beginning with political scientist David Easton's concepts of system inputs, outputs, and stress, Bert E. Swanson attempted to relate these concepts to power structure, political ideologies, and change. Unfortunately, the definitions were purely formal, not substantive, and there was given no concrete sense of the factors creating the present structure of health institutions or the forces leading to change. It is as if a scaffolding is constructed, but there is no clue as to what kind of building will be built.

Swanson argued, for example, that change in the scope of government was the important thing to study, but this change was conceived of as a purely linear process, as if the private sector contracts when the public sector expands, and vice versa. Almost every substantive study of the role of government regulation and funding shows instead that government action frequently reinforces, rather than undermines, the private sector. Moreover, Swanson treated demands upon the system (an input) as if they are not affected by the operations of the existing health care institutions, and also as if they are a purely formal property without any substantive contents. Power structures and political ideologies, too, lacked any content but were regarded as having only the formal properties of convergence versus divergence, broad versus narrow distribution, and expanded versus contracted scope of government. The result was an ahistorical focus upon abstract variables which gives the reader little sense of the specific issues and conflicts confronting any given society or community.

When examples were given (Swanson cites his own study of decision making in four communities), they were so concrete that the links to the abstract variables were not clear. Empirically descriptive terms (swimming pool, sewer system) were regarded as indicating an abstract concept (demand, scope of government), but the question remained unanswered as to how to locate these demands and their consequences within a historically developed structure of institutions and interests, operating within an environment which constrains the probabilities of certain outcomes.

The contrasting approaches of Hyman and Swanson—obviously relevant to many problems besides the politics of health care—raise many issues of theory and method underlying this analysis, a few of which must be made explicit.

3. Dominant, Challenging, and
Repressed Structural Interests

The distinction must be made between the organized action of a group to represent its interests (an "interest group") and those interests served or not served by the way they "fit" into the basic logic and principles by which the institutions of a society operate. For want of a better or more conventional term, I shall call the latter *structural interests.* These are interests which are more than potential interest groups (in David Truman's sense) which are merely waiting for the opportunity or the necessity of organizing to present demands or grievances to the appropriate authorities.[16] Rather, structural interests either do not have to be organized in order to have their interests served or cannot be organized without great difficulty. Structural interests can in turn be classified as *dominant, challenging,* and *repressed.* Dominant structural interests are those served by the structure of social, economic, and political institutions as they exist at any given time. Precisely because of this, the interests involved do not continuously have to organize and act to defend their interests; other institutions do that for them. Challenging structural interests are those being created by the changing structure of the society. Repressed structural interests are the opposite of dominant ones (although not necessarily always in conflict with them); the nature of institutions guarantees that they will *not* be served unless extraordinary political energies are mobilized.

Life can perhaps be breathed into these abstractions by identifying the principal structural interests in health care. The nature of these interests is discussed in more detail in chapters 5 and 6. An example of a dominant structural interest is that found in professional monopoly, in which existing institutions protect and reinforce the logic and principle of professional monopoly over the production and distribution of health services. Medicine is a classic case of social organization of production but the private appropriation of powers and benefits by a structural interest— professional monopoly—which through professional associations has maintained control of the supply of physicians, the distribution and cost of services, and the rules governing hospitals.

Battles occur, to be sure, between segments of those who possess such a monopoly, but these are conflicts of interest groups *within* a dominant structural interest. None of the conflicts of this type challenges the *principle* of professional monopoly—just who is going to have it. The common status of "professional monopolist" does not imply that bio-medical researchers, general practitioners, surgeons, or dentists ever have to act together in order to preserve existing institutions which maintain their professional monopoly. The concept leaves empirically open the extent to which and the conditions under which coalitions form and constitute "interest groups" in the usual sense. The central idea is that existing

institutions function for all occupations, groups, or organizations which
have the common interest signified by the classifying term.

However, the changing technology and division of labor in health care
production and distribution and the shifting rewards to social groups and
classes are creating new structural interests which I label "corporate
rationalization." The organization of health care has become increasingly
social rather than individual in character and involves a complex division
of labor between skilled persons specializing in primary care, surgery,
preventive medicine, and so forth. Bureaucratic organizations—mainly
the hospitals—are the principal agents potentially available to organize
this complex technology in a way which makes various skilled behaviors
available to patients. Hospital administrators, medical schools, government health planners, and public health agencies and researchers
constitute interest groups which share—over and above their varied
predispositions to act in concert vis-a-vis new government regulatory or
funding programs—a common relationship to the underlying changes in
the technology and organization of health care. This common relation
generates their developing structural interest in breaking the professional
monopoly of physicians over the production and distribution of health
care.

It is one of my central theses that the developing structural interest in
corporate rationalization contradicts and challenges some fundamental
interests of professional monopolies and that this contradiction accounts
for much of the sometimes muted, sometimes blaring, conflict between
doctors and hospitals, fee-for-service and prepaid practice, and health
planning and the health market. These conflicts, however, are contained
within an institutional framework which prevents corporate rationalization from generating enough social power truly to integrate and
coordinate health care. Corporate rationalization remains an ideology
and a vision linked to concrete structural interests within a market
economy.

Repressed structural interests are those of the "community population"—the varied interest groups of the white rural and urban poor,
ghetto blacks, the lower middle class just above the Medicaid income
maximum, the neighborhoods just poor enough that no doctor wants to
establish his practice there, those middle-class families rendered newly
medically indigent by sharply escalating costs, those occupations affected
by job-related diseases, and many others. These are "repressed" or
negative structural interests because no social institutions or political
mechanisms in the society insure that these interests are served. In
specific cases one or more of these interests can organize—become an

interest group—and demand a new hospital, a neighborhood health center, higher insurance coverage, or more and better care from a physician. Many instances of such successful community or individual action by equal-health advocates to improve the health care available to the community population can be cited, but none of them contradicts my point.

One important example of the community population's structural interest in health which is almost totally ignored by health institutions as they now function is occupational health. Although the Public Health Service estimates that each year 100,000 persons die, and nearly 400,000 more develop disabling occupational diseases, as a direct result of job-related illnesses or injuries, "occupational health has been virtually ignored by the medical profession, which regards it as a less-than-glamorous specialty. Only a handful of universities have departments of occupational health and fewer than a dozen physicians enter the field each year, the majority becoming company doctors" (*New York Times*, 4 March 1974, pp. 1, 21). Federal legislation has been slow and mainly symbolic in character and has established underfunded, understaffed agencies. Occupational health hazards are an excellent example of the difficulty of changing the causes of health problems either by health care institutions themselves or by any politically feasible legislative or administrative action.

Occupational health care is only one example of the broad category of preventive medicine which—in the sense of elimination of those conditions which generate illness—is highly underdeveloped in the United States and is a general instance of a repressed structural interest. Normal preventive care instead means regular checkups and examinations, which are still in the context of individual treatment.

The key difference between dominant and repressed structural interests is that enormous political and organizational energies must be summoned by repressed structural interests to offset the intrinsic disadvantages of their situation. None need be generated by dominant structural interests. Concrete and important gains produced by skilled political leadership, a united constituency, and a decisive victory can thus melt away if the structure of institutions is not changed to alter permanently the balance between dominant and repressed structural interests.[17] If attention is paid only to the visible and dramatic conflicts —the typical ones precisely because repressed structural interests must usually mobilize public opinion—then the quiet and continuous allocation of benefits to dominant structural interests will not be noticed.[18]

The terms *dominant* and *repressed* do not imply that the interests represented by these terms are always in opposition to each other. The equal-health advocates and the professional monopolists may both benefit from a government health insurance plan which subsidizes an open-ended payment plan for physicians and also underwrites extraordinary medical costs for poor families or the aged.

The distinction between interest groups and structural interests is not made in the pluralist literature because of a tendency to assume that it is a societal consensus—values, rules of the game—which creates and allows the power and privileges of particular groups to continue. Thus, several writers have argued that it is the high esteem in which physicians are held by the society which provides them with the leverage they have to influence the content of legislation, the composition of administrative boards, and the actual implementation of policy.[19] A widespread consensus in the society on the importance of health care and on the key role of physicians in performing this function provides them with the basis for the power and in effect grants them their professional monopoly.

If I am correct in asserting the importance of dominant structural interests, then the causal order may be precisely the reverse. Rather than a societal consensus giving the doctors power, it is the doctors' power which generates the societal consensus. Or, in the language I am using above, the existence of a network of political, legal, and economic institutions which guarantees that certain dominant interests will be served comes to be taken for granted as legitimate, as the only possible way in which these health services can be provided. People come to accept as inevitable that which exists and even believe that it is right. But this is quite a different argument from the one which says that because people believe in doctors, they give them power.

Thus, the formation of consensus around the provision of health services by a professional monopoly of physicians is not an independent causal force in its own right. Rather, the reinforcing and reproducing power of the institutions which guarantee the monopoly generates legitimating symbols and beliefs.[20]

4. The Implications of Theory
   for Method

A narrow concept of the pluralist political process as one of winning legislative victories and an activist image of interest groups are inadequate, in my opinion, to explain the persistence of health "crises" and the barriers to health care reform. It is also important to make clear that I reject theories which explain the functioning of institutions in terms of individual psychology of power or status, the requirements of organizational survival (the pejorative meaning of "bureaucracy"), or failures of unenlightened leadership. These attributes of individuals and organizations are probably pervasive and continuing, and thus cannot account for historically specific characteristics of social institutions.

This point needs to be emphasized because it defines the way in which I interpret data drawn necessarily from individuals and organizations—documents, reports, and interviews with leaders and officials. I cannot emphasize too strongly that I do not believe that the failures of the commission reports to face squarely the implications of their own facts stem from the stupidity of their members or from conscious attempts to mystify and deceive the public. Nor do I believe that doctors are any more rapacious or determined to maintain their powers than are members of any other privileged status group. Nor are the hospital administrators any more concerned to maintain and extend their authority over medical practice than are officials of any other type of organization. Nor are health planners unwilling to plan. The incentives—status, income, power—which motivate persons in various organizational and professional roles to behave as they do stem from the structural and cultural milieux in which they find themselves. Selfish, ignorant, venal individuals do exist, of course, but I do not assume—and it is unnecessary for my argument to assume—that they are more common among health practitioners than anywhere else. Similarly, when I use the term *ideology*, I do not mean untruthful, malicious, or manipulative assertions by individuals, but rather the continuous attempts by groups and organizations to construct symbolic presentations of their legitimate role and, by extension, the legitimate organization of the health institutions within which their role is defined.[21]

Thus, I am labeling or characterizing not *individuals* but rather social *roles* within diverse organizational and professional contexts. Individuals play multiple and sometimes contradictory roles and may function as reformers in one context and as members of an interest group in another context. An academic sociologist, for example, in his research capacity may be acting as a market reformer, in his teaching capacity acting as a professional monopolist, in his consultation to a federal agency acting as a corporate rationalizer, in his membership in a health insurance plan acting as a bureaucratic reformer. Both social conditions and personality characteristics may serve to insulate individuals from the potential contradictions in these multiple social roles, and this is a problem of some importance in social psychology. But I am concerned with the ways in which ideologies are constructed to defend structural interests composed of clusters of social roles and positions attached to only parts of individuals. This point is both a sociological commonplace and common sense, since we all know of the "distance" between our selves and our roles. I raise this point here because readers of earlier drafts of this work misconstrued some of my hypotheses—for example, those concerning the greater income and power accruing to hospital administrators who successfully built larger domains over which they had control. To recognize material motives is not to denigrate them; organizational theory has long recognized that the stability and cohesion of an organization is best guaranteed by relying upon mundane incentives rather than ideal or altruistic ones. My assumption is that our goal must be to change neither the human nature of doctors nor the communicative abilities of administrators, but rather the structure of health institutions which creates specific rewards and sanctions.

The methodological assumptions of this study flow from the theoretical perspective just stated. I am not writing a history of a single organization or analyzing a few variables which might characterize an interorganizational relationship, such as dependence, strength, extent of reciprocity, or persistence. Rather, I am concerned with how a complex *system* of organizations handles a *problem*—in this case, how the New York City health agencies handle the problem of utilizing federal and state funds to establish ambulatory care centers, and how "crises" are handled by mobilizing a commission of investigation. The empirical materials of this study are derived from only a few organizations judged to be key ones in the process of decision making. The angle of vision is thus influenced to some extent by the choice of organizations, since the specific documents available will inevitably represent the interests of the organizations which provide the point of entry or access into the system. Undoubtedly a somewhat different picture would be gained if other organizations were chosen. Theoretical assumptions about the role of the specific organization derived from organizational theory and from other studies of politics and health, provide a basis for evaluating the documents and assessing the possible biases resulting from the choice of organization. As the documents are summarized and generalizations drawn from them, the standpoint from which they are assessed will become clear.

Statements made by individuals are assumed to represent the policy position of the organization they represent and not their personal beliefs. A word or two on this assumption may be necessary in the absence of systematic samples of either documents or officials in various health organizations.

There are several logical possibilities: either the beliefs of the individual and the organizational policy expressed in documents and or at meetings coincide or they don't. If they coincide, there is no problem although perhaps the individual will state his position more strongly or pursue their policy implications more fervently if his personal beliefs in this instance are the same as those of his organization. If the two diverge, either the individual conceals his own beliefs or he doesn't. If he conceals his own beliefs, there is no problem of inference about organizational policy because his statements in fact reflect that policy. If his statements and writings are his own beliefs and contradict those of his organization, either the difference is a minor one or it is a major one. If it is a minor one, then there is no problem because the error of inference will be small.

If an individual employee's or official's expressed beliefs contradict important aspects of his organization's policy, several possibilities exist: at some point he will be removed; he will swing his organization's policy around to his own beliefs; he will be placed in a position where his beliefs are not allowed to influence decisions regarded as crucial for the organization; or he will leave. Our assumption therefore is that, over a reasonably long period of time, in hierarchical organizations, staff members' statements and writings will tend to reflect the dominant faction's position and the general policy commitments of the organization. If there is a serious split over policy and the informant is in the minority or losing faction, it is assumed that some indication of disaffection will be apparent in the interview or the document. That is, it is assumed that staff members are not likely to present their own, minority opinions as the dominant point of view.

If the statements and writings of staff members of organizations, acting in their official capacity, usually represent the majority policy position of their organization, a question arises: what does it mean to infer something about the "interests" or the "policy" of the organization? This gets into the problem of reductionism versus emergent social properties, but my position is that it is possible to differentiate among the interests of different levels of an organization, the organization as a whole, and the individuals within it. If one admits as a theoretical possibility that each level, from the individual through a department to divisions, through the organization as a whole, through coalitions of organizations, can have identifiable and distinctive interests and goals, then the problem becomes one of defining the nature of those interests and goals, establishing how different or contradictory they are at different levels, and determining their relative importance from a societal point of view. Let us assume that the only differences in interest between two departments in an organization are the status needs of its heads. This individual factor may affect the behavior of the two departments in important ways, and, depending on their importance in the organization as a whole, may affect the entire organization. Or the access of one department to information about sources of funds may be better than that of another department for structural reasons related, let us say, to the fact that the function of the first department requires it to be physically closer to the top management or leadership of the organization. In these varied ways, properties of one level of organization affect properties of another level.

To conclude, my interpretations of the data assume that there is a reasonably high correlation between ideologies and personal incentives of doctors, researchers, administrators, and the organizational interests of the medical profession, hospitals, or public health associations. That is, there is a high probability that elites will take a public position consistent with the interests of their organization. Career incentives probably require that collective myths be publicly stated, even if there is considerable private cynicism or disbelief. More detailed analyses of particular events and conflicts would require taking into account contradictions and discrepancies between ideology, personal incentives, and organizational interests.

A further distinction can also be drawn between the objective interests of an individual or group (the consequences of certain policies) and its subjective interests (beliefs about those consequences). A group may be affected in important ways by the operations of an institution, but its members may not be conscious of those consequences and thus may not act either to defend themselves or to change the structure which produces the consequences. Or even if they are conscious of the consequences, the members may be unwilling or unable to act for a variety of reasons.[22]

With these few remarks on the assumptions and rules guiding the interpretation of the empirical data derived from interviews, documents, and secondary sources, I turn to a critical evaluation of seven commissions of investigation into New York City's health institutions.

2 Commissions of Investigation, 1950-1971

1. Introduction: Reports as Interorganizational Outputs

Over twenty investigations of the New York City health system were conducted between 1950 and 1971. The reports of them (see table 1) reached a peak in 1965-68 when the municipal hospitals were under almost constant surveillance by city, state, and private agencies. Here we take these documents at face value as evidence of the serious consideration given to the problems of the New York City health system by groups of eminent physicians, hospital administrators, heads of city health and hospital agencies, outside experts and consultants, public health officials, and academics in medical schools and allied departments and disciplines.

This collection of reports constitutes an array of investigations into a major human service almost unparalleled for any other policy area, and probably for any other city at any time. Even if these reports are political documents, as is at least partly the case, expressing the balance of power of political forces—both reform and status quo—at a given time and manifesting the point of view of specific interest groups, the content of the reports warrants their being taken seriously in their own terms. The manifest content is important. What problems are seen? What are the causes of those problems which are discovered or attributed? What solutions are offered? What specific policy recommendations are made? But the latent content is also important. What is *not* defined as a problem? What assumptions are made by the logic of the analysis? What problems are seen as beyond solution? What changes, while acknowledged as important, are regarded as impossible?

Table 1   List of Reports Issued by Various
                                              Commissions of Investigation into
                                              the New York City Health
                                              System, 1950–71

Date	Title of Report	Body Issuing Report
* February 1950	Report	Mayor's Committee on the Needs of the Department of Hospitals (Kogel Committee)
* July 1960	Report	Commission on Health Services of the City of New York (Heyman Commission)
* December 1960	New York City and Its Hospitals	Hospital Council of Greater New York (Eurich, Chairman of Study Committee)
March 1961	First Class Care—or Second—in Our City Hospitals?	The Citizen's Committee for Children of New York
February 1965	Discussion and Recommendation of Public Policy in Hospitals in New York State	Governor's Committee on Hospital Costs (Folsom Committee)
December 1965	Report	Governor's Committee on Hospital Costs (Folsom Committee)
* February 1966	Report	Mayor's Advisory Task Force on Medical Economics (Haldeman, Chairman)
* March 1966	System Analysis and Planning for Public Health Care in the City of New York	System Development Corporation for the Health Research Council
October 1966	A Preliminary Survey of the Municipal Hospitals, New York City	New York State Department of Health
December 1966	The New York Municipal Hospitals: Interim Report to Governor Rockefeller of New York	New York State Senator Seymour Thaler
January 1967	Preliminary Hospital Affiliation Report	New York City Comptroller Mario A. Procaccino
March 1967	Public Health and Public Responsibility: The Task before Us	New York State Joint Legislative Committee on the Problems of Public Health and Medicare (Senator Norman F. Lent, Chairman)
April 1967	Report to Governor Nelson A. Rockefeller on Municipal Hospitals of New York City	Blue Ribbon Panel on Municipal Hospitals of New York City
September 1967	Alternative Organizational Frameworks for the Delivery of Health Services in New York City	Research and Planning Unit, Office of Administration, Office of the New York City Mayor

Date	Title of Report	Body Issuing Report
December 1967	Status of Implementation of the Recommendations of the Governor's Committee on Hospital Costs	Governor's Committee on Hospital Costs
* December 1967	Community Health Services for New York City	Commission on the Delivery of Personal Health Services (Piel Commission)
May 1968	An End to Charity Medicine: Goals for New York	The City Club of New York
June 1968	Recommendations Concerning New York City's Municipal Hospitals and the Affiliation Program	New York State Commission of Investigation
March 1969	An Investigation Concerning New York City's Municipal Hospitals and the Affiliation Program	New York State Commission of Investigation
November 1970	Geographic Boundaries, Staffing Patterns, Function of Local Planning Units	Mayor's Organizational Task Force for Comprehensive Health Planning
December 1970	Research in the Health of the City	Mayor's Committee to Evaluate the Work of the Health Research Council of the City of New York
* February 1971	Planning Public Expenditures on Mental Health Service Delivery	The New York City RAND Institute
* April 1971	Report on Health and Hospital Services and Costs	Governor's Steering Committee on Social Problems

* Reports which are summarized and their content analyzed in this study.

While the composition of the various boards and committees of inquiry may be a clue to the interests represented, the actual content of each report is just as important, if not more so, in assessing the benefits and costs of various programs and in determining the adequacy of the analysis of the causes and consequences of various characteristics of the health system contained in these reports. Despite the repeated assertions that the various investigations, reports, and recommendations never change anything, they continue to be made, and the point is then repeated in the next one. The Piel Commission of 1967 said, "Why have not earlier studies, programs, reforms, or demonstrations, met the problems with which this Commission has been charged."[1] The commission then cited a number of recommendations of previous commissions which had not been implemented. In March 1969 the New York State Commission of Investigation's report on New York City's municipal hospitals and the affiliation program said that "over the years, the [municipal] hospitals have been studied, analyzed, and investigated by a legion of government and private groups. Unfortunately, the resultant reports, findings, and recommendations have generally produced little, if any, improvement."[2] The most recent studies of the health system stress its enormous resistance to significant structural change and the difficulty of implementing the recommendations of the many reports and commissions. As Eli Ginzberg, director of the Conservation of Human Resources project at Columbia University and author of several books on the health system, put it: "Both as theoreticians and as citizens, members of the Conservation staff were intrigued with the reasons for the very slow implementation of many well-supported recommendations for far-reaching changes in the health system."[3]

The reports we shall analyze are always done by committees representing various organizations in a policy area. Therefore, the committees themselves are direct expressions of interorganizational relationships, and their product—the report—is an empirical example of an "output" of an interorganizational relationship in much the same sense as is a joint laundry program or joint cobalt bomb. But these committees and their reports are a more important type of interorganizational output than a concrete, operational service such as a joint laundry service. In the first place, these committees make, or at least recommend, policies. They are not just the creatures of prior decision-making processes. But as with almost all such processes in complex organizational systems, and regardless of the public presentation of their purpose, the formation of such committees is evidence of a breakdown or challenge of the basic agreement concerning the division of powers, resources, and functions among the various interest groups comprising an interorganizational system. The manifest function of such a committee may be substantive policy, but the latent function is to restore the equilibrium between the various social and political forces comprising the system. If the committee's operations are successful, either the existing divisions of powers and resources will be reaffirmed against challenging forces, or priorities and goals will be redefined slightly to favor a set of interest groups now more strategically located than before.

Since these reports and studies are the raw empirical data for this segment of our study of interorganizational relationships, they will be subjected to intensive analysis in this chapter, resulting in what to some readers may seem an overly exhaustive analytic summary, explication, and evaluation. Nevertheless, in order to avoid the criticism that the evidence is not given in full but only broad generalizations—a criticism made by this author of the reports themselves—each study or report will be described at considerable length so that its own evidence and argument can be made available to the reader.

The purpose of this detailed analysis is to evaluate the reports with respect to their consideration of the causes, characteristics, and consequences of, and their policy recommendations on, the "fragmentation" and lack of "coordination" of the New York City health system. Our hypothesis is that these commissions represent a temporary coalition of "corporate rationalizers" attempting to improve the level of planning, organizing, integration, and coordination of the health system without, however, really attacking the dominant interests which presently control the major resources of the health system: private physicians and the voluntary hospitals. The contradiction between the laudable goal of coordination and the unwillingness or inability to alter the power structure of the health system should lead to some clear manifestations of ideology rather that scientific or merely objective analysis. That is, according to our hypothesis, one should find in these reports ambiguities of terminology, lack of definition, lack of consistent usage, and the use of concepts for their symbolic or connotative function rather than as descriptive or explanatory tools. The "good" things—planning, integration, coordination, reorganization, affiliation—will enter the reports only to legitimate the recommendations; the "bad" things—fragmentation, duplication, uncoordination, disorganization—will simply be mentioned as "problems," but there will be little, if any, serious attention to their causes. If the reports are largely ideological in character and function and serve as a weapon in interorganizational and interest group struggles, logical gaps will appear between the "facts" mentioned and the recommendations for change seemingly adduced from the facts.

Also, if our argument is correct, the major recommendations should be "bureaucratic" in character—administrative changes and reshuffling, the establishment of new agencies and new powers for old agencies, movement from centralization to decentralization and back again, without any argument or evidence that these changes will have the supposedly desired consequences. In the absence of evidence or argument, a set of assertions will be given which rely upon plausible assumptions and inferences which assume that the reader will either accept the implicit frame of reference or be powerless to challenge that frame of reference. This is the key aspect of an ideology—the rational content is almost irrelevant to the social function of the ideas: to reassure certain groups, to convey messages of support to others, to warn still others of a potential challenge to their power.

In most of these reports, but particularly in those using the language and rhetoric of "systems analysis," the abstract and seemingly neutral tone is deceptive. As Ida Hoos remarked in her critique of systems analyses of public policy: "Precisely because systems analysis is a technique in which form takes precedence over and even determines content, the reliance on language becomes treacherous. It encourages lack of careful formalization and formulation. This leads to a chain reaction of poor conceptualization, gathering of data more because they are available than indicative, and dependence on factors only because they can be counted in the ongoing analysis and not because they are known to be important in the final analysis."[4] As we shall see later, several reports, including two by the System Development Corporation and the RAND Institute, exhibit precisely these characteristics.

2. Historical Background[5]

Throughout the 1960's, a variety of groups were raising issues, defining problems, and making demands about the health care delivery system in New York City. These groups included hospital workers, private practitioners, interns and residents, voluntary hospital spokesmen, medical students, and community groups. They represented a broad range of viewpoints about the system. Yet the policies that were developed, such as the affiliation program, the reorganization of the Health Department and of the Hospitals Department, and the creation of the Health and Hospitals Corporation, responded by and large only to a particular set of problems—the problems of financial management, structure of control over resources, the need for teaching and research patients, and staff shortages. On the assumption that it is the voluntary sector that can best deliver health services, policy makers developed plans which insured that the health care system continued to operate under the domination of the voluntary and private sectors. According to our earlier typology of the structure and alignment of interest groups in the health system, this philosophy and these policies represented the "corporate rationalizer" viewpoint.

How did this situation come about? An analysis of who identified what "crises" in the hospital system can be very useful in an attempt to understand the timing and the content of policy formation; the one employed here will be based on a summary of all of the *New York Times* articles from 1959 through 1967 that described particular situations in the health care delivery system as "critical" or as ones which so endanger the delivery of health care that remedies must be found. It will not be necessary for our purposes to evaluate the validity of these claims about "crises." In general, it was the corporate rationalizers who were the first to identify the crisis situations, and they stressed as problems those aspects of the situation that lent themselves to seeming remedies within the corporate rationalizer framework. They equated good health care with efficient management of scarce resources. The corporate rationalizers' exposure of "crises" can also be seen as an effort to promote public reorganization of the system in order to protect and solve problems in the private sector.

In 1959 the Greater New York Hospital Council warned that costs in municipal and voluntary hospitals would rise (*New York Times,* 10 March 1959, p. 72)[6] and that the examination for graduates of foreign medical schools would result in a severe shortage of interns and residents in the municipal hospitals (16 November 1959, p. 33). When Mayor Wagner established the Heyman Commission, both he and Heyman noted that the costs of hospital and medical care were rising "astronomically" and that this constituted a "very precarious financial situation" (13 February 1959, p. 1). According to the *New York Times,* the drive for the unionization of hospital workers highlighted the "constant worry in the hospital field: money" (17 May 1959, sec. iv, p. 12).

In 1960 financial problems and staff shortages were stressed. The United Hospital Fund and the Greater New York Hospital Council warned of closings of voluntary hospitals because of inadequate city reimbursement for ward patients and of the general "crisis" in the finances of municipal and voluntary hospitals (29 January 1960, p. 1; 9 May 1960, p. 14; 14 November 1960, p. 33). The Hospitals Department Annual Report was the first to emphasize a serious staff shortage (2 March 1960, p. 39), a theme picked up by the Heyman Commission (15 August 1960, p.1), the *New York Times* (6 August 1960, p. 18), and the Greater New York Hospital Council (14 November 1960, p. 33). The New York County Medical Society alleged that the sharp drop in the number of ward patients in voluntary hospitals threatened the training of interns and residents there (11 December 1960, p. 84).

In 1961 the emphasis was that the whole system faced a "crisis" due to finances. The municipal sector was in especially grave condition because of staff problems as well. The Hospital Council (9 January 1961, p. 30), Dr. Ray Trussell (2 March 1961, p. 31), and the Citizens' Committee for the Children of New York (23 March 1961, p. 40), raised these cries.

In 1962, 1963, and 1964, while the affiliation plan was being implemented in a piecemeal way, some community groups and county medical societies were questioning the wisdom of the program, but none of the groups that probed the system in earlier years were raising alarms. In this regard 1965 was also quiet until a mayoral condidate announced that conditions in one-half of the municipal hospitals were "shocking" and that the whole system was in need of an overhaul (15 October 1965, p. 30). In 1966 the "crises" returned. The system had to be reorganized. Associations of voluntary interests, members of city government, and state investigators were among those who "probed" the hospital system and found it to be in dire straits. The alarm was first sounded by the Hospital Review and Planning Council of Southern New York when it reported its findings of a survey conducted for the United Hospital Fund: New York City was facing a "major hospital crisis." All hospitals were "critically in need of [plant] revitalization" (24 February 1966, p. 1). The New York Times picked up on this theme and urged that joint financing be undertaken to ease the "crisis" (2 March 1966, p. 40). The Citizens' Committee for the Children of New York warned of sharply curtailed services due to staff shortages, inefficiency, and low morale (27 March 1966, p. 59). Councilman Modugno of the New York City Council charged that the nurse shortage (in municipal hospitals) was worse than ever (12 April 1966, p. 31). The Southern New York Hospital Review and Planning Council again stressed the urgent need for hospital renovation which should be undertaken as part of a program to develop regionalization centered around voluntary-teaching hospital complexes (23 June 1966, p. 39). Much of the concern was generated in anticipation of the forthcoming Medicare program. Martin Tolchin of the New York Times studied care in municipal hospitals and found severe staff and equipment shortages (27 June 1966, p. 1). Federal and New York State officials were preparing to review the Medicare status of the municipal hospitals in response to Tolchin's survey (16 July 1966, p. 1). Health Services Administrator Howard J. Brown threatened that staff and equipment shortages could force the major municipal hospitals to close (6 July 1966, p. 1). When State Senator Seymour Thaler wired Governor Rockefeller that conditions in several major municipal hospitals were "horrible," the governor ordered an immediate state investigation which focused on physical conditions and personnel and equipment shortages in the municipal hospitals (2 October 1966, p. 1). The Citizens' Committee for the Children of New York wrote to the governor that the municipal hospitals were in a "permanent crisis" (6 October 1966, p. 1). Senator Norman Lent reported the "inescapable conclusion" of the NYS probe that indigent patients had been treated with "cynicism and cruelty" for the past twenty years (27 October 1966, p. 29). He called the nursing shortage in the municipal hospitals a "disaster" and a "disgrace" (1 November 1966, p. 44). The United Hospital Fund undertook a study and reported "major deficiencies" in all twenty-one municipal hospitals—in plant maintenance, in personnel and supply shortages, and in too much red tape (13 November 1966, p. 70). The United Hospital Fund also reported that the voluntary hospitals were going deeply into debt because of inadequate and delayed Medicare and Medicaid reimbursements (3 December 1966, p. 1). Finally, toward the end of the year, the mayor of New York City conceded the "neglect" and "decline" of the municipal hospitals (19 December 1966, p. 1), and established a commission to review the problems (21 December 1966, p. 1).

The year 1966 was also one of continuing labor agitation which involved not only hospital workers but also physicians, nurses, veterinarians, and public health workers. Also during this time, Senator Thaler and Comptroller Mario Procaccino were making public evidence of fraud and mismanagement under affiliation contracts and were holding some of the voluntary hospitals and medical centers responsible. Although the groups that identified the "crises" were focusing on plant maintenance and equipment and personnel shortages, and were urging further regionalization under autonomous, publicly supported voluntary medical center complexes, it seems that almost every aspect and assumption of the system was problematic.

In 1967 the probes into hospital conditions and conduct under the affiliation contracts continued. The debate continued over how the system was to be reorganized. Governor Rockefeller's panel reported that the municipal hospitals "do not meet minimum standards of acceptable quality" (6 May 1967, p. 1). Administrator Brown responded to this finding by arguing that the city should turn its hospitals over to private operation or to a nonprofit corporation (18 May 1967, p. 66). By the end of the year, the Piel Commission issued its report calling the conditions in the municipal hospitals "deplorable" and "irremediable" under the present system. The commission recommended the establishment of a public corporation to solve the problems of plant contruction, purchasing, and hiring procedures.

The investigations continued in 1968, broadening into ambulatory care, as well as the deficiencies in the municipal hospitals and the affiliation programs. Calls for establishing neighborhood family care centers providing comprehensive health care, linked with back-up hospitals for in-hospital care, were heard and responded to by a variety of hospital and city plans to expand ambulatory care facilities. (See chapter 3 for a case study of the attempts to establish such centers.) Finally, in 1970, the Health and Hospitals Corporation (HHC) was formed in response to the recommendations by the Piel Commission and other investigatory bodies. It included only the nineteen municipal hospitals.

In April 1973 the so-called Scott Commission (the Temporary State Commission to Make a Study of Governmental Operation of the City of New York) reported on the workings of the city's hospitals under the aegis of the HHC. According to the *New York Times* 17 April 1973, p. 41), it "called for drastic changes to give consumers a greater voice in determining health-care priorities." The commission—established by Governor Rockefeller and resisted by city officials who "felt they were being caught in the cross-fire of a vendetta between Governor Rockefeller and Mayor Lindsay—made a number of specific criticisms of the Health and Hospital Corporation's first two-and-a-half years: (1) "Rather than decentralizing authority, as was originally envisaged, the municipal hospital system has continued to concentrate increasing power in the central office." (2) "The municipal hospitals have abdicated too much of their authority to the voluntary hospitals and medical schools that operate the public institutions under affiliation contracts." (3) "The system has been too slow to grant meaningful participation to the community advisory boards that are required at the municipal hospitals." (4) "The system's administration . . . has consistently refused to provide adequate information even to its own board of directors." Dr. Joseph T. English, president of the corporation, noted in response that while the Scott Commission called for more ambulatory-care programs, state and federal governments were cutting back, particularly on funds for neighborhood health facilities.

The major concrete recommendation of the Scott Commission was that all new hospital construction in New York City, both private and public, should be halted immediately. "The moratorium should remain in effect," the commission said, "until strong measures have been taken to shift the emphasis in medical treatment from expensive in-bed hospital care to a citywide system of what it said were desperately needed out-patient clinics."

Less than one week after the Scott Commission submitted its report, Dr. English announced his impending resignation as head of the Health and Hospital Corporation (24 April 1973, p. 30). His resignation followed by a few days a vote by the board of directors of the corporation to "review the competency of the top management of the $800 million quasi-autonomous agency that runs the city's nineteen municipal hospitals" (20 April 1973).

Early in 1974, immediately after a new administration under Mayor

Abraham Beame took office, the first steps toward a decentralizing phase of health administration began. A new commissioner of health was appointed: Dr. Lowell E. Bellin, formerly first deputy commissioner of health in the city as well as former associate medical director of the Health Insurance Plan (HIP). The mayor announced that the Health Services Administration (HSA) would be dismantled (6 January 1974, p. 21).

A special committee advised the new mayor on "a comprehensive reorganization of the city's health services, involving some decentralization of the Health and Hospitals Corporation, more authority for the Health Commissioner, and less autonomy for some departments" (15 January 1974, p. 37). A series of other organizational and administrative changes were envisaged by the committee, which included Dr. John H. Knowles, president of the Rockefeller Foundation; Martin E. Segal, an investment banker; Dr. Howard A. Rusk, head of the Institute of Rehabilitation Medicine at the N.Y.U. Medical Center; Dr. Mary C. McLaughlin, former New York City commissioner of health and now commissioner of health services for Suffolk County, as well as Dr. Bellin.

Once again in February 1974 the municipal hospitals were facing a crisis, this time caused by inflation in the costs of food and fuel, producing an anticipated $13 million deficit. The board of directors of the Health and Hospitals Corporation directed the nineteen hospitals to prepare emergency measures for cutting costs. The possibilities mentioned included delaying of hiring and postponing alterations and purchases of equipment. Harlem Hospital's executive director mentioned closing the home-care program, curtailing emergency services, and closing family-planning clinics. "Other hospitals described similar planned economies, but many maintained that they had been underfinanced to start with" (17 February 1974, p. 35).

Given the background and experience of the new mayor's committee, it may safely be predicted that its report and recommendations concerning the latest "crisis" will parallel if not duplicate those now to be summarized in this chapter.

3. 1950, The Kogel Report:
   The Needs of the
   Department of Hospitals

The earliest report to be summarized dates from 1950 and is by the Mayor's Committee on the Needs of the Department of Hospitals. It was chaired by Marcus D. Kogel, M.D., Commissioner of the Department of Hospitals, and is a brief (twelve-page) summary of some of the capital construction needs at various municipal hospitals.[7]

The report began by summarizing some of the main trends the committee perceived which should affect "future planning of medical services for any large population groups": the aging of the population, increasing medical specialization, increasing health insurance, increasing ambulatory care, and increasing home care. These trends call for careful "planning," "integration," and "reorganization" of services to make the best use of scarce resources. No discussion of how to plan, integrate, or reorganize was presented, however, nor was any indication of who might carry out such functions or when.

One main concern of the report, consistent with its all-physician membership (which, not incidentally, contrasts sharply with all subsequent committees), was to suggest that creating incentives for the professional personnel manning city hospitals was important. "It is essential in all planning to insure that the facilities, and emoluments, compensation, and recognition of professional competence, be guaranteed as far as practical in order to make available the highest quality of medical and health services" (pp. 3-4). Thus, both teaching and research opportunities should be made available in every municipal hospital. "As far as practicable, hospitals should be affiliated with teaching institutions" (p. 4). This recommendation presaged the major thrust of policy ten years later.

Another main concern was "coordination," although this (like planning, integration, and reorganization) was never defined or analyzed: coordination between the public and voluntary hospitals, coordination between the various city departments. Some sixteen to eighteen different city hospitals were mentioned, mainly with respect to capital construction or alterations. Of the twenty or so separate items, only three included any policies affecting coordination, all three of them recommending affiliation of the hospital with a medical school.

At the end, in connection with a discussion of Bedford-Stuyvesant Hospital, the committee asserted that the "needs for a hospital in this area are primarily for staff appointments for physicians for admission of their own private patients" (p. 11). The committee then said that it "believes that for the pesent, the facilities to be constructed by the city should be restricted to the primary purpose of care for indigent patients." Even patients on Blue Cross insurance, it advised, should be transferred to voluntary hospitals as soon as possible. Its final point reiterated the key importance of obtaining adequate personnel: "the problem of personnel and professional services is most important" (p. 11).

As with other reports, what was *not* included in this report is as significant as what was included. This commission (unlike the Piel Commission of 1967) clearly accepted the two-class system—the reserving of municipal hospitals for the medically indigent; it also accepted (as did the Piel Commission) the dominance of the private sector of physicians and voluntary hospitals. The concern was only with the funds available to the Department of Hospitals for expansion of existing and construction of new facilities. In 1950 the problem of community control had not arisen, and the question of whether or not the population of the area in which a hospital was located wanted certain kinds of facilities or not was never considered as even a difficulty to be dealt with. The presumption of the report was that the city agencies, within budget and political constraints, had the legitimate authority to make decisions concerning the proper allocation of resources.

The report casually assumed that affiliation of municipal hospitals with medical schools would improve the caliber of the medical staff of the former. Teaching institutions "being concerned with the training and preparation of practitioners, should endeavor to help the hospitals to obtain professional personnel of the highest order" (p. 4). Also, it assumed that voluntary cooperation between the public and private sectors and between various public agencies would suffice to insure adequate coordination. "Only through voluntary cooperation of this type [the Department of Hospitals' acceptance of the Master Plan for Hospitals and Related Facilities recently drawn up by the Hospital Council of Greater New York] can we expect to avoid unnecessary and costly duplication of facilities and services. The public is thus assured a 'hospital system' which will effectively meet the medical and hospital needs of the city" (p. 5).

This document was quite clearly, from the rhetorical tone, an internal document used by one or another administrative faction in New York City government. Its matter-of-fact taking for granted of limited resources, the two-class system, the importance of providing professionals with maximum incentives, the recognition of the low status of outpatient services, and the use of the rhetoric of bureaucratic rationality without any real analysis or content—coordination, integration, reorganization, planning—indicates that in 1950, in the absence of public clamor over the quality and quantity of health services, an incremental, "satisficing" set of assumptions could suffice as the basic frame of reference for city officials and agencies. The city could move slowly toward replacement or alteration of obsolete health facilities without causing crises for which either tangible or symbolic solutions had to be found. Nineteen sixty, the date of the next report we shall consider, marked the beginning of a decade of crisis in which a torrent of exposes, investigations, recommendations, and reorganizations flowed.

4. 1960, The Heyman Commission: Health Services in New York City

In February 1959 Mayor Robert F. Wagner appointed a Commission on Health Services, with investment banker and founder of the Health Insurance Plan of Greater New York (HIP) David M. Heyman as the chairman; Henry C. Brunie, president of the Empire Trust Company and chairman of the United Hospital Fund, as vice-chairman; and with Howard A. Rusk, M.D., director of the Institute of Physical Medicine at New York University, and thirty-six other members representing the full range of health-related private and public organizations in New York City. The report of the Commission was presented to the public on 5 August 1960.[8]

Although the charge to the Commission was to "review any of the health services in the City," most of the discussion and recommendations concern the municipal hospitals. In fact, at one point, for no apparent reason except to make clear the commitments of the commission, the report suddenly said, "A clear acceptance of the importance of preserving the voluntary hospital system is fundamental although this group of institutions is not without serious problems" (p. 13). What those problems were was not discussed, and no recommendations affecting the voluntary hospitals were made. The reader was referred to the "extensive study of municipal-voluntary hospital relationships soon to be released by the Hospital Council" (see section 5 of this chapter).[9] Thus, although charged with investigating the entire range of health services, the commission chose to consider only the municipal hospitals, and in fact went out of its way to reaffirm the integrity of the voluntary hospital component of the hospital system.

The report singled out five areas for separate consideration: standards, personnel, facilities, selected services, and organization and administration. With respect to the standards of care, the commission was most concerned with the unaffiliated municipal hospitals, although "some voluntary hospitals have very similar problems" (p. 3). As evidence of the poor care in the municipal hospitals, the commission cited the withdrawal of approvals of "various specialist programs" by the American Medical Association, loss of accreditation from the Joint Commission on Accreditation of Hospitals, very few internships from students trained in approved medical schools, and a predominance of poorly trained foreign physicians. The report's remark that "the amount of supervision given by the paid and unpaid attending staff is highly variable" is undoubtedly a euphemism.

It is striking that the remedies proposed by the commission were all "bureaucratic" in character. That is, they all were reorganizations, transfers of authority, or establishments of new mechanisms of regulation and control. But none of the recommendations referred to the voluntary hospitals, despite similar conditions in "some" of them and the general charge to the commission to consider any of the health services in the city.

Specifically, the recommendations by the commission to improve standards of care were to establish a "review mechanism," full-time chiefs of service and approval of their appointments by a "Dean's Committee," and, with respect to proprietary nursing homes, "the transfer of the medical care functions of the Department of Welfare to be supervised by an Executive Director of Medical Care in the Department of Health." How these measures would correct the shortage of well-trained medical personnel, the lack of good interns, or the deficiencies of the specialty programs was not even mentioned.

The second set of problems considered by the commission concerned the shortage of personnel, not just their quality. Instead of qualified nurses, the municipal hospital system employed nurses' aides. Although 6,157 positions were actually budgeted for staff nurses, only 1,756 were employed. But 8,451 nurses' aides were employed, despite the existence of only 5,279 budgeted positions for them. Similar, if not quite so dramatic, shortages existed for a wide variety of other personnel: dieticians, medical social workers, psychiatric social workers, occupational therapists, physical therapists, and speech and hearing therapists. For medical social workers, for example, 298 positions were budgeted, but 157 of these were vacant, although there were 40 persons on provisional appointments.

Once again, the analysis and solutions involved largely bureaucratic perspectives. The "cumbersome process of recruitment and appointment" was criticized, as well as low salary scales. While these factors were no doubt substantial and the recommendations well taken, others have much more the aura of reshuffling and yet more "studies." An "intensive examination of the entire system of personnel management" was supported as offering real "promise for the city health system."

The third set of problems considered by the commission was facilities. Again the commission was quite explicit in narrowing their focus to the municipal hospitals. The report declared that their focus was "on municipal operated or licensed facilities with full recognition that some voluntary hospitals are faced with similar problems." With this gesture, they then proceeded to ignore the voluntaries.

As with the other problems, the report advocated bureaucratic remedies and gave little or no analysis. They mentioned a study of maintenance services for the hospitals done by the City Administrator which found a "need for considerable improvement in organization, management, and planning. His recommendations for reorganizing the Department's engineering services are being implemented, but progress has been to slow" (p. 7). Their major recommendation, however, was to locate city beds at teaching centers, "both medical schools and strong teaching hospitals. The two principal reasons insofar as facilities are concerned are to implement regionalization and to eliminate costly duplication" (p. 8). The assumption, clearly, was that such a location would upgrade the quality of care and serve to further the "coordination" of the health system. Once again, however, no argument or evidence that such consequences would follow was given.

In the section on "selected services," the commission chose to deal with ambulatory care, home care, and the Homestead Plan. The 1960 commission, like the 1950 report, noted the low status of the ambulatory and emergency room services, resulting in understaffing. "It is very difficult to persuade practicing physicians to give time in the outpatient department." The Department of Hospitals was unable to secure money to pay "practicing physicians on a per session basis" (p. 10). No recommendations were made by the Commission about this "extremely important" problem, but it was noted that the area of ambulatory care will "come under university study next fall," and should be "encouraged" by the administration. Home care was barely mentioned except in a context of approval because it might save money and reduce the need for outmoded facilities. The Day and Night Hospital Program—part-time hospital care (day or night)—was approved of. The nature of the Homestead Plan was not made clear, although it was described as a Public Home Infirmary unit within the physical plant of a hospital which reduced the per diem costs of hospital care. The Homestead Plan was initiated, according to the commission, in 1957 "after a series of studies ... showed approximately *twenty percent* of the patients in municipal hospitals did not need hospital services" (p. 11, my italics). The causes of this striking figure were not analyzed nor were any recommendations made except the continuation of the Homestead Plan, although no figures on its feasibility or costs or savings possible through its extension were given.

The last section, "organization and administration," made even more direct bureaucratic recommendations. Failures or deficiencies in "communication," "coordination," and "fragmentation" were stressed (p. 12), although there was no definition of these terms or any analysis of the connection of their causes with the possible consequences of administrative reorganization.

Another structure within city government was suggested, one which could "function as a 'horizontal agency' to foster coordination of services" or could sponsor a "State Hospital Review and Planning Council which will coordinate the work of regional councils and require more of them" (p. 13). These two suggestions were merely reported by the commission as possibly helpful. Their own recommendations were for a

careful administrative review [of the health services in New York City] in terms of establishing a structure with routine policies and procedures which will improve standards, develop a series of regionalized programs with proper balance of authority between central agency and local operating units, eliminate unnecessary duplication thus conserving important personnel and expensive equipment, simplify administration, coordinate and integrate services to families, keep utilization of each type of service at the appropriate level consistent with scientific progress, prevent unnecessary construction, cut down the fragmentation of services, foster community planning, and make the maximum use of the taxpayers' investment in health protection and conservation (p. 13).

This sentence was quoted at length to give a full flavor of the bureaucratic rhetoric, containing such undefined and loaded words as "proper," "unnecessary," "important," "maximum," "scientific," "expensive," "simplify," and so forth—language which conveys an impression of rational analysis without any content.

The most specific recommendations made by the commission were: (1) raising intern and resident salaries; (2) implementing affiliations of municipal hospitals with medical schools or with "voluntary hospitals having strong teaching programs" (p. 14); and (3) appointing full-time chiefs of service in unaffiliated municipal hospitals.

At one point late in the report, it became clear why the hospitals were so understaffed. Mention was made of the "accruals" policy of the city, whereby city agencies were prevented from using their entire budget. That is, a certain amount of "forced saving" was required from each city agency at the end of the budget year, which can be obtained only by not filling budgeted positions or by not carrying out budgeted maintenance or building programs. The commission administered a slight slap on the city's wrist for this policy, saying that "the problems are more urgent than seem to be realized by those who establish policy with respect to the use of funds" (p. 15).

A few more bureaucratic recommendations were made. The Board of Hospitals should "exercise more authority" and might be "enlarged to deal with its many problems" (p.14). Responsibility for licensing of proprietary facilities "might very well be transferred to the Department of Health." Also, in a final major suggestion, the report proposed that "the Board of Hospitals, its newly invited Deans' Committee, the Department of Health, the Department of Social Welfare, the Hospital Council, the Mental Health Board, the United Hospital Fund, the Hospital Association, the Medical Societies, and several other responsible groups could begin at any time the coordination of medical and other health services usually referred to as regionalization" (p. 16). How such diverse bodies could coordinate anything, and what their incentives for doing so would be, was not discussed.

In sum, the analysis and recommendations of the Heyman Commission were either trivial, obvious, or rhetorical. What is striking is the assumption that the readers of the report would accept the implicit bureaucratic perspective and the explicit assertion that the private sector of the voluntary hospitals was inviolate and should not be invaded by public authority.

5. 1960: the Eurich Report: New York City and Its Hospitals

Less than six months after the Heyman Commission issued its report, another one was released, sponsored by the Hospital Council of Greater New York (now called the Health and Hospital Planning Council of Southern New York). It was chaired by Alvin C. Eurich.[10] Not surprisingly, in view of the overlap of about a quarter of the membership, its recommendations were very similar to those of the Heyman Commission. Greater concern for the financial stability and patient responsibilities of the voluntary hospitals was shown by the Hospital Council report.

Like the Heyman Commission, the Hospital Council report emphasized the staffing problems of the municipal hospitals, both physicians and nurses, and recommended paying physicians for outpatient services and establishing full-time chiefs of service. Both reports blamed the "accrual" system for budget stringencies, recommended the transferral of supervisory responsibility for nursing homes from the Department of Hospitals to the Department of Health, emphasized the capital needs of both voluntary and municipal hospitals for renovation and expansion, and advocated that the city pay more to the voluntaries in order to cover the full cost to them of the care of "City patients." Both reports recommended building municipal beds in voluntary hospitals. In terms of major recommendations, both reports agreed on the importance of affiliating municipal hospitals with medical schools or with voluntary hospitals with strong teaching responsibilities.

But the difference in emphasis and in a few major recommendations is striking. The Eurich report recommended limiting the number of beds in all hospitals and advocated closing municipal hospitals without affiliations, and also closing smaller voluntary hospitals and proprietary hospitals. The Heyman Commission mentioned closing some hospitals but did not link the reasons for this with the lack of an affiliation, as the Eurich report did quite strongly. Thus, the Eurich report emphasized limiting or even reducing the number of hospital beds available in New York City, a point not made or even hinted at by the Heyman Commission.

Coupled with this was a much greater concern with costs and financing in the Eurich report, particularly for the voluntary hospitals. Great emphasis was laid upon the importance of payment of bills by those persons who could afford to do so, and upon various mechanisms for increasing insurance support for the hospitals, something barely mentioned by the Heyman Commission. The Heyman Commission, on the contrary, emphasized changes costing money without considering the sources of financing: the need for increased staff, higher salaries, faster construction, payment of physicians for outpatient services, and increased payments to the voluntary hospitals.

Another major difference between the two reports was the greater emphasis given to the voluntary hospitals in the Eurich report. Care in them was simply assumed to be better without any evidence or argument, and their management was assumed to be more efficient; therefore the thrust of several recommendations was to give the voluntary hospitals "broader responsibilities." The voluntary hospitals should take over more indigent patients, and city hospital wings should be leased to the voluntaries, although how that would improve the quality of service was not made clear. With respect to the affiliation of hospitals with teaching centers, although both reports agreed on this recommendation, the Eurich report was much more hesitant about the ability of the medical schools and voluntary hospitals to take on such a major commitment and obligation as the provision of qualified professional staff for the municipal hospitals. The Eurich report, in a final difference with the Heyman Commission, advocated, at least tentatively if not as general policy, the establishing of private beds in municipal hospitals as an incentive to physicians to provide free service to ward patients without having to travel so far back to the voluntary hospital to see their paying patients.

What is striking in both reports is the casual assumption, reflected in the major recommendation, that a bureaucratic change—affiliation contract of a municipal hospital with a medical school or voluntary hospital—would have major effects upon the quality and quantity of professional staff available at the minicipal hospitals. No supporting arguments or evidence on behalf of this major change in the control of an enormous hospital system were presented. It was simply assumed that the medical schools and voluntary hospitals had the means, the will, and the resources to command a basic shift in the allocation of high quality physicians to the municipal hospitals. One important question for the analysis of the reports and investigations from further on in the decade—when the affiliation program itself became an political issue and an element in the continuing "crisis"—is whether there was ever any evidence, any serious study, or any program of research evaluating the quality of care provided by various kinds of hospitals, and the consequences of the affiliation program for the number, training, and quality and quantity of care made available to the city hospitals by the medical schools and voluntary hospitals. How many of these recommendations were followed up, studied, evaluated, or even mentioned in future reports?

Another striking similarity between the two reports is the neglect of the problem of ambulatory care. It was mentioned in both the Eurich and Heyman reports, at slightly greater length in the latter, but only in passing. The reports agreed that there was excessive hospitalization, that ambulatory care should be increased, and that one problem was the lack of physicians willing to do such low-status work for nothing. But although both reports lamented the problem, neither made any recommendations. Nothing in these reports, in other words, anticipated the great attention to be paid to the problem of "neighborhood health centers" only a few years later. This emphasis on the problems of hospitals per se seems more legitimate for the Eurich report, which only claimed to be a study of the "roles and responsibilities of the municipal and voluntary hospitals in New York City," not a study of "health services" as a whole, as the Heyman Commission was supposed to be.

In sum, despite the overlap of personnel, the Eurich report was much more committed to the voluntary hospitals as the source of high quality care, and many of its recommendations were concerned with changing the structure of control of the hospitals to place the municipal hospitals much more under the control of the voluntary hospitals. Also, the report was committed to the concept of large hospitals, rather than small ones, as the most efficient purveyor of high-technology medical care. The lack of concern with ambulatory care was consistent with the commitment of the report (and evidently the Hospital Council, its sponsor) to the problems of efficient management and funding of the larger voluntary hospitals.

These hospitals were clearly defined as analogous to corporate enterprises, facing similar problems of covering overhead costs, finding reasonable capital funding, and securing maximum fees in return for service from individual patients, third-party insurance carriers, or government agencies.

6. 1966, The
   Haldeman Report:
   Medical Economics

On 14 February 1966 the Mayor's Advisory Task Force on Medical Economics, appointed some months before, submitted its report.[11] The report of the committee on health care system requirements is of main concern to us. All members of this committee were connected with hospitals, universities, medical schools, planning councils, public health associations, and prepaid health plans. One might expect a strong emphasis on the rationalization and coordination of the health system, with relatively little attention being paid to the rights and powers of the individual physician; such is indeed the case. This brief report (28 pages) consists of an introduction, a summary of the "problems in existing patterns of health services" (thirteen numbered paragraphs), one page of "long-range goals," nine "guidelines for the future development of health services," and seven "major recommendations for future action."

The introduction summarized the scope and costs of health services in the city. The list of problems begins with the classic and orthodox statement of those groups concerned with rationalizing the organizational or corporate structure of health care:

Present organizational patterns and methods of administering and distributing services are outmoded, result in inefficient use of the City's total health resources, and are not always responsive to the health needs of the population. For the most part, the pattern of health services is characterized by uncoordinated effort; imbalance in distribution or, in some instances, critical shortages; disparity of quality; inadequacies in financing and a variety of administrative and legal barriers to the provision of coordinated and comprehensive health services. (p. 11)

These typical phrases—"outmoded," "inefficient," "imbalanced," "uncoordinated," "comprehensive"—which imply that the main barrier to the achievement of adequate health services is a failure of the organizational or bureaucratic structure indicate the ideological viewpoint we have labeled "corporate rationalization." Unfortunately, the terms were not defined nor were any empirical criteria given which might enable an assessment of the degree to which these characterizations were true. Possibly some more adequate analysis would appear in the "guidelines" section, where presumably some criteria for change were to be offered. Unfortunately, this was not the case. Most of the guidelines, not just this one, were simply statements which said "do something about the problem," without specifiying what to do or any reasons why.

Given the "problem" of a lack of "coordination" as stated in the report, it is natural that the long-range goals include the following: "The future goal for health services in New York City must be the development of a system which is a rationally financed and coordinated network of facilities and services" (p. 18). Given this "goal," the guideline follows inevitably: "Taking advantage of the fiscal relief that will be available from new State and Federal legislation, the City should move as rapidly as sound plans can be developed to coordinate existing services, fill serious deficiencies that presently exist and generally strengthen and shape medical care resources into a systematic network of services that will meet the needs of the people, especially in low income neighborhoods" (Guideline no. 1, p. 19). One could hardly expect a more helpful and concrete guideline. Let us see how this guideline is translated into a "recommendation."

The report's first "major recommendation for future action" says that "steps should be taken to achieve the goal of a coordinated hospital system in which every hospital and related health facility serves all elements of the population regardless of source of payment for care and in accordance with community needs" (p. 21). The only specific steps recommended, however, were the following: (a) a contract between the city and a voluntary hospital or medical school for total operation of a municipal hospital; (b) the opening of a municipal hospital to all patients in an economically depressed community; (c) the continuation of municipal hospital care for Medicare-eligible patients over sixty-five years old; and (d) the construction of new municipal facilities adjacent to voluntary hospitals or medical schools (p. 23).

There was no discussion of how or why these steps would contribute to rationalization, coordination, or planning. It was simply assumed that the voluntary hospitals were the model for good care, that their control of municipal hospitals would, ipso facto, constitute a move toward a more coordinated system, and, correlatively, that the public institutions lacked the capability and the resources either to become the models themselves or to take over control of the voluntaries, rather than vice versa. The grotesque discrepancy between the general, more abstract character of problem, goal, guideline, and recommendation—all defined at about the same level of vagueness—and the actual inadequate recommendations is prima facie evidence that the report as a whole was an ideological statement by one faction (or a coalition of smaller factions) in the general battle over control of the health institutions and resources of New York City.

While this particular series of statements referring to coordination may be the most glaring example of the vagueness and inadequacy typical of the wording in such reports—usually a sign either of basic disagreement among the members of an investigative committee or of their inability to think of any solutions for a fundamental problem— the other statements made by the committee were nearly as vague, in view of the similar analyses and recommendations made by the other such committees before and after this one. It is important to give them their due, however. Such reports do and did draw to at least some portion of the public's attention the pervasive, deeply institutionalized, and continuing defective character of the "outputs" of the New York City health system.

Aside from drawing attention to the highly ambiguous property of "fragmentation" as either a cause or a consequence of health care problems, this report restated many important criticisms. "In some instances" (how many?), physicians and other health professionals were "not professionally competent.... Certain areas of the City have few or no facilities" (pp. 11-12). Hospitals of all types maintained facilities segregated according to income (p. 12). Nursing home and extended care facilities were inadequate (p. 12). Of patients occupying hospital beds, about 15 to 20 percent could have been cared for in other ways, thus freeing beds for those who needed them and reducing costs considerably (p. 13). Ambulatory care facilities were "inadequate" (p. 13). Hospital emergency departments were "being overwhelmed by constantly increasing numbers of patients" (p. 13). Home care was deficient. Serious personnel shortages of all types existed (p. 13). Hospitals were concerned almost exclusively with inpatients (p. 14). Poor neighborhoods had almost no "comprehensive patient-centered medical care services at the local community level" (p. 14). All health facilities were subject to "chronic underfinancing" (p. 15). Care for the mentally ill was "inadequate" (p. 15), with a "tragic shortage" of facilities (p. 16).

Construction of new facilities had been subject to "serious delays" (p. 16).

This litany of defects and problems has been summarized merely to indicate the pathetic repetition of the same points with wearisome regularity in report after report, and to emphasize the paucity of serious analysis of the *causes* of these characteristics of health care and thus any kind of effective policy recommendations. Once again, this committee stressed the primacy of the hospital as the core service-providing institution of a "modern" system, offering the vision of a "medical health service center" of the future (p. 18). Their second major recommendation, in fact, was that the "general hospital should be the core facility for medical and related health services for a community, and services should increasingly be hospital based or related" (p. 23).

The other major recommendations can be summarized as follows: centralization of highly specialized facilities in a few hospitals; replacement of city hospitals containing fewer than 350 beds (because of economies of scale); maintenance of flexibility in facilities in order to permit inexpensive modification as medical technology changes; development of ambulatory care facilities in both voluntary and municipal hospitals; establishment of a "strong mechanism" to "achieve improved coordination of the efforts of various City agencies and voluntary institutions in planning and programming" (p. 28). How this latter recommendation differs from a guideline or a goal was not clarified, nor how it differs merely from a reformulation of the problem of fragmentation.

To summarize, this brief report was basically a restatement of the ideal health system from the point of view of corporate rationalization, emphasizing the central importance of the hospital, and specifically the voluntaries, as the organizers and integrators of health care. It can be interpreted as a weapon in the battle against both the private physicians, who are still in control of most health care, and the city bureaucracies, which still hamstring construction, hiring, and purchasing. While the affiliation contracts were mentioned favorably in this connection, they were no longer seen as the solution to the problems of coordinating the New York City health system. From the perspective of five years later, this report and others to follow seem clearly to be part of the process of political redefinition of a new medical program which would suit the political needs of the Lindsay administration. Each new regime, unable to generate enough political and social power to move toward serious improvement of the health system, must find a political formula which will hold its coalition together, fend off its enemies, and soothe the groups deprived of substantive services with slogans and promises. Judging from the internal evidence of this report, as of February 1966, no new programs, slogans, or "analyses" had yet been developed. Thus the process of redefinition had to continue in the search for a "solution" worthy of the new mayor and his reform program.

7. 1966, System Development
   Corporation: System
   Analysis and Planning

One month after the Mayor's Advisory Task Force on Medical Economics issued its report, the System Development Corporation (SDC) produced an "initial study" entitled "System Analysis and Planning for Public Health Care in the City of New York" (25 March 1966).[12] It was financed by the Health Research Council (HRC) of the city, and the directors of the study during its six months' duration were Dr. Robert B. Parks and Harvey M. Adelman, Ph. D. Dr. Parks was chairman of the advisory committee to the Task Force on Medical Economics whose report was just summarized. According to the "background" statement, the study had begun early in 1965, when officials of the HRC "opened discussions" with representatives of SDC.

One reads this system analysis with hopes that this report will at last probe beneath the surface and present, with a somewhat more comprehensive theoretical framework than that of previous reports, a truly systematic analysis of the causes of the characteristics of the New York health system. Because the study was issued under the auspices of an independent corporation, one might expect that it would be less committed to assumptions about the permanence and inevitability of certain structural characteristics of the present system. Alas, these hopes are soon dashed. Part of the report (pp. 27-60) actually contained the entire Task Force on Medical Economics report issued one month earlier, with a few differences which will be noted. Most of the rest (pp. 61-125) consisted of a sketchy "basis for system planning" which was internally contradictory and incomplete. The remainder consisted of a brief chapter on "evolution and overview" (pp. 13-26), a section of "emergent needs in environmental health" (pp. 127-45) which bore no apparent analytic relationship to the rest of the report, and a concluding chapter on the "impact of 1965 federal health legislation" (pp. 147-66), which was a useful summary of Medicaid and Medicare legislation but, again, was not integrated (in a "systems analytic" fashion) with the rest of the analysis.

Although the entire contents of the Task Force report were reproduced—facts, problems, goals, guidelines, and recommendations—one "problem" differed significantly. While problem 12 of the Task Force report read, "The physical plants of both voluntary and municipal hospitals require major expenditures for replacement or extensive modernization," clearly indicating an acceptance of the continuing existence of separate hospital systems, problem 12 of the System Analysis report read, "Excessive costs and profoundly complicated relationships are involved in the continuing tolerance of three separate hospital systems: municipal, voluntary and proprietary" (p. 41). Such a difference may indicate that a more fundamental reexamination of the system was possible for a report issued under SDC sponsorship rather than by a committee closely linked to the voluntary hospitals. (Four of the five members of the Task Force—Drs. Haldeman, James, Cherkasky, and Baehr—were affiliated with voluntary hospitals or planning agencies closely linked to them.)

At this point in the report problems 13 through 21 were inserted in the System Analysis report, additional problems in the health system which did not appear in the Task Force report. (Problems 22 and 23 in the former were the same as 12 and 13 of the latter.) Problems 14 through 21 constituted a severe indictment of both the public and the private health systems and are worth quoting in full, as background for an assessment of the adequacy of the "system analysis" which followed the listing of the problems.

14. The various departments in the health care system maintain a bewildering variety and number of expensive clinics.... 15. The city continues to tolerate wide spread duplication of expensive administrative services and appallingly archaic handling of information and records.... 16. There are a number of bad voluntary hospitals and bad clinics that continue to be subsidized with city funds because of their admission of city charge patients.... 17. City administrations have allowed vested bureaucratic practice to affect poor implementation of decentralization of health care delivery.... 18. The city has allowed its health care system departments to function so autonomously that system-wide efficiencies are, in fact, impeded.... 19. There is incredibly bad career planning and salary structuring for professionals.... 20. With the recent passage of some twenty or more significant pieces of Federal legislation affecting the health

care fields, there is no consolidated central staff to interpret this legislation and help to orient and otherwise prepare the system to institute adaptive change. 21. There is no centralized capability for planning and programming for the health care system. (pp. 42-44)

Stunning as this indictment may seem, it is nothing new; nor is it new that no criteria, no definitions of terms, no citations of research, and no empirical indicators were offered by this report to document these assertions, although the report was allegedly based on research. "Acquisitions of data" were mentioned, and "several hundred individuals" were cited (not all by name) as having "been of assistance." A possible basis for the problems, guidelines, and recommendations appears in section B ("A Basis for System Planning") of the report. However, pages 63 to 77 did not even mention the health system or New York City, except as passing illustration, and were devoted entirely to an exposition of "system planning" concepts: inputs, outputs, processes, feedback, criteria, alternatives, working plans, and so forth, complete with the neat diagrams and arrows which seem indispensable for a systems analysis. At last (pp. 78-82) five "attributes of good medical care" were named and briefly discussed: competence, comprehensiveness, continuity, patient/family centered care, early care, community oriented care. From these, "system objectives may be derived" (p. 82). The authors then noted that "both traditional and current practice still focus upon specific episodic disease (inputs), and upon specific clinical treatment (processes)," and asserted that these ways of organizing the system failed to meet the medical needs of the people. Instead, "expedient institutional forms have evolved to try to fill the gaps: community clinics of great variety, outpatient departments in various roles, emergency rooms which serve few emergencies, 'experimental' extended care capabilities, and the institutionally isolated nursing homes of poor standards, limited staffing and minimum effectiveness" (p. 83). This picture was perhaps accurate, but it was still at the level of description and criticism, not of system specification or analysis of causes. Unfortunately, the report never linked the "attributes of good care" to an analysis of why they were missing or what might have been done about it, *except* to prescribe still another reorganization at the top of the system.

At this point, apparently assuming that a serious analysis had been presented, an "institutional model" was presented and billed as a "system plan for long range implementation." This "model" (p. 85, fig. 6) simply consisted of a graph listing stages of "patient movement" through detection–prevention, diagnosis–early treatment, clinical inpatient care, extended care, and chronic care, and a list comprising the following: medical functions and facilities, community and economic factors, management factors, medical welfare support, and private sector. Following this "exposition" of an institutional model, the authors asked the rhetorical question, "Can system objectives be formulated from the attributes and from the model?" and answered it themselves: "Clearly they can" (p. 87). No arguments or evidence justifying this sweeping optimism were presented.

At this point, having presented the model for implementation, only a few steps apparently remained to transform the New York health system. The actual system plan, we were informed, remained for Phase II of the study. But the authors asserted that they could specify the additional studies needed. These are worth quoting in full in order to convince the reader that I am not parodying the argument.

First, a resolution of system objectives based upon more thorough study of the ten-element system model earlier presented. Second, refinement of, and agreement upon, the implications of the institutional model discussed above. [Note: this "model" was summarized above.] Third, completion of surveys begin in this first Phase study (section C) of the twelve 'Functional Areas of Comprehensive Planning.' [One of these, "The Structure and Role of Health Care Organizations" will be commented on below.] Fourth, the preparation of six program implementation plans—as identified in the following discussion (p. 88)

These six program implementation plans consist of the following: Five-Year Management Plan, Community Medical Service Center Plan, Plan for Coordinated Hospital System, Chronic Care Plan, Unified Information System Plan, and Leadership Coordination Plan (summarized from p. 89, fig. 7).

It should perhaps be emphasized at this point that a systems framework of analysis properly done can sensitize the analyst to complex chains of causes and consequences. But in the absense of substantive propositions linking parts of the system or some specification, no matter how tentative, of the major parameters defining the empirical system of reference, the systems language may be suspected of being ideological rather than scientific in its function, concealing the substantive interests at stake and affected by structural changes rather than clarifying them. Such is undoubtedly the case here, since the discussion remained entirely at an abstract level. None of these six plans was discussed in any detail, nor the means for generating the powers and resources necessary to implement them, nor the consequences of their implementation for any group, institution, or organization within the present health care system.

Immediately after this specification of studies and plans came the problem of implementation. According to the authors, "it is not reasonable to anticipate fulfillment of implementation programs in less than a five-year period." How this estimate was arrived at was not indicated, and it was probably inserted simply to fulfill the logical requirement of a systems analysis that the time required to change the system over to the new one be specified. But the assertion following in parentheses was even more improbable: "(Even this period would be too brief were it not for the accelerated mode of change to be induced by Medicare and other legislation.)" The assumptions in that sentence are worth pondering. It was assumed not only that the effect of Medicare would be positive—that is, in the direction predicted by the authors, although that was highly ambiguous given the abstract character of the prediction—but also that, in fact, change will be accelerated by Medicare, regardless of the direction. This faith in the 1965 federal leglislation has proved unjustified by the subsequent five years' experience and shows the shallowness of the analysis and the casual, almost unthinking nature of the prediction.

Consistent with this level of analysis was the easy prediction that all parts of the health system will simply fall in line with the "plans" as they are produced by the team of analysts in Phase II. Agreement was simply assumed, and lack of communication the chief barrier to agreement. This kind of assumption is typical of the mentality of corporate rationalization, which assumes that lack of knowledge is the chief barrier to change, that administrative mechanisms can be found to communicate that knowledge, and that quickly and easily men will fall into line behind the new "concept" of the system being offered to them. Such terms as "subsystem" and "implementation plans" were repeated in the report as if they were incantations; "system" lingo was substituted for analysis and theory. This is consistent with a faith in concepts as forces and also in the power of communication as a force for change. The reality of tough, resistant interest groups with stakes in the existing system, whose values and interests account for the system as it is, was not even hinted at in this report or in the others which take the same general point of view. Again, "each of the other plans would necessarily be correlated with the Hospital System Plan" (p. 95). Why? Can it be assumed that correlation and coordination will follow once the proper plan is conceptualized? Apparently. In and of itself this assumption vitiates the possible analytic usefulness of the entire report.

One might not criticize such an approach in this way if the distinction between an ideal system and a set of realistic policy recommendations were kept clear. One could postulate a set of key functions and institutional and organizational embodiments of those functions, and trace the interrelationships of such a complex system with the real one and ask what incentives, interests, and barriers are maintaining its present functioning. But in this report there is a constant moving back and forth from a postualted ideal scheme of relationships and functions to an implicit acceptance of major characteristics of the present system. Such analytic fuzziness can result only in the dulling of the analytic capacity of the ideal system model to serve as a basis of criticism and evaluation of the actual system and also as a way of concealing acceptance of major system parameters under the guise of abstract theory.

As was noted above, the last section of this report includes a chapter entitled "Structure and Role of Health Care Organizations." One would think that such a chapter would deal with all, or at least the major, organizations of this nature. This was not the case. The first sentence claimed that "portrayed in Figure 11 are *the four autonomous* organizations responsible for the delivery of health care in New York City." (p. 107, italics added). The authors then proceeded to list four *city* departments: Hospitals, Health, Welfare, and Community Mental Health. Why the sudden focus on city organizations? What happened to the voluntary hospitals and the private practitioners? That the voluntary hospitals and the private sector of medical practice evaded even an analysis, let alone challenge, of their role, functions, and resources, is impressive testimony to their legitimacy and power. But this ommission illustrates the poverty of this so-called systems analysis which allegedly dealt with health care organizations from the point of view of the entire health delivery system of New York City. The rest of the chapter dealt almost entirely with the interrelationships and structure of these four city organizations.

As with other reports, the *critique* offered by the SDC may well be accurate and well taken, but in the absence of criteria for description and explanation, no theory can be developed which can point to real causes and thus to serious policy recommendations for change. In the absence of such a theory—and not even a tentative one is offered—the authors resorted perforce to language which attempted to conceal the absence of serious analysis. Repetition of certain phrases—"communication," "personnel," "fractionation," "cost effectiveness"—seemingly central to the ideology of corporate rationalization, padded their report to convince the reader that it contained some substance.

One last example of one of their charts will be clarified by the reproduction showing the proposed functional organization of the ideal system (see chart).

| ADMINISTRATION |
| Interdepartmental Health Council |

Medical Information System Center —————— Program Planning

Health Research Council —————— "GSA"

| DIVISION OF MEDICAL WELFARE | DIVISION OF MENTAL HEALTH |

| DIVISION OF PUBLIC HEALTH | DIVISION OF CLINICS AND AMBULATORY CARE | DIVISION OF HOSPITAL ADMINISTRATION | DIVISION OF CHRONIC CARE |

Disease prevention, environmental health, community research, central laboratories

Hospital based, community related-diagnosis, treatment and referral

System unification and improvement

Rehabilitation, Nursing Homes, Home Care, Aged Program, etc.

Decentralized Community Medical Care Service Centers*

Fig. 1   Illustrative Functional Organization. "Conversion of District Health Centers throughout the city; activation of some Centers at or near major hospitals as possible; integration of health and welfare programs; Centers based upon Gouverneur experience to the extent possible; conversion costs partially defrayed by Federal funding."

The authors claimed for this functional organization that "it provides a basis for resolving not only the difficulties of organization discussed above in this Chapter, but those faults of institutional systems noted in Section B" (p. 120). How these new divisions would guarantee more coordination than the present departments was not discussed, nor why the same problems would not reappear, give the same allocations of powers, functions and resources. The authors simply asserted, without arguing the point or giving any evidence, that this scheme of "functional organization" would meet "all the major gaps of present capability in an orderly, rational structure. While providing flexibility for growth and alteration, the necessary features of both central integrity and decentralized authority are enhanced" (pp. 124-25).

The power of conviction of this rhetoric was undermined by several intrinsic internal contradictions in the scheme. An additional "division of clinics and ambulatory care" was proposed; such an innovation poses an intrinsic organizational dilemma, which was not even recognized, let alone discussed or analyzed. If one sets up a new agency to guarantee performance of a neglected function (in this case ambulatory care, long recognized as an underfunded, understaffed and low-status service), provision of enough resources and enough autonomy to guarantee that the staff will be committed to this function will also guarantee built-in resistance to coordination with other indispensible parts of the array of medical care facilities, such as in-hospital care. Such resistance and high degree of autonomy for an ambulatory care division would be a sign of *success*, not defeat, from the point of view of institutionalizing and protecting a particular kind of health service from attack. But from the point of view of the system as a whole, such a success would be a defeat. Such internal contradictions in a complex interorganizational system cannot be resolved by rhetoric, glistening language, or continuous manipulation of the administrative superstructure. Such deeply embedded system problems were not even mentioned by this report.

A second contradiction can also be seen. Note that in the reproduction of figure 13, arrows point from the four main divisions to "decentralized community medical care service centers." A footnote described these as follows: "Conversion of District Health Centers throughout the city; activation of some Centers at or near major hospitals as possible; integration of health and welfare programs; Centers based upon Gouverneur [a lower-East-Side ambulatory care center] experience to the extent possible; conversion costs partially defrayed by Federal funding" (p. 121). This confusing array of empirical translations of the concept of decentralized community medical care service centers failed to make clear just what functions they would perform.

But, more important for our present purpose, the authors said that "each of the six health divisions ... will [cooperate with and have representation within] the Community Medical Care Service Centers" (p. 124). Who will administer them? How will the health divisions be represented in them? Who will cooperate with whom? How do those centers differ from clinics and ambulatory care facilities? These simple and obvious questions, which raise again the basic issues of coordination of a complex system, were casually passed over by the report, which simply assumed that a recipe for reorganization would solve all of the knotty problems so eloquently summarized earlier. It is not at all clear that the system proposed will not be even more complicated and cumbersome, and more uncoordinated, fractionated, and fragmented than the one which now exists. Certainly the system analysis presented in this report gives no reasons for predicting any improvement.

But perhaps this critique has been unfair. The authors and their staff may have been operating under great pressures, with lack of enough resources and facilities to complete their analysis. Phase II of the systems analysis heralded throughout the report, may well have been more comprehensive and thorough. Unfortunately, SDC did not complete the job. Nevertheless, we still have a chance to evaluate the work of this staff. Largely on the strength of his important contribution to the Mayor's Advisory Task Force on Medical Economics and to the systems analysis, both just evaluated, Dr. Parks was chosen to head the staff for the Piel Commission, established by Mayor Lindsay on 22 December 1966, just nine months after Dr. Parks and Dr. Adelman issued their systems analysis. By this time Dr. Parks was executive vice-president of TECHNOMICS, Inc., and its staff carried out the various studies which formed the basis for the Piel Commission's report. Surely here we will see a serious and thorough analysis.

8. 1967, The Piel Commission:
Community Health Services
for New York

The so-called Piel Commission (The Commission on the Delivery of Personal Health Services) was established by Mayor Lindsay on 22 December 1966. A preliminary report was released in May 1967, and a final report on 19 December 1967. A book containing the text of the final report and the numerous staff studies carried out by the TECH-

NOMICS staff team was published in 1969.[13] The length and documentation of the volume indicate its impressive credentials. The official report occupies pages 3–97; the staff studies, pages 101–579; and six appendices, pages 583–675. Appendix A lists the names and affiliations of some 300 of the 500 persons interviewed, most of whom occupied responsible positions in New York City health institutions. Appendix B is an extensive bibliography.

The commission itself was composed of seven leading citizens: four bankers, a lawyer, a publisher, and an academic social worker. No physicians served on the commission itself, but a Medical Advisory Committee comprised fourteen physicians, eleven of whom were connected with hospitals, universities, health institutes, government health agencies, or medical schools. Only one was from a county medical society. Two were listed as representing the New York Academy of Medicine.[14] Thus, both the commission and its physician advisors were solid representatives of institutions which might be called the corporate health establishment, and would probably be predisposed toward at least the rhetoric of rationalizing the health system as a whole, with relatively little concern for the powers and privileges of the physician in solo practice. That was indeed the case, as we shall see.

As befits a commission with such a composition, the problem of fragmentation was stressed time and again with convincing examples, which it may be worthwhile for us to summarize in order to indicate again, in the words and descriptions of a responsible investigatory body, the characteristics of the interorganizational system being analyzed by these responsible bodies which themselves constitute an aspect of interorganizational behavior.

Generally the sheer complexity of the structure was stressed: "Some twenty-five City agencies administer health services to individuals in the City. They derive their charters from statutes enacted over the years for a variety of public purposes by the City, State, and Federal governments. The twenty-five agencies constitute a patchwork array of services, with different criteria of eligibility, separate medical as well as administrative records, and different methods of providing as well as purchasing care" (p. 79).

The consequences of this complexity and diversity are serious: "responsibility for personal health services is fragmented among the major health agencies and, within the agencies, among numerous bureaus that represent the historical accumulation of ad hoc programs" (p. 8). More specifically, "the district health centers and well-baby clinics of the Department of Health are located without reference to the availability of outpatient services of City (or voluntary) hospitals. As a result,

many needful neighborhoods are left entirely uncovered" (p. 24).
Moreover, in outpatient departments in both municipal and voluntary
hospitals, "the interminable waiting for appointments, the fragmentation of service into specialty clinics requiring separate appointments and
waiting times for each, the abrupt, hurried, and impersonal treatment by
the overburdened staff, the confusion of complicated regulations, the
crowded quarters, and the lack of adequate medical records—all subject
the patient to inconvenience, discomfort, and humiliation." These
characteristics are "evidence of their inadequate capacity and anachronistic geographical distribution," direct consequences of the fragmentation of the system and the absence of any planning (p. 15). The services
available in the district health centers and well-baby clinics are
similarly defective—"depersonalized, fragmented, and discontinuous"
(p. 16). Community mental health centers also suffer from fragmentation: "Principally for lack of initiative and coordination on the part of
other agencies, the Community Mental Health Board has been unable
to put into operation a single one of some fifty community mental
health centers that are to be established in New York City" (p. 17).
    The division of authority which is one of the root causes of fragmen-
tation of service was shown also in the complexity of bureaucratic
procedures. "Eighteen authorizations and clerical procedures, involving three different agencies with average total delay time of nine
months, are required to hire an x-ray technician. Similarly, fifteen
steps involving as many as four different departments are required to
make a routine purchase" (p. 25). Moreover, irrational divisions of
authority exist, as can be seen in the following instance: the Department of Welfare is charged by the state, following federal requirements, with validating Medicaid clients and signing them up when they
appear at a hospital asking for medical care. But the Department of
Hospitals provides the care. "This fragmentation of authority between
the agency responsible for the delivery of care and the agency charged
with validating claims of reimbursement has resulted in the loss of
millions of dollars of reimbursement properly owing the City from the
State and Federal governments" (pp. 26–27).
    Both fragmentation of service and its cause, division of authority,
were thus seen by the commission in the basic structure of health
services, manifest in the operations of health centers, outpatient departments, mental health centers, hiring procedures, and reimbursement authorizations—almost every aspect of the health system. Few
could argue with the impressive case made by the Piel Commission for
the existence of this pathological characteristic of the organization of
health services in New York City.

What was their solution? Let us summarize their main findings and recommendations. Their first major and most general finding was that the services available to half of the population receiving medical care at public expense "fail to meet their urgent needs for preventive and ambulatory care, on the one hand, and for long-term care, on the other. As a result, these people and the City are burdened with costs of excessive hospitalization and other costs not so easily measured" (pp. 12-13). Second, "in providing inadequate and substandard care and in serving only the indigent population in its own hospitals and clinics, the City is perpetuating a dual system of medical care with a built-in invidious double standard of private and welfare medicine" (p. 17). Third, "the City health agencies are impeded in the performance of their functions by the fragmentation of their assigned mission, by their own archaic administrative structures, and by dissipation of their authority in the system of 'checks and balances' administered by the overhead agencies of the City and mandated by both State and City law" (p. 23).

Three major recommendations were made. First, and again most general: "The City of New York should employ the authority and resources at its disposal to promote the coordination and integration of public and private resources in the development of comprehensive community health services offering medical care to all persons on the basis of their health needs" (p. 32). This recommendation, which might better be termed a goal, was deceptively simple and uncomplicated, but its implications were far-reaching, if taken seriously. Public authority was here charged with coordinating and integrating *all* resources, both public and private, into a health system serving all persons on the basis of need, rather than on ability to pay. The second recommendation, already implemented by the time the Commission report was issued, was to establish a Health Services Administration, which would consolidate all of the City health agencies—Health, Hospitals, Mental Health—into a single super-agency charged with monitoring the health status of the population, planning, coordinating, inspecting, and securing performance and fiscal accountability "of agencies receiving public funds" (p. 43). The third recommendation, later implemented in modified form by the 1970 Health and Hospitals Corporation, was that "the City should initiate the creation of a nonprofit Health Services Corporation" which would "operate the City hospitals and health centers . . . repair, renovate, and construct health facilities, . . . develop and operate system-wide data processing, communication and referral, transportation, personnel training and career development, purchasing, and laboratory services, . . . [and] promote

decentralized regional community health services throughout the City"
(p. 51).

It is interesting to note first the great differences in level of generality
of the three recommendations. The first one is not really a recommendation at all, but a vision or goal of comprehensive, accessible, and
equal health care for all. The second and third recommendations are
quite concrete examples of what we have called corporate rationalization: the shifting of administrative responsibilities with the implicit
assumption that creating new organizational forms are adequate means
for achieving the vision of recommendation no. 1. The latter two recommendations are excellent examples of the ideological perspective
which we would expect from this commission, given the makeup of its
membership. Given the proper framework of organization of powers and
functions properly divided and allocated, the system needs only the further energizing force of proper leadership to overcome all obstacles and
move forward energetically to whatever goals we set.

This point alone, however, is not yet a serious criticism, because such
an administrative reorganization might well be a major innovation which
would go far toward creating a framework within which responsible and
far-sighted political and administrative leaders and officials could
effectively operate. More important is the fundamental internal contradiction embedded in the findings and recommendations themselves: the
ambivalence which the commission's report displayed about the dual
system of municipal and voluntary hospitals, public and private control.
The commission undoubtedly was seriously split on the extent to which
these different, "dual" systems would be truly integrated and coordinated. (Some internal evidence of this split will be discussed later.)
Their analysis of the *consequences* of the dual, fragmented system (summarized earlier) was eloquently stated, but evidently they could not agree
on recommendations for the solution. The result: internal contradictions
and fuzzy, evasive language.

The contradiction is evident first in the contrast between the first
recommendation and the other two. The first, it will be recalled, called
for public authority to "promote the *coordination and integration of
public and private resources*" (p. 32, italics added). But the second
recommendation called only for consolidation of the *city* agencies in the
new Health Services Administration (HSA), and the third called for the
Health Services Corporation (HSC) to operate only *city* hospitals. It
seems fairly clear that true coordination, integration, and planning of
the *entire* health system is incompatible with the maintenance of a dual
system of control, which this definition of the powers of the HSA and
HSC calls for. These new bureaucracies might conceivably rationalize

some of the internal operations of city health institutions if they succeeded in extending the principle of the public, nonprofit corporation begun by the affiliation contracts. The latter were designed to release city institutions, at least in part, from the constraints of the checks-and-balances system in the city bureaucracies. But the new HSA and HSC certainly would lack the powers to coordinate and plan health services for the city as a whole, by definition, if they only controlled city agencies. (Another, secondary, contradiction might be noted between freeing city institutions from the checks and balances and simultaneously maintaining public accountability. How this would be done was not discussed.)

The central contradiction also appeared in the contents of a single recommendation itself. Recall that the third one called for the creation of a corporation to operate the city hospitals, but also to develop *system-wide* facilities of various kinds. How these system-wide powers would be reconciled with a dual system of control was not made clear. Then, immediately following the text of the recommendation itself came this translation and expansion: "As proposed in this Recommendation, it will be the mission of the Health Services Corporation to facilitate the transformation of the present dual system of private and public hospitals into a single, regionalized, and decentralized comprehensive health-care system" (p. 51). Does this mean that the corporation will take over the voluntary hospitals? Does this mean that the corporation will lease the municipal hospitals to the voluntaries? What *kind* of "single, regionalized" system is envisaged which would achieve the goals of the first recommendation: comprehensive, accessible, and equal health care for all? The report equivocated on these crucial questions.

This inability to confront squarely one of the key causes of fragmentation was concluded by the commission itself in its division of authority over hospitals and clinics into a dual system, and it resulted in a series of internally contradictory statements in the commission report. Some sentences implied a fully integrated system; others, the maintenance of a dual system linked only by attempts at coordination, joint services, or provision of facilities from one system to another.

Figure 1, on page 36 of the report for example, was titled "Integrated Health Services Delivery," and portrayed diagrammatically all of the different types of health service facilities in a region: ambulatory care facilities, extended and chronic care facilities, community hospitals, and a medical center. The description of this model system implied that there would be some mechanism for coordinating and planning *all* facilities in an area. The paragraph is worth quoting in full, both for its connotation of integration and for its evasive use of language.

Health service facilities in a borough or "region" should be *linked* by rational allocation of responsibility to form a comprehensive delivery system. Sites of primary care in each community are *related* to the community hospital. Each community hospital is *tied* in turn, to the teaching hospital or medical school that serves as the regional medical center. The medical center, in this model system, also serves as a community hospital *backing up* the primary care facilities of its immediate community. (p. 36, italics added)

Upon a first reading, this sounds like a description of a single system. But the rhetoric conceals and blurs the issue of control and authority. "Linked," "related," "tied," and "backing up" are terms which imply relations of cooperation and coordination, but they do not specify how these relationships will be established or maintained, nor which agencies will be the responsible authority. But, despite these ambiguities, the language clearly stresses an integrated system.

Other examples can be given showing how the report stresses the importance of a single system. After mentioning the dependence of the voluntary hospitals upon public funds, the report said that "thus, along with the former City hospitals [now under the new Health and Hospitals Corporation], they will owe much the same accounting of costs and performance to public authority. It now becomes possible, therefore, to bring about the integration of private and public resources into a single high-quality community health service" (p. 40). Later, the leverage of funds was stressed: "Through its contractual relations with the Health Services Corporation in particular, the Health Services Administration can use City operating and capital funds to promote the development of the single, comprehensive health-services system out of the present fragmented dual system" (p. 47).

The discussion of planning also implied a single system. "The planning power is central to the fruitful exercise of public authority in the development of comprehensive community health services," and that power will have increasing funds from all levels of government. "The public interest—and every principle of good government—argue that this power should be exercised by a government agency" (p. 48). True planning cannot occur for only part of a fragmented system; such "planning" is a fiction. The corporation's city-wide functions further implied a single system encompassing data-processing, laboratories, purchasing, and ambulances (pp. 58–59). And the idea of regionalization, linking community hospitals with medical centers, also does not make sense if half of the institutions providing health services are excluded (p. 59).

Thus, one part of the report emphasized, and presupposed, a disappearance of the dual system of control and organization without quite saying how this would happen or what form of authority such a single system would have. But another part, and often the very next sentence, implied the continuation of a dual system for the foreseeable future. This dilemma was never mentioned or discussed. We have already noted the appearance of the key contradiction within the content of the main recommendations themselves. But contradictions appeared in many other places. For example, the Health Services Administration is delegated the "authority for standard setting, inspection, and audit of voluntary and proprietary hospitals and other health facilities," which implies their continuation as separate types of control (p. 50). The corporation is "empowered to undertake the construction of health facilities for operation by itself or by voluntary institutions" (p. 56). The centralized purchasing system to be developed by the corporation should be made "available to voluntary institutions on a suitable reimbursement basis" (p. 59). The discussion of affiliation contracts (pp. 64-65) simply accepted their existence and continuation, and thus the dual system which created the necessity for affiliations between city and voluntary hospitals in their present form. New financing schemes (such as a Hospital Construction Authority) "would be available to non-profit voluntary hospitals as well as to the City's own Department of Hospitals" (p. 73).

The above examples indicate quite clearly that the perpetuation of the dual system was accepted, and that a variety of devices were envisaged which might have improved or readjusted the relationships between the two, but that the component units—both voluntary institutions and even city agencies like the Department of Hospitals—would continue to exist in much their present form and function. The HSA and the HSC become facilitating and, hopefully, coordinating agencies on the "top," but very few changes were presumed to penetrate to the operating levels. Given the inertia of such a complex interorganizational system, it can be assumed that the assumption of persistence of a dual system is the more realistic half of the contradiction contained in the report, since advocacy of a major transformation into a single system would require a far more intellectually serious analysis of the causes of fragmentation and possible strategies and levers of change than was presented.

Far from being a serious analysis, then, the report concealed and blurred its own internal contradictions in obfuscatory language. I have already quoted at length the paragraph describing one of the figures, referring to the terms "links," "relations," and so forth, which fail to confront the issue of the location of power and authority over the parts of the system. Another instance was the question of who would control the municipal hospitals once the corporation was formed. At least twice (p. 11 and p. 53) it was asserted that city hospitals would be "integrated into the health service system under *appropriate sponsorship* as teaching centers and community hospitals" (p. 11, italics added). The term "sponsorship" begged the question of control completely, and implied, if anything, that the municipal hospitals would be under the control of the voluntary hospitals. Thus, the commission report, despite brave rhetoric concerning the pathological consequences of a dual system of private versus welfare medicine and municipal versus voluntary hospitals, contains numerous internal contradictions stemming from its failure to confront the question of what would really be required to integrate and coordinate the fragmented health system of New York City.

But the report was also paralyzed—or, better, mesmerized—by the question of the dual system of hospital control. Without dealing with the question, it dealt with nothing else. In-hospital care was indeed acknowledged to be excessive, and corollary characteristics of underdeveloped ambulatory care, poor extended care, and inadequate emergency room facilities were even stressed. But none of the recommendations dealt with ways in which the balance between in-hospital care and ambulatory care facilities could be redressed. It seems possible that the two aspects of the report are related. Because the report could not deal effectively with the causes of the fragmented, dual system, it could not recognize the possibility that the dual system of control and service was fundamentally responsible for the inadequate ambulatory care facilities. No authoritative mechanism existed which could reallocate resources from the relatively autonomous hospitals and medical schools to the more sorely needed (for the poor, at least) ambulatory care facilities. Instead, the vision of expanded ambulatory care facilities was held up as one of the many accomplishments to be expected from the new HSA and HSC.

One turns to the part of the appendix (pp. 70-75), entitled "A Note on Alternative Forms of Organization and Implementation," hoping that some of the internal disagreements of the commission concerning the bases for their analysis and recommendations will there be clarified. Unfortunately, the alternatives listed there were not clearly distinguished either from each other or from the Commission's own ultimate recommendations, nor were any arguments presented which justified them over the others ambiguously defined and criticized. Five alternatives were given. (1) Improving government by "restructuring the relationship between the operating agencies and the overhead agencies" (p.

70). This was rejected as utopian. (2) Turning over city hospitals to voluntary hospitals. This was rejected as not contributing to system-wide integration (recommendation no. 1), although elsewhere, as has already been noted, that possibility was considered as one of the possible paths to be followed by the HSC. (3) Extending the affiliation contracts even further. This was rejected as continuing the "awkward expedient" of divided management, although elsewhere affiliations were accepted as continuing undisturbed. (4) "Total affiliation"—contracting out for all services to municipal hospitals. This was rejected as also failing to meet the goal of system-wide integration. (5) Creating an "independent Hospital Authority" in several versions. This was rejected as probably failing to meet the criteria of public accountability and service to the community at large, although it was not made clear either why this was the case, how the commission's own plan for a Health Services Corporation was structurally different from an authority, or why the HSC would be any more accountable than an authority.

In short, the consideration of alternative organizational frameworks consisted only of a series of assertions defending the commission's own recommendations, not a reasoned argument. A careful and systematic analysis would require confronting the realities of the dual system and its consequences—as set forth by the commission's own description earlier—and this the commission was unable to do, because of lack of vision, self-imposed political restrictions, or internal disagreements.

One more specific example of their lack of true consideration of alternatives may suffice. The report mentioned the study completed a few months earlier by Robb Burlage of the Institute for Policy Studies in Washington, D. C.[15] According to the commission, Burlage's recommendation was the "creation of a consolidated city-wide, extra-governmental Health Care Commission to develop comprehensive public policy for all tax-supported health services and activities and for an independent Authority, separate from existing City agencies, to implement the Commission's policies" (p. 72). The commission said that "this proposal makes inadequate provision for public accountability and for effective performance of the vital public functions assigned to the Health Services Administration in the Commission's Recommendation 2." That was all the comment on this alternative proposal.

Not only was this criticism obviously inadequate, since it did not indicate why public accountability would not be achieved by the Burlage recommendations, but it also misstated those recommendations. The Metropolitan Health Services Commission mentioned in the Burlage report would be appointed by the mayor, and therefore would be "governmental." Moreover, it would "combine the powers and functions of the Board of Health, Board of Hospitals, Community Mental Health Board, and the Chief Medical Examiner" (Burlage, p. 516). Burlage went on to describe a number of mechanisms to insure public accountability. As a matter of fact, it was not at all obvious, after several careful readings, how Burlage's combination of a policy-making commission and an operating authority differed from the Piel Commission's combination of a policy-making HSA and an operating HSC in terms of the powers and functions assigned and the goals intended to be served. Such differences may have existed in the minds of both or all parties to these debates, but they were not apparent in the texts, and they indicated once again the lack of careful analysis of the causes and possible remedies for the defects of fragmentation.

Although it is beyond the scope of this study to deal at great length with the Burlage report, it might be noted that its recommendations were essentially the same as those of the Piel Commission, and it assumed a similar ideological position (corporate rationalization) without any argument or evidence that the system of a Metropolitan Health Services Commission and Metropolitan Health Authority would succeed any better than the present system in overcoming fragmentation. For example, Burlage said that "the capacity would be greatly enlarged under the Authority for coordinating and blending State and Federal health program expenditures and for regulating and coordinating both public and private financing of the private sectors of health services according to community plans and guidelines" (p. 517). How and why this capacity would be enlarged was not made clear by subsequent explanations of the powers and functions of the authority. Our main concern here, however, is with the official commissions which exemplify one major form of interorganizational relationship concerned, at least officially, with overcoming the fragmentation of the New York City health system.

Some of the conflicts within the commission were partly exposed in the appended statement (pp. 83-96) by Professor Eveline M. Burns, one of the members of the commission.[16] Most of her statement was general and along the same lines of description and evaluation as the rest of the report. But toward the end she suddenly described the voluntary hospitals and the possible need for governmental "compulsion" in a way which evoked a one-page reply from other members of the commission (p. 97). Because Professor Burns' description of the voluntary hospitals brought up characteristics of the public-private relationships of these different forms of organizational control in a forthright way which was not typical of the rest of the report, and which exposed features of the voluntary system which were not often mentioned, it may be worth quoting her description in full.

For many years, the so-called "voluntary hospital" has not been purely, or even predominantly, "voluntary," if by this is meant supported by philanthropic contributions and fees from private patients. The voluntary hospital of today would be incapable of operating without support from the public sector. This support is not merely financial, although this is highly important, taking the form of tax privileges allowed taxpayers' contributions to the support of the hospital, tax freedom for property owned or occupied by the hospital, financial aid for construction costs and capital needs as well as the ever-growing grants for research, mainly from the Federal government. Equally important is the symbiotic relationship of the voluntary hospitals to the public system. On the one hand the City, by financing the supply of charity patients and by operating public hospitals for the poor, has provided the medical schools and voluntary teaching hospitals with badly needed teaching and research material. On the other hand, the existence of the public system has served as a screen to protect the voluntary hospital system as a whole (there are obvious exceptions) from the public criticism that would otherwise have been directed at (1) its operation of a highly selective admission system which reflects neither any rational division of labor among the various hospitals nor concern for the patient group as a whole but is determined primarily by the institutions' needs as research and teaching agencies, (2) its lack of concern with what happens to the patient once he leaves the hospital premises, i.e., an indifference to, or lack of involvement with, the community's health infrastructure, and (3) the failure of the voluntary system to give leadership in the realm of prevention (pp. 94–95).

This indictment of the voluntary hospital system is clearly part and parcel of the criticism of the dual system found in the main text of the commission report—without ever mentioning any defects in the voluntary hospitals or how their particular role is made possible by the existence of the public hospital system. It seems a safe speculation that this appended statement by Professor Burns was intended as a draft of a section of the commission report, and was rejected by a majority as too critical of the voluntary hospitals. Four of the seven members of the commission, after all, served as board members of New York City voluntary hospitals (two on Mount Sinai, one each on New York and Lenox Hill hospitals).

Her statement went on to assert that the fact that over half of the voluntary hospitals' income comes from tax money was "perhaps only the final evidence needed to demonstrate that there can no longer be such an entity as a purely 'voluntary' hospital system" (p. 95), and it warned that if the public interest could not be achieved by "discussion and negotiation between the leadership of the hospitals and the representatives of the City," then "regulation and compulsion may be essential" (p. 96). This threat of compulsion—which might seem exactly what must have been intended by the commission if it were seriously concerned with providing the new HSA and HSC with power to integrate all of the health facilities of the city into a single system— provoked the response by unnamed members of the commission to Professor Burns' statement. They stressed the importance of the teaching function and asserted that the affiliation program had attracted "first-class interns and residents" to the municipal hospitals. This teaching function was so important that government "compulsion" should be avoided, if government policies were "against what might be the judgment of the teaching hospital on what course of action it considers most consistent with its teaching function." They went on to assert that there was "nothing in the past administration of municipal hospitals either in New York City" or any other city which "would lead to the conclusion that municipal governments in general are qualified wisely to assume such power" (p. 97).

Here, without straining the interpretation too much, it seems to me that we can see the underlying strategy of the majority of the commission. They really wished to *reduce* the amount of public power and control over the hospitals as much as possible, and ultimately to turn over the municipal hospitals to voluntary control, not necessarily to existing boards, but to the same form of control by autonomous, self-perpetuating groups of private citizens—responsible bankers, executives, and attorneys like themselves. The HSA and HSC were devices not for *increasing* public control but rather for *reducing* it, in their view. Their faith lay in responsible private leadership, freed from the dead hand of encrusted city bureaucracy, and also from the conflicts and corrupt bargains of municipal politics. Such men as they would be able to act disinterestedly and to institute efficient management with the help of public funds, but funds which would be given to them without the restricting and constraining checks and balances of the multiple reviewing and budgeting agencies of the city. The judgment of the men controlling the teaching hospitals was accepted as far superior to that of any public agency as far as the "best long-term public interest" (p. 97) was concerned.

This way of understanding the viewpoint of the majority of the Commission also makes clearer the reasons for the confusing language of "relations," "links," and "ties" already mentioned. If one assumes that clear goals are defined and effective management authority is turned over to responsible, competent, and well-intentioned men, then all of this seemingly abstract rhetoric can be explained as a consequence of the assumption of consensus. The public has delegated its authority to officials who are empowered to exercise their best judgment and who must, like the stockholders of a corporation, delegate their authority to expert managers who then exercise their best judgment. Demands from the community will be transmitted through advisory committees and will be "taken into account" (p. 61) by the management to the extent that they deem it advisable. Exact relationships of superordination and subordination need not be specified, because the managers must be left free to adjust their decisions and policies according to the needs of concrete situations. To specify exactly who will control—content and structure of the relations, links, ties, back-ups, liaisons, and inputs between various health facilities— would be to fall back into the trap which already cripples the health bureaucracies of the city: establishing such a diversity of types of control and review that management flexibility is lost, delays become incredibly long, and, ultimately, the delivery of health services suffers.

This extrapolation of the ideology of corporate rationalization is plausible and almost convincing, with the single but fatal qualification that it fails to take account of the fundamental conflicts of interest between key interest groups in the health system, principally between the private practitioners of medicine and the corporate structures—the voluntary hospitals, the medical schools and universities, and the governmental agencies. Regardless of their internal differences, to some degree manifest in the commission report, the latter share a common concern with reducing the power and role of the solo physician. It is this need to maintain a common ideological front that probably accounts for the willingness of the members of the Piel Commission to bury their differences over the role of government vis-a-vis the voluntary hospitals, and to argue for the creation of the empty organizational shells of the HSC and HSA, the contents of whose operations were left to be battled out later.

The ideology of corporate rationalization stresses the centrality of the hospital as the key organization supplying and organizing health services in a modern society. The commission report is quite clear on this.

A hospital is no longer a kind of hotel for the patient and workshop for the doctor. It is no longer feasible to staff a hospital, as the City's hospitals used to be staffed, by attending physicians whose eminence would attract the necessary house staff of interns and residents to provide most of the patient care. The modern hospital is an organization of highly trained specialists supported by a skilled staff and employing instrumentation and equipment of constantly greater capital cost. To keep such an organization functioning requires an ever larger nucleus of full-time staff." (p. 18; a similar statement appears on p. 28.)

The major implicit concern of the report was to devise an administrative superstructure which would allow these extraordinarily complex organizational entities to function properly.

But totally neglected is what other public health specialists have regarded as fundamental: the provision of primary care, not specialty care. According to Dr. E. Richard Weinerman,

the ultimate effectiveness of medical care from the patient's point of view is *not* directly determined by any high-level financial or organizational medical-care system which fails to include specific and conscious efforts to reconstruct with first priority the bottom of primary level of care. In every country of the world that I have visited—not excluding those most acclaimed as having the highest forms of social organization in this field—an elaborate and complex superstructure of specialty and hospital care rests, always precariously, upon the flimsy underpinning of threadbare and often isolated services of general practitioners. This remains true in Great Britain, Sweden, Czechoslovakia, and most, certainly, in our own country—despite the affluence or sophisticated social organization which these nations represent.[17]

The issue about the primacy of general or primary care versus specialty care cannot be argued here, but the point is that the commission report completely neglected, in its concern for the "high quality" (that is, teaching and research) institutions, any specific recommendations which would take account of the shortage of general practitioners. This seems linked to their neglect of any recommendations specifically dealing with ambulatory care, despite their rhetorical show of concern. And it is linked to their unconcern or disregard of the major point made by the general practitioners: that the preservation of the personal relationship of trust and mutual confidence between patient, family, and physician is a vital part of any viable health system, one which tends to get lost in the referrals from one specialty clinic to another. Whether or not there exist the social conditions for a mass health care program which maintains such personal relationships is an important question, but it is one not even raised by the commission report in its presentation of an ideological position stressing the key importance of organizational and administrative reform.

In sum, the commission report contained a crucial internal contradiction, failed to consider alternative organizational frameworks seriously, and presented an ideology of corporate rationalization of the New York City health system which left out vital considerations and recommendations seemingly required by its own analysis—such as expansion of ambulatory care facilities. However, this criticism may be unfair, since we have not yet examined the staff studies which occupy 478 pages of the published volume. Perhaps these staff studies contain supporting documentation for the major findings and recommendations of the report, documentation which will complement and reinforce the point of view of the report.

9. Staff Studies for the Piel Commission

Chapters 2 and 3

A remarkably frank statement by the Piel Commission's staff began the brief second chapter, entitled "Summation and a Glance Ahead." They noted that a "shortage of surveys is *not* one of the problems faced" by the New York City health system (p. 101, italics in original). Each of a series of studies had "found the system as ailing as its patients." And "most of these attempted solutions failed. Those that succeeded had so little effect on the whole system that their beneficial results, from any distance, were lost to view" (p. 102). Why? The latest staff convened for the most recent investigation attempted no real answer. The recommendations by previous commissions were neither summarized nor analyzed for the reasons why their "solutions" were not tried, or, if tried, why they failed.

The staff was also refreshingly frank about their predictions for the major recommendations made by the Piel Commission itself, the studies for which were summarized in Part II of the report (pp. 101–486): "If these recommendations were followed, and if the Health Services Administration (HSA) were established under a reorganized city charter . . . the existing system for the delivery of personal health services in New York City could be somewhat revived and refreshed, with remarkably little dislocation of present structures and procedures" (p. 103). These recommendations could be brought about "with the least change in current practice" (p. 106). In some sense, they said, these recommendations were "inevitable; every survey propounds them, or something very like them" (p. 106). But, they "ruefully" predicted, going only this far would not change the system. Another survey, three, five, or ten years from now, would find the same problems: crowded wards, short-handed nursing staffs, untreated and unhappy patients jamming outpatient departments and emergency rooms (p. 104). Why? "Because the existing system for health-services delivery is not viable; there is *failure inherent in the ingredients of which it is compounded*, and all the work, talent, and benevolence in the world will not make it function well.... Current trends in the population, the economy, and the practice of medicine are at odds with the existing system" (p. 104, italics added).

With this introduction we are prepared by the staff themselves not to expect too much from the recommendations in Part II. But the staff claimed in Part III ("Toward a Successful System," pp. 489–579) to move past these limitations and to describe a "new organizational structure capable of releasing the bonds that currently paralyze the *exercise of authority* in the health-services system" (p. 105, italics added). This formulation already indicated the probable focus of their analysis, but we shall defer systematic treatment of their plan until Part II has been summarized. Hopefully, this staff, at least according to their own intentions, will deal with the "bigger issues," without deferring to "current pressures" (p. 106).

Chapter 3, "Community and Institutional Needs," consisted of a survey of the facilities and health needs of the five boroughs and a brief discussion of four "programmatic concepts" for health services delivery: shifts in public-private responsibility, community involvement, inservice education, and cost-effectiveness ratios. The summary of the borough surveys had sections on the aged, comprehensive mental health care, addiction problems, and ambulatory care. The last was basically a summary of Dr. Mary McLaughlin's plan (24 April 1967) for neighborhood family care centers.

The separate borough studies emphasized the "surprising lack of community health information," and the staff of the commission, given limited time and resources, was unable to gather any primary data. Thus, the survey of health facilities and needs was quite limited, merely summarizing demographic shifts in the age, income, and ethnic composition of the areas, listing the numbers of hospitals in each area, and reporting on a selective survey of various city hospitals by the City Hospital Visiting Committee.

Generally, the summaries made little or no connection, either implicitly or explicitly, between the health needs described and the evaluation of the adequacy of facilities. Existing institutions were mainly taken as given, and their internal operations were the only concern. The adequacy of linens and elevators, the need for ramps to the solarium and new plumbing, the shortage of staff of all kinds, and the desirability of early completion of new buildings were typical of the recommendations made for specific hospitals. It is not clear why particular hospitals were selected for mention, nor why particular kinds of problems were chosen either for observation or for mention in the report. Restriction of the surveys to the municipal hospitals indicates the limited responsibility and range of the study despite the broad mandate given to the commission to study the full range of personal health services.

One general analytic fault is found several times: *descriptive* aspects of the health system are confused with *causal* factors. Thus in chapter 2 the "real disease" of the system was found in "four factors": the waste of resources, the need for new resources, the lack of definition of goals, and the complexity and "mindlessness" of the system (p. 105). Surely these are not "factors," but aspects of the system itself which still have to be explained. The same deficiency of analysis was seen later when the problems facing Brooklyn hospitals were "attributed to four fundamental factors: multiplicity of facilities and services, maldistribution of facilities and services, fragmentation of services, and obsolescence of facilities" (p. 155). Once again these terms were merely a way of describing, at a somewhat higher level of abstraction, fragmented, obsolescent, and maldistributed health facilities; they were not an adequate explanation of *why* these characteristics existed. This failure of analysis enabled the staff to avoid looking for more fundamental causal explanations, since they apparently found one which satisfied them.

Despite the concern for the problem of fragmentation, the analysis in chapter 3 itself exhibited such fragmentation, for little awareness of the links between various programs was manifest, nor was there any attempt to consider the consequences of expanding one kind of program (mental health centers or ambulatory care facilities) for other facilities. The summary of the plan for twenty-seven new community mental health centers is a good example (pp. 179–83). The description begins auspiciously:

Traditionally, mental health facilities and services in the City of New York have been planned without consideration of regional, county, city-wide, or national objectives. Consequent fragmentation, gaps in service, and duplication of services have been recognized as critical problems, but little success has been met in efforts to solve them. (p. 179)

From that beginning one might expect to find in the summary some sensitivity to the factors which both produce and possibly alter the pattern of fragmentation.

Unfortunately, this was not the case. First, the report had faith, as many others had, in the coordinating power and consequences of federal legislation. Without giving the slightest reason why such might be the case, they said that the federal mental health center legislation of 1963–65 had "stirred movement toward revolutionary change in the field" (p. 179). In fact, the most comprehensive survey of the impact of the 1963 federal legislation in this area found that fragmentation has *increased* as a consequence.[18] The report then described the Master Plan for "coverage of New York City with networks of comprehensive community mental health centers" (p. 181) and acknowledged that these centers would "raise more problems. Some difficulty is anticipated, for example, in the changing working relationships that will be required both within and among disciplines in the new system" (p. 181–82). But no reasons or arguments were presented to justify the assertion that fragmentation would be reduced. Faith was expressed: "it is believed . . . that the program will be flexible enough to respond to these problems while achieving the desired objectives" (p. 182).

The same blind faith and failure seriously to consider the problem of fragmentation appeared in the discussion of ambulatory care facilities. Dr. McLaughlin's seemingly admirable plan for creating thirty neighborhood family care centers (later called NFCC's), each to serve a district of between 10,000 and 30,000 persons, was summarized, but it was simply asserted, with no discussion, that "the program would be *coordinated* on a district basis, with clinics operating under the medical supervision of a 'back-up' hospital depending upon the number of doctors and the measure of need evaluated for that district" (p. 193, italics added). This discussion was totally abstract because it merely presented the internal division of labor and functions of the ambulatory care center, adding, almost as an afterthought, that its services would be "coordinated" with those offered by other facilities in the area. The criteria to be used for establishing such a facility in terms of need, population composition, and density of the area were completely lacking, as well as any attempt to specify the particular areas of the city which needed such centers. Thus the discussion of community areas in New York City and their health needs bore no relationship to the plans for particular kinds of new or reorganized facilities. This intellectual fragmentation makes it difficult to evaluate either the statistical data presented on age, income, and health status of various districts, or the abstract and ideal plans for the services to be provided by particular kinds of facilities. It is as if the terms "fragmentation" and "coordination" had no content which referred to a concrete conception of the health facilities to be provided for a community. The abstract "models" of ideal systems and their interrelationships are no help (see figs. 5 and 6 on pp. 192 and 203 of the report). They assumed that arrows, lines, circles, squares, and boxes which contain or point to words ("neighborhood family care center," "district health office," "outpatient care unit," "specialty clinic," "community mental health center") convey in and of themselves adequate information about the substantive services to be offered, and how coordination will take place. Here "system analysis" has become an incantation, lacking any ability to contribute to clarification of issues and, in fact, blurring and confusing them. The desperate need for more ambulatory care facilities and some criteria for their location and character are not furthered at all by such schemes.

Another example of the lack of analysis is the brief mention of the overlapping and multiple geographic districts. For a variety of reasons, including federal requirements as well as the needs of particular agencies to define their own territories, a variety of noncoterminous administrative districts exist in New York City: mental health, health, outpatient, ambulance, welfare, and others. But the report did not describe what these districts are, discuss their rationale, provide any criteria for assessing their reasonableness in a more integrated and coordinated system, or make any recommendations for merger, abandonment, or maintenance of any of them. The report never got very specific, except with respect to simple quantitative data whose relevance for policy analysis was obscure: "Lincoln Hospital has an OEO grant," "Queens County has 26 hospitals," "New York will have 1 million persons over 65 years of age in 1970." In the absence of an adequate theoretical framework which would allow these presumably important bits and pieces of facts to be linked together for the purpose of making inferences, they provided the semblance of analysis without the reality. Unfortunately, much of the chapter has this character.

The underlying ideological character of the report was exhibited again in the chapter summary. The paragraph began by pointing, quite correctly, to the conflicts between the goals of research, teaching, and patient care, and suggested that it could not be assumed that "good patient care is a sure result of teaching and research." But what is their recommendation? *Administrative action*, which would clarify purposes, spell out goals, establish and designate functions. To quote:

"The role, or roles, of any given facility at any given time must be carefully spelled out to avoid worsening the present state of cross-purposes. While good definitions can change as need or opportunity arises, clarity of purpose for each person, each service, and each facility must be established. Certain institutions, for instance, should clearly be designated as centers of medical education" (p. 206). That statement seems unexceptional on the surface. No one, surely, could quarrel with the clarity of definitions, goals, and functions. But the hidden assumption, which makes it a component of the ideology of corporate rationalization, is that such acts have causal force. Administrative or bureaucratic decisions are assumed to "clarify," "establish," "designate," and "define." Behavior will automatically follow. Unnamed persons or organizations who do the defining, designating, and clarifying are *assumed* to have the authority and capability to enforce those decisions. In fact, it seems likely, as shown by the entire history of the inability of this long series of investigations and reports to have any substantial consequences, that the faith in corporate reorganization and rationalization is misplaced. The important forces which maintain the health system are not interested in having their goals clarified, their institutions designated, or their definitions changed. No power sufficient to enforce those changes has been generated.

The system mode of analysis, at least as expressed in this report, sometimes conceals what amounts to a requirement of fundamental institutional change in a causal assertion about "links" or "affiliations" or "intermixtures" or organizational functions. For example, in the last paragraph of chapter 3 the authors said, "The system model implies not only internal ties to medical schools but any number of other ties or affiliations between facilities. . . . Municipal and private institutions intermix. The patient who must move from one facility to another for care does not find that he *drops from one physician's responsibility and enters another's.* By and large, he enjoys continuity of care" (p. 208, italics added). It does not take much thought to realize that such a change would imply a far more basic reshaping of the physician's responsibilities—giving him, in effect, a "panel" of individuals and families to which he provides medical care, regardless of the institution in which they are located—than a mere change of the administrative superstructure would make possible. But the next sentence trivialized the change: "Implicit in this and not evident in the model shown in Figure 6 must be *improved management information and transportation programs* to tie the parts together" (p. 208, italics added). This is an excellent example of the ideology of corporate rationalization because it assumes that massive institutional changes will follow easily and readily once certain administrative innovations are established. Systems analysis, properly applied, should allow one to distinguish between those changes which have ramifying consequences for the system and those which are isolated and contained, as well as between those innovations which are so deeply embedded that they are enormously resistant to change and those which will serve the interests of powerful groups and thus will be relatively easy to install. In the absence of criteria for making these distinctions, it seems plausible to infer that a so-called systems analysis is an instrument of certain interests which have no stake in a truly systematic and revealing analysis, but rather one in concealing and blurring the real relationships of power in the system.

Chapters 4 and 5

Chapter 4 of the Piel Commission report (pp. 209-90) consisted of brief reports on nineteen municipal hospitals and the Gouverneur ambulatory care facility, derived mainly from interviews with the local hospital administrator and his staff, plus a walk through the buildings, plus a few statistics on capacity, occupancy rates, and clinic hours. According to the first paragraph, special attention was paid to the outpatient and emergency room services "since these functions represent the prime hospital interface with community health needs" (p. 209), and, in fact, descriptions of these facilities occupy the majority of the space given to each hospital.

Although the affiliation contracts were mentioned, all of the information presented was from the point of view of the hospital administrator, not from any person representing the affiliate. No attempt was made to verify the statements given to the interviewers, so that in many cases a statement was prefaced by "in the administrator's opinion," or "he reported."

The same problems reappeared with tedious repetition from one hospital to another, enlivened only by the gruesome details of a particular case or instance: staff shortages, supply shortages, lack of space, equipment, and maintenance, and so forth. With respect to the affiliations, in several hospitals (at least as reported) there were discriminatory practices in favor of the affiliate staff in such matters as offices, air conditioning, parking, and salaries. Administrators of several hospitals either felt that they could have done as well with the money themselves if given the freedom and authority which the affiliates had to hire staff, raise salaries, and improve working conditions; or they believed that the affiliation arrangement had duplicated administration and created overlapping authorities (Coler, p. 227; Goldwater, p. 250; Greenpoint, p. 255; Kings County, p. 263; Metropolitan, p. 273; Queens, p. 283). Unfortunately, the investigators did not talk to the "affiliation coordinator" at any hospital and so did not evaluate the truth of these assertions. At other hospitals administrators expressed satisfaction with the affiliations (Fordham, p. 246; Brooklyn, p. 231; Lincoln, p. 268; Morrisania, p. 279). Discriminatory practices in favor of affiliate staff were described by administrators at Harlem (p. 258) and Lincoln (p. 271). The continuous repetition of the same problems made it clear that the factors responsible were system-wide and had little to do with idiosyncratic features of any given hospital, its administrator, staffing, or those of the affiliated hospital or medical school.

Gouverneur Ambulatory Care Center (pp. 250–53) was described glowingly by the report and was seen as a model for interorganizational relationships (the Departments of Health, Mental Health, and Hospitals had "learned to work together at the community level" [p. 251]), standards of care (an appointment system was instituted there for the first time, avoiding long hours of waiting), physician commitment (a staff of full-time physicians), and relations with the community (most of the clerical staff and aides were hired locally). It remains to be seen whether or not the lessons of this successful experiment in ambulatory care will be generalized in Part III of the report.

It should be mentioned that none of the survey data provided any basis for evaluating the success or failure of the affiliation plans. The report mentioned the monetary value of the contracts and the services which the affiliate contracted to provide, but there was no indication of how many staff members were in fact provided, whether their level of training was any better than the staff they replaced, whether or how care was improved, or any other information relevant to the evaluation of the affiliation contracts. As was already noted, the only information provided was from the hospital administrator. Conceivably, a negative opinion of the affiliation could be due to his reaction against an invasion of his authority, but there was no basis given in the report for making any inferences whatever.

Chapter 5 of the Piel Commission report (pp. 291–378) dealt with "special topics": a survey of the medical records systems of five municipal hospitals; a subcommittee report on affiliation contracting; a section giving summary impressions of the municipal hospitals by patients, administrators, and professionals; a discussion of the problems of outpatient departments and emergency rooms; and a survey of the program planning needs of hospitals, both public and private, in the five boroughs. What was striking throughout this chapter was the lack of the basic data which would be necessary to arrive at the policy recommendations made by the staff and, through their studies, the commission. Apparently no data existed which would allow an evaluation of the efficacy of the affiliation contracts (and no studies had been begun or arranged for by any agency), nor were there any studies of the relationships between outpatient departments and the new concept of "neighborhood family care centers," of the requirements for a city-wide medical information system (allegedly three years in the offing in 1967), or of the criteria for closing, remodeling, or reconstructing hospitals— recommendations which dot the descriptions of the current problems afflicting the city hospitals.

Most of the discussion dealt with the city hospitals, the implicit assumption being that the voluntaries had far fewer problems, although no comparative data were given on the quality or quantity of health services provided by the dual system, nor were there any recommendations affecting the internal operations, affiliation practices, or external relationships of any voluntary hospital. At most, for example, the authors said that "changes must come about . . . if institutions such as these are to participate effectively with one another and with the city in a coordinated health services program" (p. 368). But no recommendations for changes in any hospital, or in the voluntary hospital system as a whole, were made which were analogous to the many made for the municipal hospitals. The lack of real commitment to the transformation of the dual system into a single one was clear in the kinds of observations which the staff chose to make, undoubtedly under instructions from the commission. Although all of the municipal hospitals were surveyed, only nine (of about eighty) voluntaries, four proprietaries, three government hospitals, and five (of 150) nursing homes were visited. While some kind of sampling can obviously be justified, the presumption here was that the staff should spend most of its time and resources on the municipal hospitals. Nothing is wrong with this per se, except that the study ostensibly was of "community health services in New York City," and one of the main recommendations of the commission was the elimination of the dual system.

This chapter, like others in Part II, contained a myriad of details, lists of problems, and possible recommendations with no indication of how they were arrived at. At several points, perhaps conscious of the gap between the bits of data given and the recommendations for closing or moving this or that hospital, the authors said that their general vision of the system of the future would be presented in Part III.

The studies of the affiliation contracts and the descriptions and analysis of ambulatory care facilities and needs are the principal sections of chapter 5 relevant for our purposes. The members of the subcommittee (Drs. Baehr, Barnett, and Luckey) asserted that "in almost all instances, the affiliations have been successful in raising the professional standards of the city's hospitals," but the only evidence given was the increase of Lincoln Hospital's house staff from five to fifty, undoubtedly a great achievement. "Striking improvement in staffing" also followed affiliation at Morrisania, Greenpoint, Elmhurst, and Harlem, but no details were given. The authors hastened to say that "a modest increase in the size or improvement in the professional training of the hospital staff does not in itself insure improved services" (p. 301). They noted that equipment, nurses, and other ancillary personnel remained "in gravely short supply" and that thus "the full benefits of the affiliations have not as yet been achieved" (p. 302).

But, we are told, "firm criteria are lacking for assessing improvement in the effectiveness of health care as a result of the affiliations" (p. 301). One wonders who would be in a better position to offer even soft criteria on effectiveness than the three physicians assigned to evaluate the program on such an important commission as this. But they made no attempt to offer any criteria at all, and it was clear from their own assertions and the content of the section that there was no basis for evaluating the consequences of the affiliations from any data available to them. In the absence of relevant data, fourteen of the twenty-three pages (pp. 301–24) on affiliation contracts were devoted to tables listing the cost of contracts and the services provided at each hospital.

Nevertheless, they offered "broad conclusions" (p. 317), including an assessment that "the city has failed as a partner to the contracts, far more seriously and consequentially than have voluntary agencies" (p. 317). No evidence or even argument was given for this conclusion. Nor was any reason given for the prediction that "affiliation contracts are more likely to move toward comprehensiveness . . . than toward fractionated services" (p. 318).

In the analysis of the affiliation contract provisions, the report made several points relevant to a study of interorganizational relationships, although again no supporting data were given. According to the

commission staff, the contracts existing at that time—1967—
(1) divided responsibilities between the voluntary hospital and the city;
(2) did not specify program objectives or goals; (3) did not provide for
public accountability except in post-audit form; (4) left purchasing
under the same "maze of governmental controls" (p. 318) as before;
(5) dealt narrowly only with the "original staffing crises"; (6) were oriented specifically toward clinical delivery, not toward the community;
and (7) "tended to perpetuate and amplify fractionation. (Whereas the
city fractionates administrative matters, the voluntaries have often fractionated medical delivery services.)" (pp. 318–19). These assertions
raised more questions than they answered about the exact nature of the
affiliation system and how it worked, and no more details were given
than in the above (only slight) paraphrase. How and why "fractionation" (fragmentation?) of medical delivery services was fostered by the
affiliations was not clarified, nor did they explain how a "community
orientation" differs from a "clinical delivery."

The recommendations of the staff are consistent with the ideology of
corporate rationalization. Without presenting any evidence or reasons
why these recommendations would work, they urged "clear statements" of goals, review mechanisms, and program accountability, once
again assuming that clarity of wordings would necessarily change
behavior (pp. 320–21). Considerable attention was devoted to the
contracts and their provisions: "Some motivation should be written
into the contract to cause the affiliate to scrutinize questionable cases
of patient transfer and questionable practices of patient selection"
(p. 323). This faith in contract provisions seems a little misplaced in
view of the powerful contrary motivation of the voluntaries, committed
to teaching, to select appropriate teaching "material" and cases and
reject the rest. How the major commitments of the teaching function
and its consequences for patient selection or rejection could be altered
was not discussed, and the question remains an internal contradiction
in the report, since elsewhere it accepted this primary mission of the
teaching hospitals as fundamental (p. 366). The report did not recognize in its analysis any fundamental conflicts of interests between the
municipal hospitals, medical schools, private physicians, or any other
group or organization in the health system.

The second major section of this chapter of concern to us dealt with
the outpatient departments and emergency rooms (pp. 326–39,
343–46). The main point relevant here is that planning for the establishment of "neighborhood family care centers" (NFCC's) by the city
health department was going on in isolation from the planning by

voluntary hospitals for the extension and expansion of their outpatient departments and emergency rooms—to meet the same needs, in many cases (p. 351)—and also in isolation from the planning by the Community Mental Health Board for the establishment of community mental health centers, which also responded to many of the same needs. As the report put it, "concurrently, plans are being made for family health centers that, if implemented, will relieve the responsibility of the hospital [ambulatory care] units considerably, but there is little or no communication of these ideas among those who will be affected directly.... Central planners have not yet found means for taking advantage of the experience and capability of the men and women in the OPD/ER facilities who can help them most ... wasted effort and anxieties are being poured into duplicative planning" (pp. 332-33).

Also, despite the fact that "14 municipal hospitals are all struggling with precisely the same problems and working toward precisely the same goal ... they constitute a set of competitive sub-systems, not a cooperative situation whereby problems might be solved more quickly through coordinated planning and work. Other than arrangements between emergency rooms to transfer patients, *no evidence was observed of inter-municipal-hospital cooperation"* (pp. 335-36, italics added). They add, reinforcing the importance of this observation of fragmented planning, "it bears repeating here that no coordination was observed between the central planners and the directors of present hospital ambulatory services who are closest to the problems and who have had opportunity to gain much helpful insight" (p. 336).

Unfortunately, the analysts of the commission staff were at a loss for an analysis of the causes of this "fragmentation" and thus any cogent recommendations for change. All they came up with was a pious and meaningless platitude, underlined as if it were important: "When achieved, *local autonomy must operate within the framework of overall system specification and planning"* (p. 336). This is a perfect example of the ideology of corporate rationalization: basic conflicts between the interests and incentives of particular institutions and general planning and system control are hidden in an exhortation which calls upon all participants to behave properly. The report said at this point that "there are fundamental system problems that can be dealt with only through a complete reorganization (developed in Part Three). And until long-range changes are possible, the basic problems reported here have no chance of real solution" (p. 336). Interim changes are then discussed for much of the remainder of the chapter (pp. 336-65).

The brief discussion of government hospitals is interesting mainly because of the finding that veterans' hospitals, despite being publicly owned and managed, did not suffer from some of the faults allegedly due to being subject to political and bureaucratic control: they had no nurse shortage (or at least significantly less than the municipal hospitals); the hospital administrators had considerable autonomy and control over their budgets; their physical plants were in good condition and were well equipped; and they avoided the complex and frustrating necessity of filling out eligibility forms. A simple affidavit was all that was required of those patients who were not provided all of their medical services free of charge (pp. 372–76). The commission staff concluded from this brief survey that "the basic characteristics of the V. A. Hospital system in particular contain lessons for the public hospital system of New York City" (p. 376). Hopefully, these lessons would be analyzed and taken into account in the broad picture to be presented in Part III. Unfortunately, no data on comparative quality of health care in the V. A. versus the voluntary versus the municipal hospitals were given, since, apparently, they did not exist. Such data might have been an important test of the effects of different forms of control and administration of large hospital systems.

Chapters 6, 7, and 8

Chapter 6 (pp. 379–99) of the Piel Commission report dealt with "medical manpower"—primarily the shortage of nurses and other allied health personnel—but its discussion is not relevant to a study of interorganizational relationships.

Chapter 7, "Flow and Impact of Public Funds" (pp. 400–37), summarized the provisions of Public Law 89-97 (Medicare and Medicaid), which became effective on 1 July 1966. It was noted that New York was the ninth *state* to qualify for this federal program, passing a state law on 1 May 1966, but the city program was not actually in operation until five months later. This delay cost the city about $60 million, according to the staff's estimate (p. 409).

The complex form establishing eligibility for Medicaid was reproduced in full (pp. 420-14), and one of the main recommendations of the staff was that a simple affidavit be all that is required of applicants for aid. Following this section was a comparison of hospital usage in California and New York and some statistics on income and costs of hospital care (pp. 420-27). The commission staff asserted that they "had neither time nor resources to divert to the determination of costs (and cost-analysis system requirements) for the city hospitals" (p. 426).

The billing procedures for proprietary nursing homes were then described. At this point, several recommendations for the management of Medicaid by the Assistant Commissioner of Health—mainly to centralize Medicaid administration, hire a full-time staff, "identify the total cost," and "establish an over-all budget" (pp. 433–34)—were reproduced. The new agency would handle, codify, set up, review, centralize, and introduce a variety of forms, procedures, communication systems, sources of information, programs, and operational problems (p. 434).

The Commission staff then endorsed *most* of these recommendations and added some of their own, mainly that this single Medicaid administration should be "implemented within the Health Services Administration, and specifically within the Department of Hospitals" (p. 435). The chapter concluded with eighteen staff recommendations with respect to Medicaid: to charge the Medicaid Management Agency, various Task Forces, the Board of Medicaid Administration, the Bureau of Hospital Care Services, and the Commissioner of Hospitals with conducting scheduled monthly meetings, undertaking cost accounting, preparing detailed operational programs, and establishing standard forms and procedures (pp. 436–47). Lest this paraphrase seem an unfair parody of the ideology of corporate rationalization embedded in these recommendations, let us add that there were some substantive recommendations: the affidavit of income for applicants; an "advisory rate schedule" telling physicians how much of their charges would be reimbursed; a registration system for clients; reimbursement procedures; and so forth. But none of the recommendations had to do with the quality and quantity of services, only with the administrative processing of applicants and funds.

Nothing in this chapter on the "flow and impact of public funds" rose above the narrow perspective implied above: a federal program was taken as given, and its immediate impact was the only focus of concern, since it posed problems of incorporation into an existing administrative system. This is obviously a legitimate focus, but it seems excessively narrow for a commission with such a broad mandate, and even more so for a staff with a self-chosen emphasis on the "big issues."

Chapter 8 of the Piel Commission report dealt with the "status and role of central organizations" in New York City. (pp. 438–86) Over half of the chapter (30 of 48 pages) was devoted to a description of the powers and functions of the three main service divisions of the Health Services Administration (the "super-agency" established in May 1966): the Department of Health (pp. 444–63), the Department of Hospitals (pp. 470–75), and the Community Mental Health Board (pp. 477–83). These descriptions of the formal structure of the city health agencies are a useful portrayal of the administrative complexity of the system, but they are not used as background to develop any independent studies of the actual functioning, activities, and relationships of the organizations at the operating level. The overlapping of functions, at least at the official level, is striking. All of the following names of discrete organizations are used: bureau, division, program, center, office, council, district, area, department, commission, service, project, and institution. Unfortunately, the formal description too often reads as if it were part of the official brochure put out by the agency itself, and it would be redundant to summarize the descriptions of the goals and powers of the various components of the Department of Health except to agree with the commission staff that the duplication and overlapping of an almost impossibly cumbersome structure must be described in detail to be believed. Nevertheless, no criteria or evidence were offered—except face plausibility—to justify the critique of this structure which followed. It is impossible to know whether the system exhibited healthy pluralism and competition with a diversity of types and levels of care available to the health care consumer, or was a fragmented, disjointed, and expensive system needing rationalization and reorganization. The thrust of the commission staff's description and then critique is clearly toward the latter interpretation.

The "critique" section on the Department of Health (pp. 463–70) was mainly an abstract description of administrative fragmentation, not an analysis of the causes of these characteristics of the system. The following main points were made: the twenty-two district health centers were administratively and functionally unrelated to any other ambulatory care services; the principal health data collected, mainly for health "areas" (composites of ten census tracts), were not used for or relevant to the planning of services in health "districts"; the staff of the health officer (in charge of a health district) was under dual responsibility—administratively to the health officer, technically and professionally to the central staff bureau; contacts of the operating level personnel (the district health center) with any other city departments or health personnel (Welfare, private physicians, Health, Community Mental Health Board), even though they might be serving the same clients, were "extremely limited" (p. 465). Contacts with Education and the community were more frequent partly because Health provided physicians and nurses to staff clinics within the schools. The problem of fragmentation was then summarized yet again. "There are large numbers of health and medical service agencies who do not communicate well with one another. They appear as a series of *isolated groups* generally characterized by (a) lack of adequate *funds*; (b) inadequate *personnel*; and (c) an *inability to integrate their efforts* with those of the many other agencies involved in common services" (p. 467, italics added). This description and critique of the system is becoming familiar; the question remains: Why do these situations exist? What is the explanation offered by the Piel Commission staff? Again, we must wait for Part III for their theory and consequent long-range recommendations.

The section evaluating the structure of the Department of Hospitals was also mainly concerned with organizational factors: management, staffing, building construction, capital funds, careers, and how to avoid getting people into hospitals if they do not absolutely need bed care. But in this latter connection there was no discussion of the relationships (or lack of them) between the Department of Hospitals and the Department of Health—itself responsible for ambulatory and home care facilities. For an alleged system analysis, the commission staff was itself all too likely to take existing organizational entities as given for purposes of analysis. The same point holds true for the Community Mental Health Board (CMHB) created in 1954 in response to funds provided by state legislation. These boards followed the typical pattern whereby recognition of a "problem" leads to the creation of still another agency which is, at least symbolically, a response to that problem, and yet whose establishment contributes to the increasing fragmentation of the system.

Like the other two descriptions of departments, the formal description of the Community Mental Health Board has the aura of a "public relations" job: a given set of decisions is "handled individually and evolves as appears best for the needs of the CMHB and the department involved" (p. 481), or the mission of a division is to "monitor reporting activities of all agencies funded by the CMHB" (p. 480). These are plausible as first attempts at describing the divisions of functions, but are certainly not adequate as an analysis of the actual functioning of an organization.

The section on the "problems facing the CMHB" contained a good example of the evasiveness of the commission staff in defining issues clearly. Their attempt to answer the question of whether the CMHB should itself provide mental health services or continue (as it had up to that time) to "support and guide improvement of services" provided by others was an important one (p. 483). Their discussion is worth citing in full: "The question of trend, or policy, arises again in the case of the planned mental health centers with the problem of whether these [services] should be staffed by board-salaried personnel. The tentative answer to this has so far been that it would be determined on an individual need basis, and that several approaches might be utilized if different conditions existed. Whether this degree of flexibility would lead to larger problems of coordination of mental health activities may need determination" (p. 484). Such an "answer" is obviously not an answer at all, since it does not consider what possible conditions might exist, what problems of coordination would be raised by various alternative solutions, or what the degrees of flexibility to be allowed by different arrangements might be.

To summarize, the discussion of the "status and role of central organizations" dealt only with the city departments (with a brief discussion of the recently established HSA, in addition to those already mentioned), in complete isolation from the previous chapter on public funding. There was no concern in this chapter with the dynamic processes altering the functioning of these organizations, except those administrative changes which still accepted the essential powers and functions of the city departments as given and tinkered with their internal structure. No budget data were given which would indicate the relative importance of particular components of the departments, nor any staffing information, nor the number of patients treated, nor location of facilities with respect to each other. Thus there is no basis for evaluating the general conclusions concerning fragmentation and overlapping, despite the importance given to this particular criticism of the system. More generally. from the analysis and data presented thus far, it is difficult to see what basis has been created for an overall discussion of the causes of the problems found and, consequently, any rational basis for the long-range recommendations for reorganization.

Chapters 9, 10, and 11

Chapter 9 of the Piel Commission report (pp. 489-530) was the long-awaited fundamental and long-range analysis of the basic causes and remedies of the fragmentation of the New York City health system. It began with another summary of the many studies which have been done and recommendations made to solve the deepening "crisis" of the system. The question was asked, properly: "Why have not earlier studies, programs, reforms, or demonstrations, met the problems with which this Commission has been charged?" (p. 490) Before answering this question, the staff briefly reviewed these studies.

A 1963 study by staff members of the School of Public Health at

Columbia University documented the need for chronic-care facilities. "Since 1963, the need for fulfilling the recommendations of that study has increased rather than lessened" (p. 490). (Why?) This study also found that "the city pays a high premium for operational inefficiency associated with the unnecessarily long stays of some patients, as a function of administrative factors. This problem also remains largely unsolved" (p. 490). (Why?) An early 1960s study by the Brookings Institution of the personnel and civil service system made recommendations which "if implemented, would have resolved fundamental problems before this Commission. None of these recommendations have in fact been met in any substantial form" (p. 490). (Why?) A study by Professor Herbert Klarman analyzed the professional staffing problems of the city's hospitals. The "circumstances that brought about the need for his studies, and to which he directed recommended solutions, are still inherent difficulties before this Commission" (pp. 490–91). (Why?) The commission staff asserted that "as many as 50 such special studies and reports [have been] completed since 1960—all of significance—having to do with one or more of the many aspects of health care delivery in the city. *Very few have achieved their avowed intent or have seen implementation*; only two or three have had basic influence on 'business as usual'" (p. 491; italics added). Unfortunately, the commission staff did not name or analyze those few studies, their impact, or the reasons why they were ineffective.

At this point the commission staff reported their resistance to the "great pressure" upon the commission to "focus solely upon the immediate controversy regarding affiliation contracting between the municipal and voluntary hospitals" (p. 491). They resisted this pressure because they wanted to avoid the temptation to prescribe an immediate and seemingly easy solution—the "quick fix," in their words. They also reported that they wished to avoid the temptation to recommend still another "demonstration project" because the history of these is that they either fail to achieve the great hopes placed in them, or, if successful, they fail to be implemented on a larger scale (p. 492). The comprehensive welfare medical program was cited as a case in point, as well as the Gouverneur Ambulatory Care Center.[19] A third and equally tragic case cited was that of the early-detection dental examinations begun under the auspices of the Headstart program. The dental needs of thousands of children were discovered. "However, its major result was unforeseen: the need to continue it and to do something about the dental needs that were uncovered.... A tremendous demand was the only product" (p. 492). So much for demonstration projects.

Getting closer to their own explanation, the staff then summarized the main "factors shaping system evolution" (pp. 495-98). Since they mistook trends for factors, their list was ambiguous, to say the least, as raw material for an explanation. The trends listed included the following: increasing use of paramedical personnel; increasing importance of "environmental" health delivery; increasing costs of care; increasing focus upon treatment of the population of a community rather than upon "individual clinical problems"; increasing emphasis upon group practice and salaries; a declining impact of the demonstration project as a way of monitoring and guiding change; an increasing tendency for cities to get out of the hospital-management business; and, lastly, the tendency for the dehumanized and "double standard character of welfare-oriented medicine" to conflict increasingly with the "larger social ethic."

Which of these trends are inexorable products of larger social forces; which are drifts due to a lack of strong leadership; and which are the specific products of properties of health institutions that could be changed by legal or political decisions, are not questions addressed by the commission staff, although such an attempt to distinguish between trends which are themselves *consequences* of important forces and factors and those which are *causes* of other trends would seem to be an important analytic prerequisite to a theory or explanation. Unfortunately, the trends were simply listed.

At this point, in lieu of analysis, the staff resorted to still another summary description of the problems. Their excuse was the following: "The staff looked at the manifold symptoms of 'system disease' primarily as a way to search out causal factors" (p. 498). So the same litany of problems was repeated: lack of coordination, poor quality, poor distribution of beds, lack of long-term care facilities, lack of ambulatory care programs, lack of home and day care, shortages of personnel, duplication of facilities, inadequate financing, shortage of facilities for the mentally ill, delays in construction, and requirements for replacement and modernization. It may be noted that the list is exactly the same as that given in the Mayor's Advisory Task Force on Medical Economics. A few other problems were omitted here because they are essentially duplicates, combinations, or even more general versions of the characteristics already named (e.g., the "inability or unwillingness of many institutions in the city to provide a broad range of community oriented health services" [p. 502]).

Having finished yet another summary of problems, we are now ready—together with the staff—to confront the question, Why? What, in their words, is the "common thread—a clew winding among all of these problems that will lead us to the heart of the labyrinth?" (p. 505). "The thread is there," they tell us. "It shows itself in terms such as 'uncoordinated,' 'unorganized,' 'fragmented,' 'divided responsibility.' " Here is the basic cause of all of these ills, in the staff's own italicized sentence: "*A locus of responsibility, accountability, and authority does not exist with respect to health services*" (p. 505). It is the "fractionation of authority" which causes all of these multifarious problems in New York City's health system.

And the solution? Presto: a new organization, or rather, two—the Health Services Administration and the Health Services Corporation— will combine "authority with accountability" (as prescribed in a beautiful flow chart on p. 513, fig. 20) and avoid all of the "fundamental problems of fractionation of authority" of the present system. How? Why will it work? Unfortunately, the staff didn't say. The new and rational organization was simply described in terms which imply that simply passing a law, reorganizing the powers of agencies, or redistributing authority will free leaders and officials to act rationally, and that they will immediately do so. No alternative explanations were even mentioned, let along considered in depth. The causes, and the solution, were found only in characteristics of local government administration, not in the health system as a whole, although the burden of all of the previous description and critique is that it was the entire health system which shared these flaws, not merely city government and administration.

Moreover, there was a fundamental contradiction between the assigned *cause* (the fractionation of authority), which implied a need for more centralization of authority, and the specific *recommendations* to decentralize authority into the hands of the hospital administrator and to turn over to the voluntaries more authority over the municipal hospitals. On the one hand, this contradiction was glossed over, as if the administrative machinery of HSA and HSC, given the proper powers and authority, would easily solve these problems. On the other, detailed and specific recommendations for the "disposition" of specific city hospitals were made, although from the logic of their own analysis it would seem that such specific recommendations should wait for city-wide planning, especially since, by their own description, adequate data on health needs and appropriate facilities did not exist. Thus, the staff refrained from dealing with central policy questions but jumped in with specific recommendations on matters which by their own logic should have been left either to the hospital administrator or to HSC.

The flow chart for the ideal system is a model of system analysis jargon, assuming the solution of problems which have yet even to be defined. Policies are decided, goals are established, programs planned, plans reviewed, authorizations issued, operations initiated, expenditures incurred, and results produced. Then, beginning the feedback process, as in any properly functioning system, results are assessed, cost-effectiveness is analyzed, programs are modified, and expenditures are audited (pp. 512–14). Since the cause of all of the problems is fractionation of authority and since this new system has both authority and accountability, the problems will be solved. Why or how the system will change, in fact, remains to be seen, since the entire model is completely abstract.

Despite the fact that alternative explanations had not been considered, the staff then considered alternative courses of action to the HSA and HSC: (1) decentralizing city agencies; (2) turning city hospitals over to the private sector; (3) keeping the status quo of partial affiliations; (4) moving to total affiliations; and (5) creating an independent "authority" (pp. 514–16). These were all rejected for various reasons which were obscurely discussed: lack of accountability, lack of authority, and abrogation of governmental responsibility. These are all bad things, of course; "an entirely new alternative is needed" (p. 516).

But what is this alternative? Unfortunately, the structure of the proposed reorganization, creating the Health Services Administration and the Health Services Corporation, was completely obscured in a fog of rhetoric. The central question of the powers which these new agencies would have over the voluntary hospitals was left entirely open at the theoretical level—and entirely closed at the operational level. That is, when describing the powers and functions of HSA and HSC, the system models (p. 521, fig. 21; p. 523, fig. 22; and p. 526, fig. 23) sounded as if the entire health system would be encompassed. HSC would "operate facilities" (p. 521) and engage in "facilities management: hospitals, ambulatory care centers, district health offices, and others" (p. 523) as if the entire health system would be within their purview, and, seemingly, as would be required by the elimination of the dual system which is regarded by the commission itself as the cause of such deficient health care for the majority of New York City residents.

But in the description of the actual content of the powers of HSA and HSC, the all-too-familiar dual system appeared, and in nearly unchanged form. Never were any regulations or controls on any voluntary hospitals discussed; quite the opposite: the emphasis was on selling or affiliating the municipal hospitals with the voluntaries. In spite of the fact that the voluntary hospitals are now largely supported by public funds or public tax support, how they would be brought into a system of publicly accountable authority was never mentioned. The assumption in the entire discussion was that the reorganization scheme presented, complete with flow charts and organizational diagrams, would convince the reader that this was a solution to the problem of fractionation of authority. Neither evidence nor argument was presented which linked the alleged explanation to the purported cure, and in fact a tremendous gap existed between the possibly well-founded description and critique of the functioning of the system and the causal analysis and recommendations which allegedly followed from that analysis. Such leaps from facts to poorly justified and illogical analysis and recommendations are typical of an ideological rather than scientific analysis, and, in this case, are an excellent example of the specific ideology of corporate rationalization.

Chapter 10, "Some Related Recommendations" (pp. 531–59), continued in the same vein. The chapter started by asserting that "poorly defined goals are at the heart of the recurring conflict between teaching, research, and patient care." Such a formulation minimized the conflicts of interest between the groups involved by assuming that if they would only communicate with each other properly and clarify their goals, the conflicts would disappear. Who was going to do the defining, and who would persuade the others to accept *their* definitions, was not made clear, because the problem of power and authority in the system, despite all the rhetoric, was never confronted squarely.

The same lack of concern with the issue of power was found in the next paragraph. "A role for each institution must be worked out within a planned and coherent framework. A focus of purposes and resources will make of each hospital a truly effective instrument for its system role." A beautiful vision. But would HSA or HSC have the authority to define the role for each institution, including the voluntary hospitals? Remarkably, the staff never said; it evaded the issue completely by presenting at this point—believe it or not—still another repetition of the problems which beset the system: duplications, fragmentation, compartmentalization, waste of available resources, et cetera, et cetera (pp. 531–34). Seldom has it been so clearly shown how repetition can substitute for analysis.

Immediately in this chapter began the list of concrete recommendations for *city* hospitals (again, the voluntaries were never mentioned except as they might take over or run a municipal hospital): convert Coler; operate Fordham; merge Sea View; relinquish Coney Island; affiliate Bellevue; build Cumberland; renovate Goldwater; administer

Lincoln. The details do not matter (although there were nine pages of specific recommendations for the city hospitals), because there was no justification, no discussion of how "public accountability" would be maintained—simply an assertion that it would be—and no indication of how "integration and coordination" would be achieved. One might even suspect that these decisions had been made before the commission had begun its work, and that the entire 500 pages were merely scaffolding around them, so inconsistent were the specific recommendations with the fundamental argument about coordination and planning of a *single* health system for New York City. The very fact that any *specific* recommendations were made at all seems to contradict their general thesis concerning the basis for coordination and planning.

The next-to-last section of chapter 10 dealt with "public funding: financing the corporation" (pp. 546-52) and presented a "cash flow cycle," assuming a single operational entity. The last section (pp. 552-59) was a brief discussion of a "management data system," which elaborated the concept of an "information system" without, however, discussing what specific data would be needed for what purposes or how they would be collected and used. The ideology of corporate rationalization was manifest: the rhetoric of a modern system of data processing with no substance or content. The discussion was couched at a level of generality to which no one could take exception: viz., "To a significant degree, the delivery of health care is inherently based on timely, accurate, and useful information from many sources to support many functions" (p. 556). Amen.

It might be noted here that nowhere in Part III did any discussion of specific programs for improving ambulatory care facilities appear, nor any analysis of how the Veteran's Administration hospitals—heralded as a large-scale hospital system without many of the problems plaguing the New York City hospitals—function and what aspects of their structure might be adopted.

Chapter 11, the last chapter of the Piel Commission report, is titled "Policies for HSA" (pp. 560-79). Much of it (pp. 561-69) is taken nearly verbatim from the Mayor's Task Force on Medical Economics, including all of the guidelines and recommendations from that document with only minor variations in wording, with the addition of fourteen policies.

The report's distinctions between a "guideline" and a "recommendation" have already been criticized as ambiguous. The addition of "policies" compounds the confusion, as another summary will make clear. Most of them are trivial, obvious, overgeneral, or contradictory. The guidelines (each summarized here into a key phrase) consisted of advice to (1) coordinate services; (2) strengthen municipal-voluntary hospital partnership; (3) maintain existing operating budgets; (4) reduce hospital beds; (5) modernize budget and personnel policies; (6) complete capital projects; (7) avoid delays in construction; (8) develop standards; (9) support cost reimbursement (pp. 561-63). The recommendations (paraphrased and summarized) were to (1) take steps to coordinate the system; (2) develop coordinated "medical service centers"; (3) limit specialized facilities and centralize other services; (4) close small hospitals; (5) design facilities for flexibility; (6) develop ambulatory care centers; and (7) create the capability in HSA for improving coordination (pp. 563-69).

Lastly came the fourteen policies for HSA, the essence of which is given here to indicate concretely the lack of clarity and specificity of the report's analysis.

1. Develop the full range of health services for New York City (hospitals, public health services, ambulatory care facilities, long-term care facilities).

2. "Integrate and consolidate in reasonable and productive ways the historically separate, if not sometimes competitive, urban systems of health care delivery in the City of New York" (p. 572).

3. "Disengage the City of New York from its historical but unnecessary and inappropriate role in the direct management of health care delivery support activities" (p. 573).

4. "Make functional throughout the city an objectives-oriented system of health care delivery operations for the entire health system" (p. 573).

5. "Develop and promulgate major planned programs having to do with prevention, early detection and treatment, ambulatory care, intensive clinical care, extended care, and chronic care" (p. 574).

6. "Encourage the decline and ultimate removal of the impeding effects of professional schisms in health sciences and delivery" (p. 574). (The casual way in which a fundamental problem of the social organization of health care is raised and glossed over is striking.)

7. "Bring about a sound, effective, and accountable system of control and operation for all public funds" (p. 575).

8. "Bring about the regionalization of public health care delivery through localized administration and activity" (p. 575). (Here is another contradiction, compounded by the next sentence of the report,

which urges a "reduction in the role of central administration." How "regionalization" is reconciled with "localization" simultaneously with an increase in public accountability, centralized planning, but decentralized administration, poses problems of analysis and policy that were not even raised in this report.)

9. "Develop an 'optimum formula' for the development, change in, and application of, health care services at the regional level and within the communities of the city" (p. 576).

10. "Assure an effective linkage between research advances and improved patient care" (p. 577).

11. "Formulate, stimulate, and (if necessary) itself [HSA] carry out innovative training programs" (p. 578).

12. "Effect the use of support technologies to every reasonable and feasible extent" (p. 578).

13. "Provide comprehensive strengthening of traditional programs of environmental health" (p. 579).

14. The "operating policy" of HSA should be to "bring about realization of sufficiently improved health care delivery that New York City will not only achieve appropriate delivery for funds expended but will achieve an outstanding rank in the nation and in the world for the delivery of health care to its citizens" (p. 579).

How a goal of this stupendous magnitude can be an "operating policy" is not clear, because the staff studies ended at this point, followed by a list of 300 interviewees, 367 bibliographic items, and four other appendixes. We are left with the overwhelming impression that all of the problems have been dumped into HSA's lap. Given the ambiguity with which authority, accountability, leadership, resources, autonomy, goals, guidelines, recommendations, and policies, as well as all of the other weapons of justice, were placed at the disposal of the wise and far-seeing leadership of the new administration and corporation, we can be once again reassured that there has been a symbolic and meaningless response to the health "crisis."

10. 1971, the RAND Institute:
Mental Health Service
Delivery

A recent study by the New York City RAND Institute provides another opportunity to assess the state of research and planning on the subject of the coordination of mental health services.[20] The RAND Institute was "established in 1969 by the City of New York and the Rand Corporation as a center for the continuing application of scientific and analytic techniques to problems of urban life and local government," according to the blurb on the cover of the report. This particular study "is part of a program of health research ... undertaken for New York City's Health Services Administration. The objective of the program is to furnish the health-service policymakers of New York City with information necessary for the efficient operation of public programs" (p. iii).

The study itself and the program it evaluates—the community mental health centers funded by 1963 federal legislation—are examples of complex interorganizational relationships concerned with increasing the coordination of presumably fragmented systems. The federal and state legislative context can be summarized in the report's own words: "The essential purposes of the series of legislative enactments, beginning in 1963 at the federal level and followed by enactments at the state level, have been 1) to develop an alternative and a supplement to the state hospital for the treatment of the seriously mentally ill, 2) to ensure citizens with low income an access to mental health services, inpatient as well as ambulatory, and 3) to integrate, using a structure of formal arrangements, various deliverers of care" (p. 1). Thus, the federal legislation aimed at coordination of services, as well as increasing the number of services available to the poor. And this report itself is an instance of relationships between New York City, the RAND Institute, and the "Eastside" Community Mental Health Center in New York City (the subject of the case study).

The striking thing about this report is that, despite its emphasis upon the intent of the federal legislation and its stress upon the "lack of coordination among producers" as one of the main characteristics of the supply of mental health services, neither the theoretical discussion nor the empirical data gathered from two community mental health centers (the other is in California) even attempted to measure the degree of coordination, discover the causes of fragmentation, or suggest any policy recommendations for changing those causes. In fact, the basic theoretical framework adopted by the author permitted him to ignore this problem, and his methodology prevented him from even seeing it as a meaningful problem. The author argued that "the community mental health center represents a response of policymakers to the well-known lack of coordination among producers, as well as a means for providing new types of treatment units to accommodate patients at all levels of impairment" (p. 19). That the original 1963 federal legislation, in fact, required that a mental health center "contain five components—inpatient, outpatient, partial hospital, emergency, and consultation and education services—and the recommendation that they offer diagnostic and rehabilitative services, precare and aftercare services in the community, training, and research and evaluation reflect the notion that mental health services should be coordinated" (p. 2).

However, none of the data presented by the author bears upon these seemingly major problems and intents of the legislation. The data which were presented consisted of allocations of time by the staff to various activities (administration, patient care, etc.), the services provided to outpatients for a sample week, the numbers of staff members in various occupations (medical records librarian, vocational nurse, physician, etc.), and the earnings per hour for different occupations. All of these bits of data pertain to the activities of the staff members of each separate center, analyzed as a free-standing entity. Some of them might pertain to the problem of coordination of patient services, but they were neither described nor analyzed with this problem in mind.

In fact, the whole thrust of the analysis is away from a focus upon the health system—or even the *mental* health system—as a whole. Data were gathered for separate units, and formulae were discussed for "program performance scores" which took as their basic data the number of program units (methadone, inpatient care, etc.), the number of patient-contracts or patient-days, and an "effectiveness parameter" for which adequate data did not exist. Although the author continuously noted the inadequacy of the basic data which could be inserted into his formulae, the point here is not that he was simply proposing abstract formulae but that the theoretical framework is one which makes it impossible to consider the problem of fragmentation. The author said that his scheme for the development of program performance scores lacked the necessary data. Nevertheless, "in the short run, the method's major contribution will be a framework into which the necessary pieces of information may be fitted" (p. 39).

Later, in discussing the data requirements in more detail, he noted the main questions of concern in studying each provider unit. "What and how much does each produce? What types of inputs and how much of each are employed to produce a given output?" (p. 41). This language implied that each organization would be analyzed as an independent entity, and, in fact, that was the procedure he followed. In discussing alternative measures of output, the author discussed services provided, cases treated, and mental health status indicators, settling upon the first as the "most satisfactory output for a study of mental health services production" (p. 45). A list of various therapeutic and other mental health care activities was given in table 7 (pp. 46–47). The point here is not to criticize this list, which may be perfectly comprehensive and adequate, but to observe that nowhere are the problems of coordinating mental health services taken by themselves and nowhere are the problems of coordinating mental health services with other health services mentioned, either as a theoretical or policy issue, or as questions requiring empirical data to answer.

This lack of concern for a problem which the author himself has indicated is of importance leads to some curious methodological decisions. Discussing the relative merits of "cases treated" versus "services provided" as measures of output, the author noted that "one Westside ward treats large numbers of patients, but the ward is used essentially as a way station to the state hospital" (p. 44). This observation was used as evidence for rejecting "cases treated" as an indicator of output. The clear assumption was that the single center was the unit for which services were being measured, not the complex set of facilities available for the treatment of an entire population. One would assume that if fragmentation of services was a key problem for study, the criteria for outputs would include the ease of transfer from one type of agency or institution to another, the conditions or criteria under which transfers took place, and their consequences. None of these considerations appeared in this report.

The section on possible economies of scale might have considered the contribution of different-sized health centers to the problem of fragmentation, but it did not. Again, the perspective was one which considered size as a property of a single organization and thus as a factor which affected staff morale, the amount of specialization possible, and the amount of random demand as a factor influencing capacity. All of these were properties of the single organization. And the policy recommendation was basically that "large centers should not be funded" (p. 91), although the author's point was slightly more complex than that. But clearly whether one large center or many small centers are established is a decision which involves the problem of coordination of fragmented health services in a central way, and the discussion never mentioned this issue.

Despite obeisance to the problem of fragmentation, then, the author never considered it empirically or theoretically of importance. In fact, the only reference, after the initial ones, where fragmentation was seen as a problem occurred in a section in which the author speculated that attempts at coordination might be excessively expensive in terms of staff time and suggested trying to find ways of maximizing staff time spent in actual patient care, rather than in coordination efforts (p. 18). No data were presented, nor even any speculation on the possible findings of data on the relative importance of various uses of staff time. What accounts for this internal contradiction in the report? Surely if fragmentation were an important problem, the author would have been required to deal with it in a more substantial way by the sponsor of the study—New York City. It is possible that this problem is merely a symbolic one with which no involved interest group is really concerned, since a really substantial attempt at coordination would inevitably involve changing both the balance of power between agencies and a significant increase in centralization.

But quite aside from this factor—which may well underlie the absence of any real demand for substantive research on the extent and consequences of fragmentation, and any serious policy recommendations which could result in the generation of enough power to impose some real coordination—the analytic framework used by the author of the RAND report impedes a serious definition of the problem, let alone a solution. The author drew from academic economics an abstract model of a competitive market economy. In such an analytic context, the assumptions may be useful. But, when applied to a real problem of policy research, the model becomes almost meaningless and, worse, a barrier to effective policy planning. Without going into great detail, a few examples may make the point.

The author of this report assumed that health care providers are like firms, meeting demands and producing commodities for a market. Demands arise when patients arrive at the door of a provider wanting services. The health market, like others, functions well only when consumers possess the necessary information about the availability, cost, and quality of services. Only then will there be incentives for the producers continually to seek to improve their efficiency and productivity, since under conditions of poor information, inefficient, expensive, and poor quality services will continue to exist.

Although the author admitted that no data exist on the effectiveness of mental health services and that very little information exists on the availability and cost of those services (regardless of how ineffective they may be even when you get them), he failed to consider the extent to which lack of information is a systematic structural characteristic of the system and not just an accidental, temporary defect of a normal market to be corrected just by providing consumers with information.

In fact, even the health professionals and social workers in the New York and California community mental health centers he studied had little information on the services available to their clients (p. 6). And it would seem that the staff would have little incentive to increase the supply of information, since that would just sharply increase the focused demands for services and, consequently, their work load. Moreover, if accurate information on high quality subsidized services were available to the poor, this would reduce the access to those services by the upper middle class. Thus, for both organizational factors (staff interests) and social class factors, it seems that a lack of information serves important functions. But information is a necessary part of a market system and therefore must be of concern in an analytic paradigm which stresses an open market.

Another aspect of the theoretical framework which would seem almost laughably naïve if it weren't such an intrinsic part of the economic paradigm, concerns the role of government. The author assumed that government actions are either a response to the aggregate preferences of a majority of consumers or a reflection of society-wide values. The structure of powerful interest groups seeking to maximize their interests—which may be inconsistent and contradictory with either or both majority preferences or society-wide values—was totally neglected as an empirical possibility.

For example, the author asserted that "alcohol is taxed because of the commonly held view that alcohol had deleterious effects" (p. 13). However, many things which have deleterious effects are not taxed, and vice versa. The structure of taxation is a result of the historical victories of various pressure and interest groups, not of society-wide values. Another example: "Individual A may make B relatively wealthier by taxing himself and subsidizing B, using government as an inter-mediary" (p. 13). The metaphorical language reflects a real underlying assumption about the nature and causes of governmental action as a response to aggregated preferences, which is probably false with respect both to the causal direction of the relationship and to its basic character. Government action shapes preferences as much as vice versa, and the whole formulation neglects the complex process through which groups and organizations form with interests of their own.

Further, attempting to distinguish the market for mental health services from others, the author said, "an individual's demand for mental health services is not fully predictable and stable, unlike his demand for such commodities as food, clothing and shelter" (p. 14).

This seems plausible on the face of it: we cannot predict when an individual will become mentally ill, but we can predict that he will always need food and shelter. But this approach is wrong and stems from the focus on the individual as the ultimate unit, possessing preferences and making demands. Although we certainly can't predict when a given individual will get sick, neither can we predict when he will buy a house. Conversely, we can predict the aggregate market for mental health treatment for a given population with probably the same level of accuracy that we can predict the demand for new cars in a given year.

The shallowness of the analytic framework of this report is also shown by its numerous tautologies. For example, attempting to explain why a nonprofit sector has emerged in health care, the author suggested that the "best explanation" is that "seriously ill patients or their families have not been able to pay for care" (p. 16). The system is nonprofit because there is no profit to be made. Again, it seems unlikely that such profound explanations are due to any logical or theoretical inadequacies on the part of the author, but rather are due to implicit assumptions of the theoretical paradigm, which caused the author simply to fail to see certain phenomena as relevant data and certain relationships as important.

This report is a depressing example of policy research sponsored and paid for by New York City. Its theoretical paradigm is incomplete and naïve, applying academic models and assumptions where they are inappropriate. The data analyzed are sketchy and inadequate even for the narrow context proposed, and even the data proposed as necessary are irrelevant to the problems of the health care system which are allegedly the inspiration for such research.

More generally, the very focus of the study on community mental health centers feeds into and further reinforces the fragmentation of the health system. If these centers were successful in "integrating" inpatient, outpatient, emergency, and consultation services, as required by federal law, they would fragment the system as a whole. "Mental" health cannot be separated from "physical" health by administrative rulings, professional specialization, and establishment of separate free-standing clinics or centers. The very attempt to establish "comprehensive" centers is thus an internal contradiction in the basic legislation. Undoubtedly, the legislation was seen as a "forward step," since it was not politically realistic to reform or reorganize the whole system, and an attempt to coordinate "part" of it was seen as a progressive, liberal advance. Once again, this is a dilemma of the strategy of piecemeal reform, if the coordination and integration of the entire health system is the goal.

11. Summary and Conclusions

A sampling of the reports of various commissions of investigation of the New York City health system between 1950 and 1971 has been summarized. The sponsorship, membership, content, analysis, and recommendations of others are substantially the same as those evaluated here. Only length and redundancy, although certainly more evidence, would be added if more of these reports were summarized here.

In the course of this investigation no study or report was located which evaluated the impact or the influence of previous recommendations by other commissions. Nor have we found any other follow-up studies or attempts to consider the specific impact of a previous policy recommendation. Given this lack of responsiveness, it is possible to say that these commissions are themselves instances of the fragmentation of the system. Each study and report stands alone with only a gesture toward the previous ones, acknowledging their existence, noting that the same problems persist, but giving no analysis of the previous recommendations, the specific state of affairs with respect to their implementation, the effect on the system of their implementation, the reasons why they were not implemented, or why the consequences of implementation were different from those anticipated. Each study and report is thus a response to a "crisis" in the same sense and in the same way as the Mayor's establishment of the Health Services Administration is a response to a "crisis." The reports are not part of an integrated, coordinated, and continuing program of research and evaluation. The result is a lack of a cumulative body of data which could be used for continuous monitoring of the outputs of the health system. Each new report must rely on the same sketchy body of data: income and age composition of areas of the city, hospital beds and occupancy rates, hospital costs per patient-day, funds spent by city, state, and federal agencies. None of these data, unfortunately, are aggregated or related to each other in ways which bear upon the crucial analytic or policy questions.

Given the inadequacy of analysis and recommendations, it is almost too easy to predict that administrative reorganizations, whether to centralize or decentralize operations, will not solve all, or even any, of the multiplicity of problems consigned to their care. Rather, the "innovations" introduced, far from integrating and coordinating the system, will further complicate and fragment it. The reason is that the dual system not only is perpetuated but is more deeply embedded than ever, because the public funds provided to private institutions become even more safely guaranteed and legitimated by still another layer of public bureaucracy. Yet—and this is evident more in the concrete recommendations than in the generalized rhetoric—the new bureaucracies will *not* be given the necessary powers, functions, and resources to achieve the laudable goal of overcoming "fractionation of authority."

Division of authority is *not* the cause of the multifarious problems faced by the New York City health system but is yet another manifestation of those problems. The failure of any of these commissions of investigation to confront these problems squarely and to probe deeply for their causes is also a manifestation of the functioning of the system. These reports are not part of the solution, but part of the problem. They serve as symbolic, not tangible, responses—to use Murray Edelman's terms—which produce public quiescence in the face of deeply embedded structural problems of the health system.[21]

The political incentives to set up such commissions are clear. As Ida Hoos has observed, public officials can have their cake and eat it too by appointing task forces. "The mayor of a large city, for example, wins his election by pledging to do something about the bad conditions of housing, transportation, health, crime, and so on. Among his first official acts is the signing of contracts with consultants to do 'urban analysis' and 'plan rationally.' From then on, he has a ready-made rationalization for any position taken, any decision made or avoided." She gives an example from New York City, "where $75 million was paid to outside consultants in 1969, it was discovered, late in the game, that *ten different studies of one bridge* had been made since 1948, that the current Transportation Administrator was unaware of six of them, and that not one of them was implementable or implemented. A sequence of administrations had reaped the benefits of public display of concern over the situation without making a further attempt at its amelioration." She concludes that "with New York as a model, the lesser cities of the nation cannot be far behind. The political advantages are evident, the temptations are great."[22]

3 The Planning Council and the Coordination of Neighborhood Health Care

1. Introduction

Our analysis in chapter 2 of the reports of a number of commissions of investigation in New York City from 1950 to 1971 has shown that the lack of adequate outpatient or ambulatory care facilities is a chronic feature of the health care "crisis." In fact it is so chronic that the term *crisis* does not seem appropriate and may be misleading if it implies that the causes of the lack of ambulatory care facilities are to be found in decisions made in the immediate past and thus that the situation is one which has only recently come into existence.

The reasons for poor ambulatory care facilities are fairly well recognized: (1) the low-status character of such facilities, requiring low levels of medical skills and therefore not attracting ambitious and highly qualified doctors; and (2) the fact that these facilities largely serve the poor, who use emergency rooms and outpatient clinics as a substitute for the family doctor. These facilities are therefore regarded by both the hospitals and their doctors as part of their charity public services.

What has been the response to this "crisis"? The neighborhood health center program was the response in the mid 1960s. This program provides material for case studies of the interrelationships of city, state, and federal agencies with municipal and voluntary hospitals in New York City. Applications for federal grants are a key instance of interorganizational relationships, and their fate, in terms of both approval and implementation, as they wend their way through various city, state, and federal agencies, illustrates the complex interorganizational relationships in the health delivery system.

Local attempts at coordination are vitiated by what some theorists of interorganizational relationships call a "turbulent" environment. Unfortunately, most research on organizations has regarded each organization as a separate entity and has seen properties of the environment as a part of the "field" with which leaders or elites must deal, not as persistent characteristics of the society. In the case of federal programs in the health field, and probably in other fields as well, a complex environment seems to be a persistent characteristic of the system. Federal legislation in the area of what is now called "comprehensive health care" is a good case in point. Generally, the impact of the diverse, uncoordinated, and even contradictory federal agencies and funding has been further to fragment the already uncoordinated health system at the local level. A detailed case study of attempts to establish comprehensive neighborhood health care centers will illustrate some of the consequences of the complex problems for local health agencies created by vacillating and uncertain federal commitments to programs and funding.

Neighborhood health centers have a long history in the United States, rising and falling in popularity as a response to ever-new definitions of health care as in a state of crisis. The same themes and goals reappear over and over again—location in neighborhoods so as to provide comprehensive care to an entire population, community participation in governance, coordination of many different services under one roof to improve the efficiency of care, and an emphasis on preventive rather than "crisis" or emergency health care.[1]

Efforts to establish neighborhood health centers also have a long history in New York City but have usually been linked to battles over administrative jurisdiction between heads of functional bureaus and heads of district health offices. The first two comprehensive health centers (to use one of the current terms) in New York City were established, as might be expected, as demonstration projects in the 1920s in East Harlem and Yorkville, funded by the Red Cross and the Milbank Memorial Fund. The centers were supposed to show "how health and welfare work in a given area could be co-ordinated, and to initiate such services as might be wanting" (p. 7).[2] These demonstrations apparently worked well, and "a small group of leaders in the private health and welfare field ... began to visualize a system of neighborhood health centers throughout the city, the buildings to be provided and maintained by public funds, in which their private agencies would have both space and a voice in local planning" (p. 7). In 1929 the Committee on Neighborhood Health Development recommended that the city be divided into thirty health districts, each containing such a health center. Although delayed by the depression, seven centers were opened in 1934 under LaGuardia's new administration of the city. Funds from the federal Public Works Administration built seven buildings. By 1937 the entire city was divided into thirty districts clustered into twenty administrative units. There was practically continuous conflict between 1914 and 1958 (the date of my source) over the allocation of authority between functional bureaus and geographical districts. Depending on the general political situation in New York and also on the beliefs of the Commissioner of Health, authority vacillated back and forth, and the distinction between adminstrative responsibility officially held by the district health officers and technical responsibility officially held by the bureau chiefs continuously broke down in practice. The solution sought in 1959 was to upgrade the borough level of adminstration and to place in the borough director's hands responsibility for coordinating the system.

What is striking about this history is the repetition of the same problems *and* the same solutions. The first challenge (1914) to the functional bureaus contained language and reasoning practically identical to much of the recent reports. The separate units within the Department of Health were "almost completely uncoordinated," but simultaneously the bureaus themselves were "over-centralized." The specialization of departmental personnel led to an inability to perceive problems in their broad context. Existing procedures led to "costly and irritating duplication." City-wide statistics hid "alarming contrasts between various sections of the city." Public health administration was still too negative, and what was needed was "new ways of organizing and administering health work."[3]

The solution for the last fifty years has been the administrative juggling of power and authority, which have either constantly been reallocated among officials or assigned to newly created ones, hopefully more capable of doing the job. Accusations of lack of cooperation, a willingness to compromise, failure to communicate, and inability to define goals were frequent and led to attempts to create new channels of communication, new sets of rules defining goals and procedures, and new officials responsible for coordination.

The issue is whether this long history is the result, as Kaufman argues, of problems "generic to organization"—mainly an inherent conflict between areal officials and functional officials—or whether (even if such a universal tendency is admitted) the particular form and intensity of organizational conflict are particularly likely to be found in a society with political and economic institutions like those of the twentieth-century United States. There is no easy answer to this question, although I lean to the latter and advance an argument along those lines later on in this book. Kaufman summarizes the actions of high New York City officials over the years by saying that "primary emphasis was placed on changing in various ways the formal hierarchical relationships between the functional and areal officers." Kaufman's explanation deserves some attention, because it displays the assumptions of an alternative analytic framework. "There was little or no attempt to modify attitudes and win compliance by education or other means, partly because the pressure of other official business prevented successive commissioners from giving their full attention to this possibility, and partly because there was a fundamental lack of agreement on—perhaps understanding of—the objectives of the Department" (p. 18). Surely the "pressure of other official business" was institutionalized into both political and administrative behavior. What he is saying is that the establishment of comprehensive health care centers was such a low priority item on the agenda of New York City's political leaders, and therefore of its top administrative officials, that other matters constantly took priority, and a long-standing internal struggle between the bureau heads and the district health officers could be allowed to continue for fifty years because there was no constituency with enough numbers and political resources to demand that that conflict be resolved. Also, the "fundamental lack of agreement on objectives" was also institutionalized into political and administrative behavior. The Department of Health could not possibly define its goals and embed them into an appropriate set of administrative machinery precisely because of the basic conflict over whose interests that machinery was supposed to serve. In the absence of political mechanisms which could enforce the translation of stated public policy into administrative implementation, no group or component of the array of health organizations and services provided by the city had the power or resources to impose its own definition of what those goals meant. Kaufman retains a voluntaristic image of what motivated, responsible, and competent leadership might have accomplished and ends with a kind of qualified optimism. The successive commissioners of health did have "various choices open to them in a number of different fields. . . . At the end of 45 years, it is conceivable that a viable form of areal administration is at last emerging, but the experience of 45 years compels the observer to be cautious, if not skeptical" (pp. 17-18).

This study adds another chapter to the continuing story of neighborhood health care in New York City but rejects Kaufman's explanation in terms of endemic features of complex organizations. While it is undoubtedly true that specialized functions, the tendency for professionals to contact each other across hierarchies, the cohesion and traditions of long-established bureaus, and the technical expertise of staff would exacerbate the conflicts Kaufman describes, it is also true that under some political and economic conditions those organizational *tendencies* can be successfully combated. Under other conditions they are endemic. Neither the analytic question of how to explain why organizational and professional conflicts supersede political capabilities and goals, nor the political question of how to mobilize enough resources successfully to force a resolution of those conflicts, is answered by suggesting that it is possible for administrators to make choices.

Thus, the new federal programs of the 1960s just revived an old solution to some of the problems of health care delivery in New York City. The beginning of the war on poverty with the establishment of the Office of Economic Opportunity (OEO) in 1964 marked the availability of federal funds for a variety of health-related activities to local institutions. And because of the general political popularity of fighting poverty at that time, other federal agencies, notably the Department of Health, Education, and Welfare (HEW), began to initiate poverty programs of their own, partly as a way of increasing their own budgets by winning congressional favor for innovative programs. One of the emerging health programs for poverty areas went under a variety of names—comprehensive health center, comprehensive care center, neighborhood family care center—but was essentially conceived of as an outpatient or ambulatory care facility, linked to a back-up hospital which would provide in-hospital care where necessary. The assumption was that it would be cheaper and quicker to build these centers in poverty areas rather than either expanding the outpatient clinic facilities of existing hospitals or building new hospitals in poverty areas.

In 1965, when the funds became available, thus stimulating discussion among New York City health leaders about what might be done with them, plans developed to remodel the old district health stations which originally had been set up in the 1930s under the LaGuardia administration to perform the same functions of a neighborhood health center. Then it was decided that it would be better to build new facilities rather than remodel old ones, and the Neighborhood Family Care Center (NFCC) program was born. Seventeen centers were originally planned in 1965; fifteen were mentioned in the next capital budget; and the Health and Hospital Planning Council—charged with a preliminary review of the adequacy of the plans and their coordination with existing health facilities—received eleven "letters of intent."

The Health and Hospital Planning Council approved eight of those (the ones which mentioned a back-up hospital and a specific site). In December 1970 the city announced that fifteen were still being planned, but now mainly with city funds rather than state or federal funds, and by 1971 four more had been "withdrawn without prejudice" by the state, upon the request of the Health Services Administration, because of lack of a site or lack of funding. By early 1971 ground had been broken for exactly *one* Neighborhood Family Care Center.

The total picture is not quite this bleak, however, because there were successful attempts to establish ambulatory care facilities, which are not counted as part of the Neighborhood Family Care Center program. By March of 1970, according to a Planning Council memo, thirty-one health centers of various types which had been approved by the council were pending, in operation, or in planning. These had already been or were going to be funded from a variety of sources—private, federal, state, and city—ranging from private foundations to the Office of Economic Opportunity, Title II of the Children's Bureau of HEW, section 314e of Public Law 89-749 through HEW, the Health Services Administration through the New York City capital budget, and ultimately, partly by the state of New York. By 10 March 1970 sixteen of these were in operation, seven under OEO funding, five under Title II, two under HEW 314e grants, and two under NYC capital budgeting. This constituted all of the proposed health centers under the first three sources of funding, but only a small proportion of the fifteen proposed centers under New York City funding. Six of the remaining thirteen were "pending," and seven were "in planning." All except two of the thirty-one projects were in the boroughs of Brooklyn (12), Manhattan (10), and the Bronx (7).

It is beyond our scope here to consider the specific differences in the programs of these various types of health centers, but the very overlapping of their concerns, the lack of any coherent data on the populations and areas they would serve, and their relationships to other health care units in the area are significant in themselves. In the rest of this chapter, case studies of attempts to establish particular NFCC's are presented which take the broad background of federal legislation and its translation into specific local programs as given and focus upon the operations of the Health and Hospital Planning Council of Southern New York insofar as it operated as a mediating agency, a clearinghouse for information, and an official body charged with establishing guidelines for coordination between health agencies in New York City.[4]

2. The Health and Hospital
   Planning Council of Southern
   New York

The Health and Hospital Planning Council of Southern New York is itself an example of an interorganizational relationship, and not just an organization in its own right. It is a link between relatively independent and autonomous organizations—hospitals and city and state governments—but is itself dependent, by its budget and by its charter, upon those organizations. It is composed of member organizations, and its board of directors is largely composed of representatives of organizations, save for a few physicians. Most of the positions on its board are quite explicitly reserved for representatives of organizations, and when a person leaves an official position with that organization, he is replaced on the council also. The Health Services Administrator of the City is regularly on the board, as are representatives of Catholic Charities, Blue Cross, and so forth. (For the 1969-70 members, see the accompanying list.)

Member Organizations, Health and
Hospital Planning Council of
Southern New York, Inc., 1969-1970

Associated Hospital Service of New York

Association of Private Hospitals, Inc.

Catholic Charities, Archdiocese of New York

Catholic Charities, Diocese of Brooklyn

Commerce and Industry Association of New York

Community Council of Greater New York

The Coordinating Council of the First District Branch of the Medical Society of the State of New York

Federation of Jewish Philanthropies of New York

Federation of Protestant Welfare Agencies, Inc.

The Greater New York Fund

Greater New York Hospital Association

The Hospital Association of Southeastern New York

Long Island Federation of Labor AFL-CIO

Metropolitan New York Nursing Home Association, Inc.

Nassau-Suffolk Hospital Council, Inc.

The New York Academy of Medicine

New York City Central Labor Council AFL-CIO

Public Health Association of New York City

State Communities Aid Association

Teamster Joint Council No. 16

United Hospital Fund of New York

Westchester County AFL-CIO Central Labor Body

The Westchester County Association, Inc.

Westchester County Hospital Association

Source: Health and Hospital Planning Council of Southern New York, Inc., 1969-70, *Annual Report.*

The Planning Council is thus an important organization to study, not only because it is an example of a type of interorganizational relationship or linkage which is probably increasingly important, but also because it publicly defines itself as responsible for the "coordination" of health services. The inscription printed on the inside front cover of each of the last few annual reports of the council reads, "A non-profit organization incorporated to *coordinate* and improve hospital and health services and to *plan* the development of these services in relation to community needs" (italics added).

The Health and Hospital Planning Council began in 1938 as a voluntary planning agency, established by the United Hospital Fund to consider needs for ambulance service. (Its name has changed several times during its history, but the details are not important.) It provided a forum and a place where the needs and interests of the voluntary hospitals for expansion could be discussed and thrashed out. In 1965, under the Folsom Act, it assumed quasi-legal responsibilities for review of all new hospital and out-of-hospital facilities for Southern New York, thus becoming eligible for state funds and becoming at least in part a state agency linked to the New York State Department of Health in the review process. In 1968–69 the Council fought to become the Comprehensive Health Planning Agency under Public Law 89-749, but it lost to New York's city government, becoming only one of the myriad of health agencies and consumer groups represented in the Mayor's Organizational Task Force for Comprehensive Health Planning, which became the official planning agency in October 1971.

These changes of funding, function, and powers have, according to staff members, made the Planning Council mainly a review agency. Its research and planning functions have dwindled, and, aside from its review function, its character was very much in flux in 1970–71. Its staff members report that many of the area-wide planning councils in the United States under voluntary auspices have lost out to public agencies organized under Comprehensive Health Planning auspices.

The review process of ambulatory care facilities conducted by the council, as outlined by staff members, can be summarized briefly. (These procedures were in flux in 1971, and the following description and case instances applied mainly to the 1967–70 period.) The sponsoring agency submitted a "letter of intent," which included only a general statement of the program, mention of the back-up hospital, and a brief discussion of the facilities, staffing, and funding. At this point, a meeting was to be called between the council and representatives of the sponsoring agency, and an informal discussion was held about the project. Staff members of the council observed that once applicants got copies of the guidelines, they were usually smart enough to observe the guidelines, at least verbally. The council was under the pressure of time, since it usually had to act within sixty days in order to get the proposal to the state within 120 days, and it was mainly interested in assessing the commitment and the resources of the sponsor and the general need of the area. But the council did not require that extensive documentation or research supporting the guidelines be submitted. Rather, informal assurances were accepted, and the general reputation of the agency, hospital, or other organization was regarded as evidence of commitment. As one staff member put it, "the Council was supposed to recommend on 'ballpark' needs" and provide advice on the feasibility and desirability of the proposed project. The guidelines, then, were not regarded as "regulations," since the council had no police powers and could not require modifications.

Thus, the council review process consisted of informal meetings with the various involved or affected organizations in which suggestions were offered to the sponsor; then, quite routinely, a letter recommending approval would be sent to the state. According to council staff members, no other materials were sent to the state except the letter recommending approval—no supporting documents reporting the staff work of the council and no grounds for the recommendations. According to one man on the council staff, the state had a variety of agencies with their own staffs doing evaluations of the proposals, and they neither wanted nor needed the council's staff documents.

It was the impression of council staff members that the council was actually *more* interested in the actual program of the ambulatory care facility than was the state, which was concerned with making sure that minimum standards of safety for the building and minimum qualifications of the staff were met. In fact, according to a staff member, the state revised its own review guidelines to reduce the amount of attention necessary to the substance of the proposed health program. If this is so, then at no point in the review process was any serious attention paid to the mechanisms of coordination of one new program with another. It is important to contrast this account of the normal functioning of the council review process with the substance of the council's own guidelines, which are summarized in the following section.

3. Guidelines for Coordination

In 1966 the Health and Hospital Planning Council adopted "guidelines for evaluating proposals for neighborhood clinics and health centers."

These contained, from a layman's point of view at least, excellent and comprehensive criteria for adequate comprehensive outpatient facilities which would be linked to a hospital for more specialized in-hospital treatment.[5] Those guidelines of primary interest to us—the interorganizational relationships of various health-care providers—were detailed and numerous. Under the heading "demonstration of need for facility," the guideline requested information concerning "the proposed facility's arrangement with other ambulatory care facilities in the area in respect to redelineating service areas and to selection of patients" (p. 38). Under "location" was mentioned the requirement that the new facility should be "accessible to the sponsoring hospital." Under "scope of services and estimates of volume," information was asked for concerning "arrangements for assuring availability of health services not provided at the proposed neighborhood center." Under "facilities" a "description of arrangements for obtaining laboratory examinations not provided at the ambulatory care facility" was asked for. Under "emergency services" it was noted that "provision should be made for night and weekend emergency service either at the backup hospital, or at the neighborhood health center if feasible." Under the heading "organization" the guidelines asserted that while an ambulatory care facility must often be outside of the physical facilities of the back-up hospital itself, "it is nevertheless essential that close functional integration of staff structure and services of the clinic and of the associated general hospital be maintained" (p. 41). Under "auspices" it was stated that "a neighborhood health center must be developed under the auspices of a voluntary or public general hospital with an operating certificate from the State of New York and accredited by the Joint Commission on Accreditation of Hospitals, or by a voluntary agency established in accordance with New York State law which has established an affiliation with a suitable general hospital." Lastly, under "consumer participation," the guidelines noted that approval of proposals would "take into consideration evidence of consumer participation in the planning process," and that "mechanisms" for that participation should be described.

These guidelines seem clear, comprehensive, and necessary for the coordination of a new neighborhood health center with existing hospital and ambulatory care facilities. However, according to staff members at the Planning Council, almost none of the proposals for neighborhood health centers met the guidelines in these particular respects involving coordination with existing services. Examination of the letters of intent and allied documents submitted to the Planning Council to secure their approval, as required under New York State's Folsom Act, supports their statement. Almost none of the coordinating mechanisms suggested or required by the guidelines were spelled out in the detail seemingly indicated. At the most, a back-up hospital and some indication of its willingness to play that role were specified. But, even here, according to staff members at the Planning Council, the commitment of the back-up hospital at this point was casual at best and did not involve a binding commitment to provide in-hospital services for the envisaged population of 55,000 persons in a specified neighborhood.

Almost all of the proposals except those by the Health Services Administration of the City were directly sponsored by hospitals. It seems likely that the Planning Council relied upon the general reputation of a hospital to provide a basis for its evaluation. A hospital which was not overcrowded and which had a reputation for adequate staffing and administrative capability was assumed to be able to exercise enough good judgment not to allow a proposal to go forward which ultimately might strain its physical or financial capabilities. Whatever the specific reason for the council's trust in the hospitals, none of the files examined contained any documents which (1) analyzed existing outpatient facilities in the area to be served or documented how the new center would fill a need not presently being served; (2) presented specific plans for providing laboratory examinations or emergency room services at some other health facility in the area if they were not to be contained in the health center; (3) suggested how "functional integration" of the staff structures of the two organizations was to be achieved; or (4) spelled out mechanisms for "consumer participation."

An example or two of the kind of links to the back-up hospital specified will illustrate the point. The Rousso Community Health Center, under auspices of the Albert Einstein College of Medicine and funded under Title II, Children's Bureau, HEW, submitted a letter of intent on 4 January 1968 to Dr. Donald G. Dickson, Associate Commissioner for New York City Affairs, New York State Department of Health, for approval of the project. The only mention of relationships with any other health facility was in the following sentences: "Consultants in the various medical and surgical specialties will be available on a regularly scheduled basis within the Project and also at the back-up facilities of the Bronx Municipal Hospital Center. Hospitalization, when required, will be in the Jacobi Hospital of the Bronx Municipal Hospital Center." But, the letter continued, a "secondary goal" is the "development of a viable model for satellite comprehensive health care units, which ultimately would serve for the reorganization of the Pedia-

tric Out-Patient Department of the Bronx Municipal Hospital Center."
Although no details were given on how or why the proposed comprehensive child care program would be related to, would replace, or
would supplement or complement the existing outpatient department
of the back-up hospital, the new center was nevertheless regarded as a
potential replacement for it.

On 21 February 1968 Dr. Dickson of the New York State Health
Department's city office was sent another letter modifying the first,
from Irving Starin, M.D., Assistant Dean of Albert Einstein College of
Medicine, indicating that the new facilities would contain not only the
child care project, but also "several other ambulatory care clinical
activities." A mental health ambulatory care program in Bronx Municipal Hospital was to be moved to the new facility, a hard-of-hearing
clinic, a postgraduate dental program, and others were to be established. Once again, nothing was said about relationships to existing
services and how they met the needs of the community. On 8 February
1968 Jack C. Haldeman, M.D., president of the Planning Council,
wrote to Hollis S. Ingraham, M.D., Commissioner, New York State
Department of Health in Albany, approving on behalf of the council
the "comprehensive child care project." The only mention of any other
facilities included was the following: "The ambulatory care services
will be provided by the staff of Jacobi Hospital, of the Bronx Municipal
Hospital Center, which will also provide inpatient care when necessary." Thus, the proposal was approved without any of the supporting
evidence and information related to "coordination" having been provided.

If lack of concern with mechanisms of coordination was typical of
the proposals submitted by hospitals, it was even more true of those
submitted by the Health Services Administration in its Neighborhood
Family Care Center (NFCC) projects, announced in early 1967. In this
case there was no attention paid in the proposal to the way the facility
would be related to existing neighborhood facilities; furthermore, only
one model or prototype was developed to be built in all high priority
poverty areas. When required to submit a plan for approval, the city in
each case submitted exactly the same proposal, the "prototype 55"
plan. (See the summary of this proposal in section 4 of this chapter.)

Pressed by the Planning Council to submit specific program characteristics and not just building plans, the city replied, through the person
of Lloyd H. Siegel (AIA, Acting Deputy Administrator, Health Space
Planning, Architecture, Construction, and Equipment, of the city's
Health Services Administration) in a letter dated 27 January 1969, to

Mr. Saul Ellenbogen (architectural consultant of the Planning Council):

We understand that there is some confusion on the functional program for each of our Neighborhood Family Care Centers.... All of these centers will be constructed in accordance with the program (both functional and architectural) set forth in our publication "Neighborhood Family Care Center-55," dated November, 1967.... This program applies to all centers proposed by the Health Services Administration, unless you are notified of specific exceptions for individual cases.

To repeat, the "Program" referred to contained no references to any other health facilities at all, except for a quite general mention of the "back-up hospital." It was designed to be a general prototype, and no specification was given of community needs, other facilities, or even the general requirements of facilities which should be present in the back-up hospital.

4. "Prototype 55" and the Planning Council

The character and difficulties of coordination between various local agencies in New York City and state and federal bodies are well illustrated by the history of the attempts to develop neighborhood health centers, neighborhood family care centers, ambulatory care facilities, or similarly functioning facilities under whatever name. Because the availability of OEO funds early in 1967 spurred many applications and created problems of coordination and planning, the records at the Health and Hospital Planning Council are more complete from that time on, and it is convenient to start at that point.

A meeting on 17 March 1967 between representatives of the New York City Health Department and those of the Hospital Review and Planning Council of Southern New York, Inc., considered some of the problems facing various city agencies confronted with new federal funding sources. At this meeting were a number of high officials: Paul Densen; Jack Haldeman, M.D., President of the Planning Council; James Haughton, M.D., Deputy Health Services Administrator; Beatrice Kresky, M.D., then on the staff of the Planning Council, later Deputy Director of the Mayor's Organizational Task Force for Comprehensive Health Planning; Edward O'Rourke, M.D., Commissioner of Health; Lee Podolin of the Hospital Planning Council; and Leonard S. Rosenfeld, M.D., also of the council staff (but later to become an official of Flower-Fifth Avenue, a voluntary hospital). Most of the meeting was spent dealing with problems of horizontal and vertical interorganizational relationships, although obviously not in these terms. The immediate problem was what to do with eight OEO grant applications for ambulatory care projects which had to be approved and submitted to the municipal Community Development Agency by Monday, March 20, and to OEO by March 30. "The consensus of committee opinion was that adequate review was impossible in this short period of time" and that OEO should be contacted to "remove the pressure and allow time for adequate planning and review on the part of the Council and the Health Department."

The assessment was made by the committee that "OEO does not appear to have a knowledgeable advisory committee and mechanisms for implementation and long range planning are not well established" —quite understandable in view of the speedy development of OEO's health services program and the distance of the Washington agency from local needs. Thus the procedures to be followed were quite ambiguous. For example, a poverty area had to have an incorporated community health council, with by-laws and minutes, presumably to indicate organizational stability. According to the minutes of the meeting, "no one is sure of the method of incorporation or the channel of distribution of their recommendations." It was also unclear at that point as to who was eligible to apply for OEO funds. "May any group of physicians apply for an OEO grant in a poverty area, or must application be submitted by an accredited hospital?" someone asked. "No clear answer was forthcoming." Wisely anticipating financial cutbacks within a few years, some of the persons attending raised questions about "long-range financial commitments and responsibility for the projected ambulatory care units," but some present felt that "federal funding for these projects will be available for an indefinite period."

The Health Department was developing tentative guidelines for approval of the OEO grant application. As in most cases, the funds became available quickly, as a result of political pressure upon OEO to prove its capability by developing innovative programs, and there was little time to develop any coherent plans to integrate these facilities with others or to consider their implications for the clientele, funding, and organization of other health care providers in possible areas. Thus, criteria presumably normally applied were relaxed.

The Health Department is not insistent on hospitals with approved residencies and is not inquiring too deeply into "hospital back-up" for inpatient care. Criteria for service area and population estimates are established, and comprehensive care units staffed by pediatricians, internists, obstetricians and psychiatrists are required for Health Department approval. Criteria for location of the project in terms of population at risk and availability and adequacy of other facilities in the area have not been developed, chiefly because OEO is insisting on identification of possible sites in the grant application and there is no time for sensible planning.

Given the time pressures, it was inevitable that coordination should become one of the first victims, although the meeting ended with a discussion of "methods of setting up an effective coordinating mechanism of the Health Department and Hospital Council for the purpose of establishing criteria and standards and reviewing grant applications. . . . The necessity of liaison with the Community Mental Health Board was discussed."

The essentially reactive role of the council became clear in a report of a meeting held on 17 August 1967 between two representatives of the council (Dr. Rosenfeld and Dr. Kresky) and Mr. Harold Light of the New York City Department of Health. The memo by Dr. Kresky noted that "neither renovations in existing District Health Centers nor the construction and planning of new ambulatory care units (New York City Budget, OEO, Title II) are brought to the Health and Hospital Planning Council for approval in the early planning stages. These sponsoring hospitals appear to proceed each at his own pace according to individual needs. Polite or politic people . . . ask for consultation with us, listen to our opinion and then probably do what they please. Other administrators and physicians will probably do what they please."

At this point, the city was already planning some fifteen neighborhood family care centers, but details about these do not appear in the minutes. Mr. Light did say that "the standards drawn up by Dr. McLaughlin will be the program prototype of the neighborhood health centers funded by New York City. The prototype for construction will be the schematics and specifications drawn up by Mr. McIntyre who is on loan from the Council to the Department of Hospitals. At present the Health Department has no plans for individualization of either program or construction of new facilities." At this early point the question was raised about "individualizing" the structure and the program to the specific needs of the community. Although the minutes do not say this, it seems clear that, anxious to get something started, the city agencies attempted to define a building which would serve generally for all areas.

In November 1967 concrete proposals for a prototype neighborhood family care center were issued by the Health Services Administration.

This plan is worth summarizing in some detail, particularly with reference to its attention to interorganizational coordination.

The Health Services Administration's plans were contained in two lengthy booklets which described in great detail a "Program for a Neighborhood Family Care Center" (NFCC), one for a "population at risk" of 30,000 persons, the second for 55,000 persons. The booklets were credited to the Health Facilities Planning and Construction division of the Department of Hospitals of the city. Acknowledgements were made for the assistance of Robert L. McIntyre, Senior Architectural Associate, Health and Hospital Planning Council of Southern New York; Dr. Mary McLaughlin, at that time Associate Deputy Commissioner, New York City Department of Health; Robert Derzon, First Deputy Commissioner of Hospitals; and Mrs. Marjorie H. Frank, Assistant to the Commissioner for Comprehensive Service Units, New York City Community Mental Health Board, as well as to the Montefiore Medical Group and Meridian Management, Inc. Thus, most of the city health agencies were involved, although no doubt their commitment and involvement varied greatly. The key person may well have been Lloyd H. Siegel, AIA, an architect who was at that time Assistant Commissioner, Health Facilities Planning and Construction of the Department of Hospitals. Mr. Siegel figured frequently in the later correspondence and meetings between the city and the Health and Hospital Planning Council concerning the criteria to be used in gaining the council's approval of the city's plans for neighborhood family care centers.

The general perspective of the NFCC program is indicated by the credit given to Dr. Sidney Garfield, "principal founder of the Kaiser Foundation" in California, whose "experience and fund of knowledge has been of extreme value to the authors" (p.ii). The proposals were signed by Howard J. Brown, M.D., Health Services Administrator; Joseph V. Terenzio, Commissioner of Hospitals; Edward O'Rourke, Commissioner of Health; and Marvin E. Perkins, Commissioner of Mental Health Services—the three of whom represented the major arms of the newly established super-agency: the Health Services Administration. The announcement of the availability of OEO funds in March 1967, the enactment of Medicare and Medicaid in 1965, and the availability of funds through Regional Medical Programs and Comprehensive Health Planning legislation enacted by the federal government in 1966 undoubtedly provided a tremendous impetus to the development of plans for ambulatory care facilities in the city.

These neighborhood family care centers were envisaged as nearly complete outpatient or ambulatory care facilities, and the program made no mention of any proposed link to a back-up hospital for more specialized care or for in-hospital treatment. This omission was one of the major concerns of the Health and Hospital Planning Council in its correspondence and official reactions to the plans for neighborhood family care centers submitted to them by the city for their approval, as provided for by 1965 New York State legislation (the Folsom Act). The program was actually a detailed specification of plans for the layout and functions of a building, complete with schematic drawings for three floors of a 45,000 square foot building. Administrative facilities were allotted 12,000, diagnostic and treatment facilities 25,000, and adjunct and mechanical facilities 7,000 square feet. Included were family care, obstetrics-gynecology, opthalmology-optometry, psychiatry, and other specialty clinics, as well as space for dentistry and multiphasic screening. Since the proposal was regarded as a general prototype of a facility, no mention was made of funding requirements, specific site location, or details concerning a possible back-up hospital. Some general requirements for location were given, however.

The Center should be situated in a position of optimum availability and accessibility to the population it will serve. Ideally this would be at the demographic center of its health district, but this criterion must be modified by considerations of adequacy of public transport vehicles, land cost and availability, zoning, convenience to other public agencies and institutions, and avoidance of those sites where neighboring structures and uses would impair its effectiveness. (p. 59)

The facility, the introduction indicated, was "designed for a theoretical 30,000 population in a building that would be open 12 hours a day for five and a half days per week, fifty-two weeks per year."

No details were given on how the new center would be linked to any other neighborhood health facility. In fact, the only mention of any other institution was, for example, that contained in the provision for the "referral [of the patient] to back-up hospital services" included in the list of "activities" to take place in the "intake" section, and in the statement in the "medical records" section that the "record...will accompany the patient to the back-up hospital whenever the patient is referred there for specialty ambulatory or in-patient care."

Even though there was no discussion of specific centers, it was clear that a number of sites were under concrete consideration at that time. The "30,000" proposal included schematic site plans for Mott Haven and Brownsville Family Care Centers, locating the buildings in specific sites: on the corner of St. Ann's Avenue and 144th Street for the former, on the corner of New Jersey Avenue and Pitkin Avenue for the latter. The "55,000" proposal includes schematic site plans for the Riverside, Central Harlem, and Morrisania health care centers, again with specific locations (Morrisania at Prospect and East 152nd; Central Harlem at Lenox Avenue in the Stephen Foster housing project; and Riverside at Columbus Avenue and West 81st Street).

Later, as the city developed plans for its fifteen NFCCs, these prototype proposals were all (according to Planning Council staff members) that was submitted to the council, which objected on several grounds: mainly that no consideration was given to the facilities available at the back-up hospital which might make certain services either necessary or superfluous at the family care center and also that the multiphasic screening system, being recommended by Garfield as highly successful at Kaiser, was unproved and should not be built in as standard equipment in every center. The council also found these prototypes upsetting because their Facilities Planning Committee had not been consulted and because this failure to communicate with the council seemed to be becoming a typical pattern for city agencies, although not for the voluntary hospitals. The assumption underlying some of the council staff's reaction to the city prototype was that the neighborhood family care centers should not be regarded as "freestanding" agencies, but closely linked to the back-up hospital. One might note here that the difference in the choice of words used to describe the linkage between hospital and neighborhood family care center probably indicates a basic difference in viewpoint. The city usually used the phrase "back-up" hospital, implying that the hospital was there in case of need, but that the primary and responsible agent was the center itself. The Planning Council frequently used the word "sponsoring" hospital, indicating that the primary organization and agent was the hospital itself.

The growing concern of the council was documented in a memorandum, prepared by Dr. Rosenfeld of the staff on 5 February 1968, concerning the "status of planning of ambulatory care." He noted that "a rapidly increasing awareness of the need for more adequate facilities for ambulatory care services during the past couple of years is self-evident. During this period, a number of agencies have entered the field of financing and planning of ambulatory clinic facilities." He cited most of those agencies already mentioned at city, state, and federal levels. "Also, the voluntary hospitals have indicated a greater interest in ambulatory care than has been anticipated largely by virtue of the fact that, for the first time, there is promise of reasonably adequate financing of this form of service." The memo went on to "assess some of the obstacles that have been encountered to planning and progress." First he listed "poor liaison between the responsible agencies," including "inadequacies in communication between the Health Department and hospitals" and "problems in following procedures under the Folsom Act," mainly the failure of the city Health Services Administration to submit proposals to the Council for review and recommendation. Several instances were cited. Dr. Rosenfeld inferred that "on the one hand the Health Services Administration is less than enthusiastic about clearing plans with the State Health Department, and on the other it seems that the State Health Department is reluctant to bring the matter to issue." Assuming Dr. Rosenfeld was correct in his inference, this is probably an instance of the strategy whereby one agency attempts to push its plans beyond the point where they can be easily stopped by another agency, even a nominally or legally superior one.

But the role of the Council was also in question here. The memo continued, "On the other hand, this leaves the Council in rather an anomalous position with regard to discharge of its responsibility under the Folsom Act." The legal power of review and recommendation provided to the Planning Council by the Folsom Act had apparently become the main sources of leverage available to it to influence the policy-making process.

The question of council strategy was then raised. "The direct approach would be to ask for a meeting with representatives of the State Health Department and the Health Services Administration in an attempt to work out a modus vivendi. Although attractive, this may be hazardous in that it would bring issues squarely to the fore, which might result in hardening of adversary positions rather than in resolutions." Alternatives mentioned were informal approaches to both the state and city as a "preliminary to more formal discussions" and simply to "continue current procedures" while awaiting the arrival of Dr. Bernard Bucove, newly appointed Health Services Administrator for the city. Apparently whatever informal mechanisms were available or were tried did not work, for on 4 June 1968, a kind of United Nations meeting of almost all of the organizations involved in the planning of ambulatory care facilities was called. The character and outcome of this meeting are summarized in the next section.

The June 4th meeting did not solve the problem. On July 19 Planning Council president Dr. Haldeman wrote to Dr. Bernard Bucove, the new

Health Services Administrator of the city, questioning the seeming inflexibility of the "Prototype 55" programs now in the capital budget of the city. He noted that the back-up hospitals named in the proposals "would not appear to be of the size or to command the resources that would be necessary to function in this capacity. Furthermore, advice from several of these institutions indicates that they were not consulted in the course of development of their plans." He pointed out that the council "feels that in planning medical facilities of any size, plans should be individualized in accordance with the characteristics, needs and resources of the community, the program projected and the pattern of agreements among the various responsible parties." Dr. Haldeman called for a meeting between the HSA, other city departments, and the council. It is clear that, quite aside from the substantive merits of the points raised, the council was concerned to reassert its role in the review process.

Another meeting parallel in goals to the June 4th one was held on 30 July 1968, with some thirty persons present, representing city, state, federal, and voluntary health agencies. As the minutes indicate, and as subsequent reports by persons attending the meeting confirmed, the discussion seldom confronted any issues directly. Instead, representatives of agencies spoke from their own points of view. Since the meeting had no authoritative status and no decision-making authority, there was no incentive for any group present to do more than to attempt to express its perspective and defend its own interests as forcefully as possible. At the meeting Dr. McLaughlin did summarize the status as of that time of the eleven "Prototype 55" freestanding centers then planned by the Health Department and also the "additions and renovations on seven district health centers." These were all included in the current capital budget of the city, but had no operational funding.

On August 8 a memo written by a Planning Council staff member summarized the situation of the neighborhood health centers vis-a-vis the council: Fourteen of twenty-five letters of intent for such centers were pending review, thirteen of the fourteen being city projects, with eleven of those in turn being called "Prototype 55" freestanding centers. The memo noted that "all of these reviews are pending because no program has been submitted for review. It is apparent, however, that sites are being selected, communities are being consulted, and plans are being developed for construction for some of these projects." In other words, the city was moving ahead without consulting the council.

On August 8 Dr. Bucove of HSA and Dr. Mary McLaughlin of the Health Department met with three representatives of the council, Drs.

Haldeman and Rosenfeld and Mr. Williams. The memorandum prepared on August 19 seems to indicate that there was almost complete agreement by the city officials with the position of the council. According to Dr. Rosenfeld,

Dr. Bucove described the review of city policy in discussions with the Meridian Corporation which has been retained by the city as a consulting agency. As a result of these discussions, it was decided to abandon the policy adopted by the city of constructing a series of centers designed according to prototype plans developed by the Health Services Administration calling for construction of centers with a capacity for care of 55,000 patients each. It was agreed that plans for these centers would be individualized according to the characteristics, needs and resources of each community.

Dr. McLaughlin then advised the attendees that "a program for each center would be prepared by the committee made up of the health officer, representatives of the community and representatives of the back-up hospital." The council memorandum then noted that "the Council will defer review of each proposal until such time as a program has been prepared. No review will be initiated until a site and a back-up institution have been identified." The meeting was seemingly a victory for the council's viewpoint that rigid "prototype" health centers should not be imposed on all neighborhoods.

After this meeting Dr. Bucove wrote to Dr. Haldeman on August 14, indicating his feeling that "many of the questions have either been resolved or we have a mutually clear understanding of what needs to take place." On August 19 Dr. Rosenfeld of the Council sent fifteen copies of the council's guidelines to Dr. McLaughlin, "in accordance with the understanding reached in Dr. Haldeman's office on August 9." But by the end of September no word on the individualized projects was forthcoming to the council, and Mr. Williams sent a letter to Dr. McLaughlin: "We understood that the District Health officers of the several districts where centers are being planned would prepare programs for discussion. Since we have had no further word, I thought I would drop you this note to say that we would be glad to get together with you and any of your health officers to discuss preliminary plans and to do whatever we can to help expedite the planning process." Dr. McLaughlin replied on October 4: "I have yet to hear of any of the Health Officers' sitting down with the communities and back-up hospitals to detail programs in individual areas with the exception of a pediatric program in Brookdale. I'll make sure they touch base with you when they do." Her letter neatly avoided taking any responsibility for calling such a meeting. The council made another try on October 31 via a letter from Mr. Williams to Mr. Robert Derzon, First Deputy Commissioner of the Department of Hospitals, with a copy to the Department of Health (Dr. McLaughlin): "It occurred to me that programs and plans may be sufficiently advanced on three Neighborhood Family Health Center projects to warrant initiation of the Folsom review procedure. . . . We would appreciate your putting us in touch with the proper persons to discuss this."

In November, an entirely new set of factors entered the situation. According to a *New York Times* article on 1 November 1968, a new state corporation, the State Health and Mental Health Facilities Improvement Corporation, was going to build four new hospitals, two housing projects for hospital staffs, and, of most concern to our discussion here, eight neighborhood health centers, all of which were included in the city capital budget. The eight included three in the Bronx (St. Francis, Morrisania, and South-Bronx-Longwood), four in Brooklyn (East New York, Greenpoint, Brownsville, and Bedford), and one in Manhattan (Washington Heights). According to the story,

all of these facilities already have been programmed by the city and sites have been acquired or are in process of acquisition. . . . A spokesman for the city administration said these would have been built with city funds, but that the new state corporation, which can bypass many of the steps legally required for municipal projects, will make the facilities usable so much sooner, a major consideration because of the city's acute shortage of hospital and health care facilities.

According to Mayor Lindsay, the city would eventually pay off the construction costs, but the new plan would place the facilities in use by five years, as against ten to fifteen years if the city were to build them. (The ground was broken for the first one, across the street from Morrisania Hospital in the Bronx, on 17 February 1971 [*New York Times*, 18 February 1971], even though funds for their construction were in the 1968–69 and the tentative 1969–70 municipal capital budgets [*New York Times*, 1 November 1968].)

This announcement placed the council in a quandary, since, as indicated in a memo dated 6 November 1968, it was still apparently the intention of the city to build "prototype 55" facilities at all of the projects, "even though they have not indicated this intention in all the Letters of Intent. It has been the Council's position . . . that these projects would not be reviewed until a site was identified and a program presented. Many of the Letters of Intent do not identify the back-up hospital. Whether, in fact, sites, programs and hospitals are now part of the package has not been, up to now, made known to us."

The dilemma of the council was underlined by their belief that it was important, of course, that "the Council not hold up in any way the decision to build any or all of these neighborhood centers. The need for facilities is apparent and should not be hard to document." The controversy over whether or not the general prototype plan submitted by the city fulfilled the requirements of sound planning for facilities suitable for a particular community continue to be described in the Planning Council documents, but no new points relevant to our concerns emerged.

A bit more history was mentioned in the report of a meeting held on December 5, attended by representatives of the Council, at which Dr. Mary McLaughlin spoke. According to the report,

the Lindsay administration reacted enthusiastically to innovative proposals she made in 1966 that District Health Centers provide treatment as well as preventive services. The Capital Budget of 1967 earmarked funds to renovate existing health centers as well as to construct new family care centers where needed. . . . At this juncture Lloyd Siegel, recognizing that the architectural plans he had previously developed for Montefiore's ambulatory unit was potentially useful as a model for the new health centers, decided that his planning department would draw up prototype plans, one for a population of 30,000 and one for 55,000. Dr. McLaughlin did not explain, this evening, how the decision was made to expand her simple program to the creation of some 18 projects all based on the Prototype 55 model. She did say that the architects demonstrated to her that the high cost of renovation made alterations of a health center almost as expensive as new construction.

Why such expensive renovation was necessary was also apparently not made clear. This little example is another instance of how relatively simple needs of the community for improved health services become escalated into multi-million-dollar building projects, and the result is that nothing is done.

On January 3 the council's appropriate staff held a policy discussion on city projects, and it was decided that "a desirable posture for the Council to take—in light of the urgent needs of the community—is not to stand in the way of allowing these projects to proceed, but to put on the record the serious and substantial questions we have raised concerning the program."

On 27 January 1969 Lloyd Siegel sent a letter to the council, confirming that the "prototype 55" model would be constructed for all of the Neighborhood Family Care Centers, "unless you are notified of specific exceptions for individual cases." Without quite saying so, the administration had rejected the authority of the council to review and approve. On February 13 an internal memo from Rosenfeld to Haldeman indicated that "it may be difficult to reconcile the policies of the Health Services Administration and of the Council."

As the months passed, first one neighborhood center and then another ran into difficulties of one kind or another. On 4 June 1969, the *New York Times* wrote that the plan for eight health centers (originally seventeen) was now down to four: Brownsville, Morrisania, Longwood, and Washington Heights.

5. An Attempt at Interagency
   Coordination

The dilemmas and difficulties of establishing interorganizational coordination between diverse agencies comprising New York City's health facilities are illustrated rather well by the attendance at, and character of, a two-and-a-half hour meeting held on 4 June 1968 at the Health and Hospital Planning Council offices on East 54th Street, in the middle of the controversy between the council and the city over the "Prototype 55" plan.

Dr. Leonard Rosenfeld of the council staff prepared a set of "notes on progress and problems in neighborhood health center planning and development" for discussion at the interagency meeting attended by twenty-eight persons representing from twelve to twenty agencies—city, state, federal, and private—depending on which level of any agency is counted. The accompanying list shows the persons present at that meeting and their affiliations and should give some concrete idea of the complex organizational interests represented. Seven persons representing various branches of New York City government attended; six from voluntary hospitals, medical schools, and associations; seven from the Planning Council; one from New York State; and four federal officials from HEW, HUD, and OEO. One city and one federal representative were invited but were unable to come. These notes and the available summary of the discussion are worth treating at some length.

Meeting of Representatives of Agencies Responsible for Planning and Development of Ambulatory Care Facilities (Health and Hospitals Planning Council Headquarters, June 1968)

New York City

Health Services Administration
Dr. Bernard Bucove, health services administrator (co-chairman of the meeting)
Mr. Robert A. Derzon, deputy commissioner of hospitals
Dr. Mary C. McLaughlin, associate deputy commissioner of health
Dr. Edward O'Rourke, commissioner of health
Dr. Herbert Freilich (representing the Honorable Joseph Terenzio, commissioner of hospitals)
Human Resources Adminstration (Model Cities Program)
Mrs. Roberta Spohn (representing Miss Alice Brophy, assistant deputy administrator)
Community Development Agency
Miss Jano Whelan, coordinator for the Neighborhood Health Program
Catholic Charities, Archdiocese of New York
Mr. Thomas McLoughlin, co-director, Division of Health and Hospitals (representing the Right Rev. Msgr. Christopher G. Kane, co-director, Division of Health and Hospitals)
Catholic Charities, Diocese of Brooklyn
Dr. Thomas Gocke, director of community medicine
Mr. Robert Murphy (representing the Right Rev. Msgr. James H. Fitzpatrick, director, Division of Health and Hospitals)
Federation of Jewish Philanthropies
Dr. Morris Hinenburg, medical care consultant
Associated Medical Schools of Greater New York
Dr. Vincent dePaul Larkin, program coordinator
Association of Directors of Ambulatory Care
Dr. Benjamin Wainfeld, president
Health and Hospital Planning Council of Southern New York, Inc.
Dr. George Baehr, member, Board of Directors
Dr. Jack C. Haldeman, president (co-chairman of the meeting)
Dr. George Reader, member, Ambulatory Care Advisory Committee
Dr. L. S. Rosenfeld, director, Medical Services Division
Dr. Cecil G. Sheps, chairman, Ambulatory Care Advisory Committee
Mr. Herbert Williams, planning associate
Mr. Barry Halber

New York State

Department of Health
Dr. Donald G. Dickson, associate commissioner for New York City Affairs

Federal

Department of Health, Education, and Welfare
Dr. C. Robert Dean, associate regional health director
Office of Economic Opportunity
Dr. Gary London, OEO
Mr. Daniel Zwick, Community Action Program
Department of Housing and Urban Development
Miss Linda Broderick (representing Mr. Morton Isler, acting staff director, HUD Representative Program)
Human Resources Department of Columbia University
Mrs. Miriam Ostow, observer

Invited but unable to attend:

Federal

Department of Health, Education and Welfare Children's Bureau
Harriet Felton, M.D.

New York City

Community Development Agency
Jack Aquerros, deputy commissioner

It must be kept in mind that from the council's point of view the main purpose of the meeting was to reaffirm the review powers of the council. The first paragraph of Dr. Rosenfeld's notes indicates that the attendees were reminded that "about a year ago [1967], on the basis of an interpretation of the Folsom Legislation by the State Commissioner of Health, the Health and Hospital Planning Council assumed responsibility for review and recommendation of plans for development and expansion of ambulatory care facilities in addition to its traditional responsibilities in planning of inpatient facilities."

The memorandum went on to summarize the division of labor among the numerous city, state, and federal agencies concerned with planning and developing ambulatory care agencies. As Dr. Rosenfeld put it, "because responsibility for planning of ambulatory care facilities is divided among a number of agencies with limited mechanisms of coordination, no one agency has a full perspective of the progress and problems in this field."

It was apparent from Dr. Rosenfeld's summary that the stages of development of an ambulatory care facility were extraordinarily complex, involving many agencies at all levels of government, not to mention many voluntary agencies. This meeting was devoted *only* to ambulatory care facilities, not hospitals, mental health centers, or preventive care, yet Rosenfeld devoted a paragraph or at least a sentence to *each* of the following: the Department of Health (city); the Department of Hospitals (city); the Health Services Administration (city); the Department of Health (state); the Department of Social Services (state); the Health and Hospital Planning Council of Southern New York (regional); the Community Development Agency of the Office of Economic Opportunity (federal); the Children's Bureau of the Department of Health Education and Welfare (federal); the Office of Comprehensive Health Planning of HEW (federal); the Neighborhood Facilities Grants programs (federal); the Model Cities Program (federal); the Regional Public Health Office (federal); not to mention the Neighborhood Health Councils established under OEO requirements; as well as neighborhood associations, hospitals, and medical associations.

The words used to describe these organizations and to indicate their functions and actions included the following: planning, funding, administering, standard-setting, approving, reviewing, licensing, consulting, studying, supervising, supporting, guaranteeing, appraising, sponsoring, articulating, formulating, applying, allocating, incorporating, documenting, improving, participating, and training. Note that only a few of these functions and actions referred to the actual process of *operating* a health care facility; almost all referred to stages of a bureaucratic process, involving relationships between organizations located in both horizontal strata and vertical hierarchies. Furthermore, Dr. Rosenfeld's list of the "problems" in the planning of ambulatory care facilities provided an excellent summary of the complexity and lack of coordination of the health care system from the point of view of an agency with a stake in maintaining a role in the review process—a role which was currently being challenged by the city. His first major point was that "while medical care and mental health facilities are often developed to serve the same populations, compartmentalization of responsibility for planning, organization, administration and evaluation is institutionalized in public policy. There are separate channels for review of proposals, and limited opportunities for coordination of effort." In other words the fragmentation of the system was not an accident or a by-product of haste in attempts to solve or meet crises, but, as he put it, was "institutionalized in public policy." Therefore, the causes are not to be found in the motives of officials seeking to extend the power and prestige of their organizations, although those motives may indeed be the proximate causes of fragmentation, but rather are found in more fundamental features of the political economy of the society. Why is it that this compartmentalization occurs?

The way in which mental health and general health centers were set up illustrates the way in which fragmentation is built into public policy. To quote Dr. Rosenfeld again, "under the provisions of State law, financing and supervision of mental health centers flows along channels that are independent of those for general health facilities. Clinic service areas and catchment areas for community mental health centers are designed without reference to each other."

Thus this meeting, attended, no doubt, in good faith by concerned members of various agencies, could not even address the problem of coordinating mental health with general health facilities without attempting to change state law. Even with the best of intentions, the participants were hamstrung not only by their own organizational commitments but also by an institutionalized and legalized framework which guaranteed the continuation of fragmentation and prevented the raising of questions or solutions in a context which would allow even the definition of a solution, let alone the possibility of accumulation of enough power to carry that solution into reality. What is interesting about the rhetoric used by participants is that no one justified the fragmentation of the health system in terms of pluralism, democracy, diversity, and the other language used by the liberal democratic theorists to justify this mode of operations. The participants in the system felt trapped by their inadequacy and helplessness, but their only response was to hold meetings such as this one, believing that "communication" would help.

The second major point which Dr. Rosenfeld made was that

the numbers of agencies involved in review and approval of proposals, each with its own requirements, imposes delays and frustrations on institutions that wish to develop needed facilities. There is widespread ignorance and a good deal of confusion among institutions with regard to the requirements of the various reviewing and funding agencies. The confusion is heightened by the fact that communications among reviewing and funding agencies and with local sponsoring organizations are often inadequate. Furthermore, there have been examples of conflicting requirements by different agencies.

Again, let us assume good faith on the part of all of the actors involved. The picture is one of a highly pluralistic system in which it is difficult for operating agencies to find out where to find money to establish a new program, facility, or function and hard to know how to get the money. The federal and state agencies in no sense can be regarded as standing above this diversity, but rather are part of it, since they have many different programs with sometimes "contradictory requirements."

This pluralistic diversity can be hailed as providing many points of access to the system, and the variations in funding source and requirements can be regarded as allowing many different kinds of programs a chance to develop. But the problem is that there is very little evidence that these are in fact the consequences. As Dr. Rosenfeld pointed out, it is partly as a consequence of the operations of this kind of pluralism that "there has been no systematic assessment of relative need for service in neighborhoods throughout the city." This is a remarkable statement. Consider its implications: "facilities are being developed on the basis of interest and initiative of institutions and local groups." This might seem to be the way that such facilities should be developed; and yet there has been *no assessment of the need for services* in neighborhoods. New facilities are being established under diverse auspices, sources of funding, and control. If there has been no assessment of community need, but only an assessment by a local institution or group that *funding* is available for a new program, then it may well be that the organizational needs of the already established hospitals which are the primary applicants for new ambulatory care facilities will be the main ones being served by the application. In turn, are the needs of the local institution likely to be consistent with, related to, or contradictory to those of the local community? From a superficial point of view, it may seem that addition of another clinic or another neighborhood health center of any kind would almost always serve community needs, particularly in poverty areas. This in many cases may be true.

Dr. Rosenfeld's notes described a third major feature of the way in which ambulatory care facilities are established which also was probably not accidental and therefore cannot be cured by improving "communication" between the interested parties:

> While the State legislation assumes early advice to the State Health department and in turn to the Health and Hospital Planning Council of the intention to develop facilities, such advice is often submitted late, long after local interest and support has been mobilized and plans are well formulated. This results in reducing flexibility and latitude for negotiations, and frequently limits discretion with regard to both site selection and approval of questionable plans.

This description of the process, although intended as a criticism, was undoubtedly exactly what was planned by the applicants for a new ambulatory care facility. They *wanted* to reduce flexibility and limit negotiations and discretion, and thus increase the chances that their plans and site would have to be approved because of the lateness of their submission for review. This process may be a deeply institutionalized property of the political economy of the United States. Political bargaining takes place in a context in which the participants have a stake in *reducing*, not increasing, the information available to the competitors for scarce resources. Also, participants want to form a potentially winning coalition as early as possible, in order to increase the costs of information and mobilization to other participants who might wish to enter the market for the same political commodity at the same time.

The same point about the lack of communication was made by Dr. Rosenfeld in connection with city and Planning Council relationships.

> City policies with regard to program development and the development of specific projects are sometimes adopted not only without consultation with the Council, but also without consensus among the relevant branches of the City government. An example is the recent adoption of a capital budget by the City for neighborhood health centers [the NFCC's] without consultation with branches of the Health Services Administration responsible for program and also without consultation with the Council regarding needs and priorities, or potentialities with regard to staffing and organization.

This sentence, casually inserted, obviously refers to one of the central reasons for the meeting—the failure by the city government to recognize the state-mandated (under the Folsom Act) review role by the Planning Council.

A fourth major point made by Dr. Rosenfeld concerned the "confusion" about the role of neighborhood organizations. Generally speaking, the use of the word *confusion* by one participant in the political process usually means that there is conflict over goals and procedures. This seems clear from Dr. Rosenfeld's specific discussion of the powers of neighborhood organizations. Originally, the Office of Economic Opportunity

took the position that neighborhood health councils should assume the role of boards of trustees. In the New York City metropolitan area, this brought about confusion and conflict by virtue of the fact that it is a generally accepted policy in this area, and one adopted in the guidelines of the Health and Hospital Planning Council, that neighborhood health centers should be developed not as independent free standing facilities, but under the aegis of and as part of the organization of general hospitals.

This is by now a familiar conflict between established institutions and the abortive attempt, through federal OEO legislation, to institute effective and "maximum feasible participation" by the poor. As Dr. Rosenfeld put it, "this created a situation in which on the one hand the Neighborhood Health Councils expected to assume responsibility for policy determination, budget and the like, while on the other hand the administration and boards of responsible hospitals could not relinquish responsibility in these areas." The outcome was a defeat for community participation and power. "While the Office of Economic Opportunity has since amended its policies, confusion still persists among neighborhood groups with regard to their roles." In other words, the neighborhood groups had lost their slim statutory grasp upon power in the controlling boards of the health centers, but they maintained the hope and vision of some meaningful participation.

The rhetoric used to define the issue of community control is clear from Dr. Rosenfeld's posing of the dilemma for those possessing organizational control of the health resources of the community: "Although the need to allocate greater responsibility to the community for the planning of health services than has been traditional in the past is now widely recognized, it is not yet clear how this can be accomplished without loss of effectiveness in organization and channels of accountability." Note the assumption that present modes of organization were reasonably "effective" and "accountable" and that greater community participation would reduce those laudable goals. Parenthetically, in a later comment on this manuscript, Dr. Rosenfeld said that "I believe that the Council was not reluctant to accept the idea of allocating responsibility to a community body, but no legally chartered body of this sort existed. Boards of institutions have the legal and fiscal responsibility for provision of services and for maintaining quality. Within this framework, the only way that I can see that community representatives could be given responsibility, would be by bringing them onto boards of trustees. This I think would be both equitable and sound. The issue is one of organizational principle and legal responsibility rather than ideological."[6] My comment in turn is that the significant point is that in fact—as Dr. Rosenfeld's comment itself indicates—no organizational or legal mechanisms have been established which allow community bodies significant power. The reasons for that will be considered in a later chapter.

Since there exists no research which demonstrates the differences in levels of effectiveness and accountability of various modes of organization of the health delivery system, such a statement—a familiar one in the writings of heads of or spokesmen for the major corporate groups (the hospitals, the medical schools, the city agencies) seeking to fend off invasions of their power by patients, communities, students—is clearly an ideological one, offered with the assumption that the basic validity of the present mode of organizing health services and the basic powers of those who now control the major health institutions would be accepted by their reader. It probably was true that few or none of the meeting's participants, who represented established health agencies, would have challenged this assumption. But note that this casual assumption that the present system was reasonably "effective" and "accountable" contradicts all of the other major points made by Dr. Rosenfeld concerning "compartmentalization of responsibility," "conflicting requirements," lack of "consultation," and "delays and frustrations in developing needed facilities." This connotative language fails to indicate the criteria by which one or another system of delivery and its control could be judged for "effectiveness" or "accountability." Such vagueness of language conceals the quite concrete struggles over the allocation of powers among established health institutions which this meeting represented and the exclusion from the meeting of representatives of community groups.

In attempting to explain why all of these various problems in the development of neighborhood health centers existed, Dr. Rosenfeld concluded that they "seem to emanate from the fact that in the aggregate these projects have the charateristics of a crash program. In a rather desperate effort to meet patient needs and to satisfy mounting community pressure, the lead time normally required for planning, organization, and development of services has not been provided. Furthermore, most of these plans involve innovations in organization and staffing, which would suggest the need for more rather than less time for planning and development." He summarized four problems arising from this "haste and urgency." Again, these are worth giving at length, because they portray the definition of the problem of coordination encountered by one important interorganizational link, the Planning Council: "(1) Inadequate opportunity for discussion among responsible agencies to develop common understanding and concerted effort. (2) Multiple and often conflicting approaches to the community without sufficient time to develop an orderly system of relationships. (3) Levels of financing that are not commensurate with the goals set for the program. (4) Inadequate consideration to manpower requirements, medical, administration, and ancillary."

The assumptions of this analysis were that discussion would lead to agreement; that more time would result in more orderly relationships; that organizations did not have to inflate their goals in order to increase their chances of getting admittedly inadequate funding; and that programs were not usually, if ever, applied for without guarantees of available manpower. An orderly and rational environment with maximum information available to all parties and agreements reached through calm and rational discussion was assumed to be possible *if only* the various organizations involved would act in good faith. Stampeded, however, by "community pressures," the organizations lose their collective heads, and move, still in good faith and with the best of motives, to respond to "patient needs." It should be recalled, however, that even before community pressure developed for participation in planning or policy-making of health care facilities, ambulatory care facilities were underfinanced, overcrowded, poorly staffed, poorly located, and inadequate in numbers, by the accounts of all of the various commissions of investigation already summarized. The haste and urgency with which health agencies responded to the patient needs newly manifested by community pressure was surely not necessary in these earlier years. Agencies presumably had all the time they needed for "planning, organization and development of services." The absence, acknowledged by Dr. Rosenfeld, of any serious assessment of community needs for health facilities cannot be attributed to community pressures, but can only be explained by the fact that no organization, not even those charged with planning and research on health needs, had a serious stake in developing such an assessment. Each organization was concerned with maintaining and extending its own autonomy, resources, and functions, and with engaging in only those coalitions, relationships, and exchanges with other organizations which its elites perceived as beneficial to the organization in general or to their own careers.

In concluding his notes, Dr. Rosenfeld suggested that the meeting of 4 June 1968 might well consider establishing a "coordinating body to meet periodically for mutual advice on policies and assessment of progress, and for discussion of needs, problems, and disposition of individual projects." Thus, yet another coordinating body is proposed. Here again we see the impossible dilemma which the corporate rationalizer, assuming his good faith, faces. It is unrealistic, given the situational constraints—both organizational and political—to reconsider the institutionalized bases of power which have produced fragmentation at the bottom and bureaucratization at the top. The natural, almost inevitable, proposal is that still another organization be established to coordinate all of the previously established ones. As it turned out, this particular group, according to the records available, held only two meetings.

The minutes of the first one, held on 4 June 1968, are sketchy, and do not convey either the spirit or much of the contents of the meeting. What is significant, however, is what was *not* discussed at the meeting: namely, the major contents of Dr. Rosenfeld's notes, which were circulated to all invited persons prior to the meeting. Regardless of possible criticisms which we may have of his assumptions, Dr. Rosenfeld's memo did raise the key issue of coordination and planning for interagency discussion. But although Dr. Rosenfeld reviewed his memo contents at the beginning, much of the discussion, according to Herbert Williams of the Planning Council (who prepared the minutes from which this description is taken), was concerned with the "role of the Neighborhood Community Groups in the organization of a local health center." And from his brief summary given it seems clear that most of the agencies represented were threatened by the demands of the community groups and were seeking some way to defend or insulate themselves from those demands. Such language as "responsibility," "partnership," "communication," and "information"—implying an ultimate consensus of goals which it was the duty of community groups to realize and to share—was used by the city and state officials present.

The two persons present who apparently represented, to some extent, "community" sentiment were Miss Jano Whelan from the OEO-financed Community Development Agency and Mrs. Roberta Spohn from Model Cities; both emphasized the need to link medical care to the "larger economic issues, such as housing, jobs and training," and warned that this committee would "invite attack by community groups" unless it made those connections. Two persons commented that representatives of neighborhood community groups should have been invited to the meeting and suggested that they be invited in the future. Why the community should come to meetings of an ad hoc group with no decision-making power was apparently not discussed. The role of symbolic representation—mere attendance at a meeting—in reducing conflict and demands by providing the semblance of power without its substance is quite clear from examples such as these.

The meeting probably performed the symbolic function of meetings of organizations which have no intention of relinquishing any power if they can help it. Meetings which have no official status and at which no decisions can be made which threaten anybody's power are meetings which are necessary to preserve the amenities of civilized discourse and the illusion that communication of relevant information is taking place. The participants thus "agreed that one of the values of this meeting would be that representatives of the several agencies would get to know each other and that they could facilitate development of effective channels of communication." Given this imperative goal, the meeting endorsed a proposal "that agency representatives meet regularly, until some of the current urgent problems have been resolved." This proposal, be it noted, was itself one of the main outcomes of the meeting, rather than any moves toward resolving urgent problems of the planning of ambulatory care facilities. The second proposal endorsed was "that ad hoc groups be organized to discuss and recommend approaches to such problems" as manpower, finances, and priorities. Under priorities, it was noted that "there is a need for assessment of relative priorities of need, not just for the poverty areas, but for the entire city." Why these priorities had not already been the high priority task for *some* agency was an embarrassing question which apparently was not asked. Lastly, the gathering "recommended that each agency prepare a brief description of its program, its legislative base, its limitations, and its application procedures. This would be incorporated in a packet for neighborhood community groups, and hopefully this would reduce misunderstandings and confusion."

The internal contradiction beneath the smooth rhetoric and surface plausibility of these proposals deserves some comment. The last recommendation assumes that communication to the community of information about the programs of all of the agencies will "reduce misunderstandings and confusion." This naive statement is no accident and is not a characteristic of persons inexperienced in organizational bargaining but rather is an ideological characteristic of certain kinds of interorganizational relationships. Such a recommendation of a course of action avoids challenging any organization's role, identity, and distinctive interests. It assumes the possibility of consensus on a wide range of programs, each sponsored by a different organization—or, if not consensus, then at least the possibility of an array of programs as a whole which will resemble the achievement of the public interest. It is assumed that the programs are, in the aggregate, responsive to the needs of a constituency or clientele which has demanded them. Each agency in this process of pluralistic activity has a valid role to play, and all that is required is a coordinating organization to communicate to the various agencies their role in the complex division of labor.

But there is a second assumption behind the preparation of agency packets for community groups which is worth emphasizing. Recall that the participants at this June 4th meeting have just agreed that there are serious problems of manpower, finances, and priorities for the city as a whole in the development of ambulatory care programs. But now they have also recommended that community groups be given information on the full array of agencies ready to supply money, to establish new programs, and to build buildings for them. If manpower and funding are inadequate from a citywide point of view, and if there are no mechanisms to assess the health care priorities of the city as a whole versus the needs of a particular neighborhood, then the only result of telling any given community group that Model Cities, or Comprehensive Health Planning, or OEO, or the Children's Bureau stands ready to offer them money will be to *increase* the demands coming from community groups which have no basis for judging relative priorities and no interest in doing so. Thus, the net effect of increasing the information available to community groups is to decrease whatever coordination and control exist at the time.

There is one final note on this meeting which, according to the summary, never dealt with any substantive issues. The question was raised by Dr. George Baehr (director emeritus of medicine at Mount Sinai Hospital and a member of the Planning Council's board of directors) concerning the relationship of the group meeting on June 4 to the Comprehensive

Health Planning committee which was in the process of being formed under Public Law 89-749. According to the minutes—and the speaker is not identified—the agency formed under this law would "eventually take over this job; . . . this was an emergency arrangement to cope with urgent problems and decisions concerning effectiveness of service."

6. Knickerbocker Hospital and
   Neighborhood Health Care[7]

The contradiction between the relatively simple and inexpensive needs perceived by community groups for some ambulatory and outpatient health facilities and the expensive needs of hospitals in poor areas for capital and operating funds is illustrated extremely well by a case study of a Manhattanville community group and Knickerbocker Hospital (which became Logan Memorial Hospital in February 1974). A request for a dental chair and some optical services was converted into a proposal for a comprehensive health center to be built and run by the hospital.

Sometime in March of 1969 Mrs. G. Francis Ladson, a representative of the Manhattanville Health Services Committee, sent a letter on the stationery of Public School 161 in Manhattan to President Nixon, asking for help in meeting the needs of "those who are in desperate need of medical and dental attention" in the Manhattanville community. According to her letter, "within the past two years the health services in the Manhattanville Community have dwindled to less than minimal. Medical and dental centers once catering to the needs of the community have closed their doors." Her letter suggested some of the adverse consequences of the federal programs of Medicare and Medicaid for the availability of health care.

At the inception of Medicare and Medicaid, the Guggenheim Dental Clinic closed up shop because they felt there would be little need for their services. Medicare and Medicaid provided that patients use private dentists. The fees would be paid by federal funds. Red tape prevented prompt payment of fees and dentists began refusing Medicaid patients. The community was then left without proper dental services. A dental chair was installed at P.S. 125 and now there is a six month waiting list for these services. In the meantime, many children are being denied proper dental care.

Optical services were also reduced because of new federal programs.

Mrs. Ladson's letter to the president continued: "At one time the community availed itself of the optical services of the Red Cross. These facilities were withdrawn because of Medicare and Medicaid. Under these programs an eye examination and a pair of glasses were made available to those in need. No provision was made for lost and broken glasses. As a result, many children have gone without proper optical accommodation for months." Mrs. Ladson asserted that "for the past two years, we have asked political leaders for some recognition of our problems." Finally the group decided to approach the president of the United States. They asked for full-time dental and optical services in the community and full-time medical facilities, social workers, and psychologists within the schools.

The Manhattanville Health Services Committee was clearly asking for what is now called a "comprehensive health center"—ambulatory health facilities for fairly routine dental, optical, and medical services. This letter stimulated a sequence of transmittals to various offices and levels of government. President Nixon's office sent the letter to the New York regional office of the Department of Health, Education, and Welfare. This office in turn—in the person of William J. Putnam, D.D.S., Assistant Surgeon General and Regional Health Director—sent a letter to Hollis S. Ingraham, M.D., Commissioner of Health, New York State Department of Health in Albany. Putnam's letter (actually signed by C. Robert Dean, M.D.), dated 8 April 1969, said, "Attached is a copy of a letter from Mrs. G. Francis Ladson of the Manhattanville Health Group to President Nixon indicating their need for health services. We would appreciate being advised of any action which you might take with regard to this problem."

This letter was received by the executive office of the New York State Department of Health on April 10, and Deputy Commissioner Robert P. Whalen, M.D., sent it on to Donald G. Dickson, M.D., of the Community Health and Hospital Affairs division of the New York State Department of Health, via a memo reading, "Will you please handle?" Dr. Dickson received the memo, together with the attached letters, on 11 April 1969. On April 15, via courier service, Mr. G. Rosettie of Dr. Dickson's office in Albany sent the accumulating file to Dr. Matthew A. Vassallo, Associate Commissioner, New York City Affairs, New York State Department of Health, at his New York City office on Madison Avenue, with the following memo: "Dr. Vassallo: Dr. Dickson sends this down to you for handling. Thank you."

Dr. Vassallo ultimately replied to Mrs. Ladson, at the P.S. 161

address, 499 W. 133rd Street, in answer to her first communication with
President Nixon. The letter, dated April 25th, invited Mrs.
Ladson and one or two other members of the Manhattanville Health Services Committee to meet in "our office" at 270 Madison Avenue sometime in May.
Dr. Vassallo indicated that he intended to invite "representatives of
other interested agencies." A copy of this letter was sent back to Dr.
Putnam at the New York City regional office of HEW. At this point, the
letter from the community group had gone through two federal offices or
agencies (the Presidency and HEW) and several layers of the State
Department of Health, in both Albany and New York City. Mrs. Ladson
replied to Dr. Vassallo on 1 May 1969, accepting his invitation to attend
a meeting on 12 May 1969.

At about the same time, Knickerbocker Hospital, serving the Manhat-
tanville area, was working with a planning consultant, Alfred Kurtz and
Associates, to develop a proposal for a 314e grant ("Partnership for
Health" under the Comprehensive Health Planning Act) for a family
health center satellite. In a memorandum prepared by Mr. Herbert
Williams, Planning Associate of the Health and Hospital Planning
Council, and dated 4 March 1969, it was indicated that

Mr. Kurtz will be conferring with the City Health Department, the
Mental Health Board and various other agencies, but he made us
his first stop. He wanted to know whether we had any data to help
him demonstrate medical need in this area. I gave him a copy of our
Guidelines and the legislative references to Letters of Intent and
construction. I will also be sending him whatever demographic data,
population statistics, welfare data and other indices that are readily
available. I will indicate on a map the location and capacity of other
outpatient facilities that serve this area.

The material provided by Mr. Williams allowed Mr. Kurtz to prepare a
proposal evaluating the need for a comprehensive health care center in
Manhattanville which will be described later.

Very quickly the community group's request for relatively simple
increases in full-time staff in the schools and a few full-time doctors,
dentists, and opticians in the community, simply requiring some medical
offices, thus became transformed into a consideration of new construction of buildings housing a "comprehensive health center" or the
remodelling of a hospital. The minutes of the May 12th meeting
illustrate this point.

The meeting, held at the 270 Madison Avenue offices of the New York

City office of the New York State Health Department, was attended by eight persons. Two persons, Bernard Weisl, M.D., and Raymond Tobia, represented the New York State Health Department. (Dr. Vassallo did not attend, having, apparently through yet another memo, turned the matter over to Dr. Weisl.) Mr. Herbert Williams represented the Health and Hospital Planning Council, Mr. Daniel O'Connell the New York City Health Department, and four persons were present from the Manhattanville Health Group (Mrs. Francis Ladson, listed as the "Director," Ruby Ward, Juanita Attmore, and Gary Berman, listed as a teacher at P.S. 161). Mrs. Ladson repeated the needs detailed in her letter to the President two months before. The urgency of the needs was reaffirmed. According to Mr. Berman from P.S. 161, "when a child who has a reading problem is not furnished with corrective lenses, the child becomes a problem in the school and is not able to keep up with the school work." The group said that P.S. 161 was a new building and had four rooms available for medical purposes. They wanted to have a dental unit installed in one of those rooms.

The history of their attempts to get this relatively simple request granted is revealing. According to Dr. Weisl's minutes, the group had "discussions with Dr. Daniel O'Connell of the New York City Department of Health [present at the May 12 meeting] and Dr. Schindelhiem, the dental representative of that department. Dr. Manberg, the supervising dentist associated with Riverside Health Center, informed the Manhattanville group that he could furnish a dental chair. Apparently this dental chair was to come from the central Harlem Health Center which was being discontinued, but the date of availability of the chair was not certain. Dr. Manberg indicated that while the Health Department could supply the chair, they could not install it in the school. When Mrs. Ladson spoke with Mr. Felix Berman, the principal of P.S. 161, he suggested that the group get the commitment for the dental chair in writing. Mrs. Ladson stated that they had not been able to get this confirmation in writing. Dr. O'Connell indicated that the installation of the chair would be a responsibility of the board of education, and apparently that was where the matter stood at that time.

This brief summary obviously is only a glimpse of the difficulties involved in securing a change in available services. Dr. O'Connell did respond to their description of their problems. The informal minutes continued: "he indicated that he would check into the matter of the dental chair and find out when it would be available. He will also try to get a letter from the Department of Health to the Manhattanville group indicating that a chair would be available so that *they might present* the problem of having the chair installed to the proper person in the Board of Education" (italics added). Note that it was now up to the community group to attempt to find the "proper person" in the board of education who could approve or arrange to have the chair installed in P.S. 161. (The Manhattanville group also said that they had "tried vainly to have meetings with the representatives of the City of New York," but had not succeeded except for the meetings with Dr. O'Connell and his staff.)

At this point, Mr. Williams of the Planning Council "stated that he would recommend the Manhattanville area as a site for the building of a neighborhood health center. He indicated that this was a recommendation that would take several years in implementing since it was not on the schedule of proposed neighborhood health centers. He further stated that he could see that there is a definite need for such a facility and would make this recommendation. Besides quite specific responses, then, such as Dr. O'Connell's, which involved considerable initiative on the part of the community group, there were also the escalated plans of the representative of the Planning Council, who saw the needs as requiring the long-term building of a neighborhood health center, rather than simply hiring a few dentists, doctors, and nurses and setting up a community health facility in existing buildings.

Mr. Williams' own memo summarizing the meeting, indicated that he "discussed briefly some of the long range plans for neighborhood health centers to the East, North and South of this area. It is apparent that present plans do not adequately cover this area and some provisions should be made . . . . " (the memo breaks off at this point). From the evidence of Mr. Williams' statements to the meeting and his own memo, it seems clear that there had been no sense of a need for a neighborhood health center in this area prior to the visible emergence of the Manhattanville Health Group and its letter to the president. Obviously no additional research had been done which might have demonstrated need, and no explicit criteria for adequate health service facilities apparently existed. A demand thus defines a need, which is consistent with basic tenets of economics. In his previous memo of March 4 concerning the Kurtz request, Mr. Williams said only that he would provide data and did not indicate anything about the council's own independent evaluation of need for the area. The criteria seem to be sufficiently ambiguous and flexible to be adjusted to fit almost any institution which has raised some money and/or has political support.

The desires of the community group meshed nicely with the needs of

Knickerbocker Hospital for additional funding. At this point, according to another memo by Mr. Williams dated 21 May 1969, the incipient new proposal for a Manhattanville comprehensive health center began to be considered in relation to other areas and hospitals.

Steve Jonas suggested that the municipal project for Washington Heights give up Health Area 9 to Knickerbocker and add (to the North) Health Area 5. He also suggested that Manhattanville Project be extended from its present 125 Street Southern border to 114 Street; this is on the periphery of the St. Luke's area and takes in Health Areas 14 and 18. While Sydenham Hospital presently serves HA's 14 and 18, they will be focusing their main efforts to the East in Health Areas 15, 19, 24, under a Ghetto Medicine program.

His memo on "latest developments" goes on:

Knickerbocker has met with a community group (the same PTA group that met with us at the State Health Department a few weeks ago) to enlist their help in involving other community sponsors to the North and South of Health Areas 9 and 11. The 'gimmick' Knickerbocker would like to use in applying for PHS [Public Health Service] funds is that they would combine this health center with a school for emotionally disturbed children. This would of course have to be financed with Mental Health funds.

It should not be inferred that Knickerbocker officials were being either cynical or self-serving in seeking a "gimmick" (regardless of whether that language is that of Knickerbocker officials or of Planning Council staff members). Hospitals are the key initiating agencies for projects which then come to be complex affairs, partly because the externally funded projects are seen as providing indispensable overhead support for various parts of the hospital operation as well as providing additional services. Given the constantly shifting number and content of federal and state programs of various kinds, both hospitals and allied organizations such as the Planning Council must be constantly seeking for new formulae which will successfully bring forth federal or state funds. With these interests at stake, community groups come to be seen as instrumental in providing the legitimacy of "sponsorship." The community group will be told, as these memos indicate, "help is several years off; wait until we can get money to build a building; meanwhile lend us your support." From the point of view of the institutions, this position is perfectly rational; they must survive, and these programs are part of the necessary planning for the future capital and operating costs of the institutions. The more programs and projects the hospital can incorporate into its structure, the more stability it has achieved. To some extent this is done by renaming existing underfinanced programs according to the latest fundable project grant; it is also done by actually expanding physical plant and hiring more staff.

At this point, internal consultations among the Planning Council staff began. Mr. Williams drafted a memo to Leonard S. Rosenfeld, M.D., director of the Medical Services Division of the Planning Council. He mentioned the proposal for a 314e grant being developed by Alfred Kurtz, who was named as a "planning consultant for Knickerbocker Hospital." After working on the proposal for Health Areas 9 and 11, Mr. Kurtz apparently "learned that Health Area 9 is part of the present Washington Heights N.F.C.C. [Neighborhood Family Care Center] project. Steve Jonas suggested, however, that Knickerbocker might expand southward to take in Health Areas 14 and 18." Mr. Williams then offered some general evaluations of the needs of the area.

This has been one of the relatively quiet poverty areas in the city. While it has not attracted much attention, there has been a recent large migration of people from Santo Domingo. There are no adequate health facilities in the area which is just out of reach of St. Luke's, Columbia University and Mount Sinai. The Physician Affiliation Study, however, did show a surprisingly high ratio of one private practice physician to 1,500 population.

The question of the appropriateness of Knickerbocker Hospital's serving the back-up function for the proposed community health center was then raised, in view of its lack of resources.

I have serious doubts whether community people, if they had a choice in the matter, would choose Knickerbocker. If the Council continues to encourage Mr. Kurtz in developing these plans, we will soon be called upon to write letters of endorsement and recommendation to the funding agency. I hinted at this problem and Kurtz understood exactly what I was saying. He thought it might be more helpful to make our position clear at an early stage. He suggested that perhaps Knickerbocker should draft a letter to the Council asking what our opinion would be, in a preliminary way, if they were to undertake this proposal. I told him that I would discuss this with you so that he could decide how to proceed.

This memorandum indicates several important things. First, it is clear that the council acts mainly as a screening mechanism for proposals initiated by hospitals, with planning consultants and community groups defining needs or making demands (similar processes insofar as a need is not visible until a demand is made). But more important is the further indication that the fairly simple request by the Manhattanville Health Group for a few more medical, dental, and optical services had become transformed into the issue of whether or not Knickerbocker Hospital should be chosen as the back-up for a new community health center to be built with federal funds. Given the facts that a community health center would be three to five years off, by Mr. Williams' own description, and that a new Knickerbocker was even more years away, the immediate but prosaic needs of the community could not possibly be met by the council's getting involved in those lengthy negotiations for funding and sites.

Dr. Rosenfeld scribbled a memo back to Mr. Williams: "HW—agree with your position. Long-term financing, among others, will present problems. Preliminary request for Council opinion would seem in order." In an important sense, the council was not about to get involved in the seemingly minor issue of hiring a few more doctors and dentists in the Manhattanville area. Its procedures were geared toward "brick and mortar" construction proposals and toward those kinds of programs and projects directly definable in ways which could secure federal grants to hospitals.

On 5 June 1969, Knickerbocker Hospital itself finally contacted the Health and Hospital Planning Council, via a letter from Executive Director Alvin J. Conway to Dr. Rosenfeld. It said that

Knickerbocker Hospital is interested in developing an ambulatory comprehensive health care center for the residents of Health Areas Nos. 11, 14, and 18. . . . We are not aware of any ambulatory comprehensive health care center being planned for the Area outlined above. However, before initiating a letter of intent, we would appreciate your opinions at this time regarding such a facility in the Area desired. Since we have retained the services of a consulting firm to assist us in preparing an application for a grant under Section 314e, U.S. Public Health Services Act as amended by Public Law 89–749, an early reply would be appreciated.
    We realize that such an undertaking would require full cooperation from Sydenham Hospital. Both Sydenham and Knickerbocker Hospitals would be needed as back-up facilities for in-patients and special ancillary professional services. As soon as you have rendered your opinion, if favorable, we would proceed to develop such cooperative efforts with Sydenham Hospital.

Mr. Williams responded to this letter two weeks later. On June 18 he wrote to Mr. Conway: "The largest portion of the target area you outlined for a projected ambulatory health center is not now, as far as we know, being planned for by any other agency. A possible exception is on the southern portion from 114th Street to 123rd Street which might more suitably be served by current St. Luke's Hospital projects." He continued: "I would suggest as a next step that there be a small informal meeting between a member of your staff, your consultant and us to explore your proposal in terms of the needs of the community and the resources of the back-up hospital." Suggesting a meeting in early July, he enclosed a copy of the Planning Council's "Guidelines for Evaluating Proposals for Neighborhood Clinics and Health Centers." (See the summary of these guidelines in an earlier section.)

The suggested meeting was held on 3 July 1969. Attending it were Mr. Alfred Kurtz, the planning consultant to Knickerbocker; Mr. Norman Harrison, Associate Executive Director of Knickerbocker; Dr. Doris Wethers, Director of Pediatrics of Knickerbocker; and Mr. Williams of the Planning Council. Mr. Williams' memorandum summarized the recognized community need: "Knickerbocker Hospital realizes that to make a strong grant application to HEW (section 314-e) they will have to demonstrate: 1. Strong backup capabilities. 2. Organized community support." He noted that the 90 percent occupancy rate of the hospital (80 percent Medicaid patients) "leaves little available for supporting a new population." According to his report,

Mr. Harrison said that he hoped the projected comprehensive care center would supplant the Hospitals' OPD. Dr. Wethers said that in Pediatrics Knickerbocker has made arrangements with Presbyterian, Sydenham and other hospitals for referrals in specialities lacking in Knickerbocker. In order to overcome these weaknesses, Knickerbocker has approached Sydenham Hospital to be a co-sponsor for the project. Sydenham would also supply the necessary OB in-hospital beds which are lacking in Knickerbocker.

The weaknesses of capacity at this hospital are apparent here.

At this point, the question of community support was raised.

Efforts were also made [by the hospital] to develop community support. At first, the community was cool to Knickerbocker, until Knickerbocker promised a large role to the community. There was discussion of forming an "open membership" planning board which in turn would elect a Board of Trustees for the project on a proportional basis for each area. Implied was that the community would eventually be the direct sponsor. They also discussed creating a Coordinating Committee of Board members and hospital members.

Other proposed community committees were finance, professional care, and personnel. Mr. Williams summarized the outcome of the meeting: "Since this was an exploratory meeting, no present action is required of the Council. I offered whatever help we can give in the planning phase to the community members particularly. When a program is drawn up and an application submitted to HEW, then a Letter of Intent will be submitted to us for action."

On July 28 Knickerbocker wrote another letter to Dr. Rosenfeld at the council, having heard no word from the council since the July 3rd meeting and being "anxious to proceed with the project"; they asked that the council "render an opinion as soon as conveniently possible." In addition, they reported that they had told Mr. Williams at the previous meeting that they had already contacted the Sydenham and St. Luke's hospital staffs to solicit their support. According to Mr. Alvin J. Conway, who wrote the letter, they

received support from the Medical Board of Sydenham Hospital to proceed with the project. . . . an ambulatory comprehensive health care center for the residents of Health Areas #11,#14, and #18. . . . We were also informed by both Dr. Paul Torrence [Project Director, St. Luke's Neighborhood Health Care Center] and Mr. Garry Gambudi of St. Luke's Hospital Center [Assistant Director] that neither short nor long range plans of the Neighborhood Health Care Center of the Hospital Center include expansion of the existing or addition of another Neighborhood Health Care Center which would provide comprehensive health care to the residents of Health Areas #14 and #18.

Officials at Knickerbocker were concerned lest their demonstration of community need, and the capability of Knickerbocker to fill that need independently of the plans of presumably better equipped hospitals, be considered inadequate.

On 31 July 1969 Mr. Williams of the council replied to the executive director of Knickerbocker. He repeated that "these health areas do not now have adequate organized ambulatory care facilities to serve the medical care needs of the community. Furthermore, as of now, no potential sponsor has submitted a Letter of Intent to develop a project for these health areas." Mr. Williams went on to reaffirm the council's interpretation of the July meeting.

Our July 3 meeting with your staff identified financial funding as an important hurdle to planning. Should the Knickerbocker Hospital wish to proceed with this project, we would be glad to review a proposal submitted to the New York State Department of Health as a Letter of Intent for the establishment of a facility to meet these needs. In addition to need and location, such factors as the organization and scope of services, the degree of community support, the medical resources of the back-up hospital and plans for financing both capital and operating expenses would be evaluated as indicated at the meeting. The Council would provide whatever help it can in developing a plan for the project.

The situation placed Knickerbocker in a double bind. On the one hand, they could not raise the money for the project without a reasonable plan of operation and without some endorsement from organizations such as the Planning Council. On the other, they could not get the endorsement of the council without some concrete evidence that they could fund both capital and operating expenses. This situation has necessitated repeated applications both by Knickerbocker and by other hospitals, according to Mr. Williams in a 1971 interview.

On the same day that Mr. Williams wrote this letter to the executive director, Mr. Kurtz, the planning consultant for Knickerbocker, also wrote Mr. Conway a letter in which he transmitted his report on a "plan for delivering comprehensive health care services as needed by the population in Manhattanville to meet requirements for obtaining financial support from Federal sources to develop and operate initially the proposed project." The title page of the report included the following sentence: "This is a confidential report and intended solely for the information of the Hospital." But on 5 August 1969 Dr. Wethers, director of pediatrics, sent a copy to the Planning Council with a mimeographed letter: "I am enclosing for your information an Interim Report on a Comprehensive Health Services Project." Mr. Kurtz' opening letter also said, "We are indeed sorry that this project is now at a standstill awaiting a decision by the Health and Hospital Review and Planning Council of Southern New York, Inc., regarding approval to provide services to Health Areas #11, #14, and #18."

The report itself was thirty-seven pages long. The two major sections, besides a brief introduction, presented population and health data for Manhattanville (25 pages) and a plan for consumer organization for representation in a consumer health care association, and a consumer policy and planning board (9 pages). The report noted that "the scope of the study followed, as a minimum, the points covered in the guidelines for development of comprehensive health service projects issued on June 25, 1968, by the Office of Comprehensive Health Planning Program Development Branch, United States Public Health Service. These guidelines result from legislation under Section 314 (e)1, United States Public Health Services Act as amended by Public Law 89-749."

The population and health data given were of several types: census data on the characteristics of the population of the area (education, income, employment, marital status, etc.); health statistics such as live births, early infancy diseases, and accidents; Knickerbocker hospital statistics on outpatient clinic visits; school health data on immunizations and the age and sex of patients; and the like. None of the data were analyzed, nor were any inferences drawn about their implications for the community need for more or different types of health services or for any kind of organization of either hospital or ambulatory care facilities. That the inadequacies of the data were realized by the authors of the report is apparent in their concluding statement:

Health care statistics from external and internal sources are generally limited and frequently not coordinated. Trends and information regarding deficiencies in programs and services are not provided by the Health and Hospital Review and Planning Council of Southern New York, Inc., Department of Health, or Community Mental Health Board. . . . Further, the limited statistics accumulated by each of the agencies mentioned are not coordinated so that it frequently requires a search of raw data to make comparisons. Also, the Department of Health maintains records by Health Areas, the Community Mental Health Board by Catchment Areas, and the Board of Education by School Districts which seldom, if ever, coincide. Thus the data as reported have limited usefulness and minimal value for planning comprehensive health care programs and services since it is difficult and sometimes impossible to determine the needs for the population in Manhattanville.

Despite this disturbing evaluation of their own data, which would seem to lead to the conclusion that nothing could be concluded, the report went on:

From a review and analysis of the limited data, however, it is questionable whether a separate comprehensive health care center for families residing in Manhattanville should be planned. At 17,210 patient visits to the Outpatient Clinic of Knickerbocker Hospital, it appears that even the 1970 projected population of 40,170 in Manhattanville will be served adequately, especially since the population residing in Health Area #9 will probably require fewer services from such a facility.

No indication was given of how this conclusion was arrived at, either from the data given or from any other argument or evidence.

The report also said that the education, income, and employment data "indicate that private physicians would probably provide a substantial amount of the medical care needs in Health Area #9. This interpretation is substantiated still further by considering the favorable ratio of physicians to the popultion in Health Area #9." (This was mentioned earlier as 1 : 1,500.) In contrast, the poorer population of Health Area #11 "would probably require such services as provided in existing and proposed health care centers."

The report went on to summarize the contacts with the Planning Council and other hospitals already described above. The recommendations of Mr. Kurtz and associates were as follows: "1. A separate comprehensive health care center for the families of Manhattanville should not be planned. 2. Consideration should be given to reorganizing the outpatient clinic of Knickerbocker hospital for delivering comprehensive health care to the families of Health Area #11. 3. A study should be conducted to determine health care needs of the population residing in health areas #14 and #18." Once again, no evidence or argument supporting these recommendations appeared in the report, save the sole statistic that income and educational levels in Area #11 were somewhat lower than in #9. No criteria for need were given, nor did the report consider whether or not reorganizing the outpatient clinics of Knickerbocker was likely to meet those needs.

Following these recommendations were nine pages of detailed recommendations for consumer or community participation in the proposed Comprehensive Health Care Center. Quite aside from the fact that the report had just recommended that plans for such a center be dropped, it is significant that so much space (nine of 37 pages) was devoted to quite concrete mechanisms for the functioning of community representation. Such details as the suggested frequency of meetings of the Consumer Health Care Association (quarterly), residence qualifications (one year), and dues (one dollar for persons not covered under Medicaid or Medicare) were not ignored. Likewise, the structure and functions of a consumer policy and planning board, to be elected from members of the association, were described in minute detail: membership composition (half over the age of 26, half under), the number on the Board (a maximum of 15), and requirements for attendance of members (a minimum of 75 percent of the meetings).

This detailed discussion of the operations of agencies for consumer or community representation was given despite the absence of any substantive analysis of community needs for health care facilities and possible ways of supplying those needs. Instead symbolic "democratic" representation of the "community" on the boards of the Comprehensive Health Care Center was provided. This section of the report was obviously an attempt to respond to the requirement that community support be demonstrated, but it is significant that no mention was made of either the original Manhattanville Health Group which had sent its letter to President Nixon back in March, or any other community group which had been offered a chance to participate in the making of these plans. Nowhere was there any evidence that the alternatives of a new Comprehensive Health Care Center outside of Knickerbocker or the reorganization of outpatient clinics had even been considered by any community group of any kind.

This proposal was never completed, and the file ends at this point, without the Planning Council ever having to pronounce judgment on the workability or feasibility of Knickerbocker Hospital's sponsorship of a Comprehensive Health Care Center. According to Mr. Williams of the Planning Council in an interview in 1971, there has been little change in the availability of services in Manhattanville from the spring of 1969 to the summer of 1971, and since there are no new proposals being considered, no change is likely for several years. The needs in the area still exist, but the original community group has disappeared, either from frustration or apathy or because the organizing nucleus has left the area.

On 16 July 1970, more than a year after the submission of Mr. Kurtz' ill-fated report, Dr. Wethers, Director of Pediatrics at Knickerbocker, wrote to Mr. Williams at the Planning Council to thank him for his "past support of the Manhattanville Comprehensive Health Care Project." She said that "the temporary suspension of planning brought about by the exhaustion of planning funds will now be continued indefinitely. The hospital has been led to believe by numerous advisors that the chances of getting such a program funded through federal funds under the existing administration are slim indeed." But Knickerbocker had lost neither its hope nor its vision. Dr. Wethers went on:

However, on the positive side, and the major reason for the suspension of planning, is the fact that the hospital has been approved as a recipient for funds under the New York State Ghetto Medicine Act. This means that we will be able to expand and remodel our existing OPD, and will be able to incorporate into it most of the features necessary to make it a comprehensive health facility. Certain features, however, such as the psychiatric treatment center, and the close relationship planned with school health will have to wait until the creation of the new hospital projected to replace Knickerbocker Hospital and Sydenham Hospital provides new space and funds.

Thus the cycle continues.

To summarize, the Knickerbocker application was never completed, and therefore the council did not have to decide whether or not to endorse it. It was the opinion of Planning Council staff interviewed that no significant improvement or even change in the health care facilities available in the Manhattanville area had occurred since this episode in 1969. The community group had disappeared from view, and no other group had appeared to express the needs of the community for health services. The Planning Council did not, it might be repeated, take any initiative to encourage other groups to prepare proposals for ambulatory care facilities, since it did not define that as its role.

Knickerbocker actually applied for still another ambulatory care facility in May 1971, but no commitment of money was attached, so the proposal was withdrawn. According to a Planning Council staff member interviewed in June 1971, Knickerbocker Hospital had the commitment to carry out a comprehensive health center program, but it lacked the resources. The reservations which the Planning Council had about its capabilities did not mean that they would not have supported Knickerbocker's application. On the contrary, the staff member interviewed believed that they would have strongly supported it on the grounds that there was a community need and that Knickerbocker should be strengthened to meet those needs. The council might have asked, however, that Knickerbocker give up its OPD's and convert that space into sorely needed expansion of in-hospital facilities in return for being allowed to develop a new comprehensive health center.

Council staff noted that, in general, grant proposals had formerly been put in by hospitals primarily as a way of "preempting a franchise" for a program or project in a certain area, without any secure funding or even planning of proposed facilities. In 1970–71, as a result of a proliferation of pending applications (and not from any change of its legislative powers), the state Department of Health tightened up its procedures and began to require definite statements of need, plans, and , most importantly, commitments for funds. If funding commitments are not part of the proposal, it automatically is withdrawn after thirty days. As a result, the Planning Council works with applying units to try to get funds, assurances from back-up hospitals, and definitions of community needs. If the proposal seems to be a good one, the council will write a letter endorsing it, thus helping to raise funds. Programs tend to develop according to what is available in grants. Thus, since there was money in 1971 for methadone clinics and mental health programs, these have become a standard part of grant proposals. A "package" will be created, like Knickerbocker's tentative plan to combine mental health money for a school for emotionally disturbed with "314e" money.

There seems to be a great difficulty in getting under way a "small" program, like the one that the Manhattanville Health Group wanted, mainly because of the lack of organizational incentives. Knickerbocker

Hospital had nothing to gain from it. Because of its financial straits, the hospital wanted to "get," not to "give." A small program—sponsoring an outpatient clinic—simply didn't involve enough money, community legitimacy, or authority to allow Knickerbocker to become "the" hospital for that section of the city. Knickerbocker needed dollars in order to be bailed out. Unfortunately, nobody else made out an application for the project. In their attempts to initiate a "small" program, people sometimes go directly to the City Health Department, but they "can't dislodge anybody," according to the council. "Small" programs do not have the visibility, the political or administrative payoffs, or the financial and organizational incentives to induce enough interorganizational coordination to get past the enormous hurdles which must be jumped before they can be established.

By the end of 1971 Knickerbocker Hospital was again in a financial crisis, and the board of directors announced that nothing "short of a miracle" could keep the institution from closing within thirty days. The hospital was in debt for overpayments which the federal government had made to it for Medicaid and Medicare patients in 1966 and 1967; it could not rely any longer on philanthropic gifts; and it had increasingly devoted its expensive beds to elderly patients who had no place to go for after-hospital care. According to the late Dr. Arthur C. Logan, a visiting surgeon at Knickerbocker and a member of the Health and Hospital Corporation board (and whose wife was a member of the Knickerbocker board), "the state was looking into the possibility of getting a state-guaranteed commercial loan" (*New York Times,* 4 December 1971, p. 29).

This footnote to the story is a tragic commentary on the inability of New York City and, more generally, American society as a whole to devise some viable organizational and financial mechanisms for providing health care to the poor. The whole concept of treating such a fundamental instrument of health care as a hospital as subject to closure because of debts is an incredible one and testifies to the total lack of control over such basic institutions necessary to community life by the population residing in that same community. One wonders why the impending closing of the only hospital serving one of the poorest areas of the city does not constitute a health care "crisis" worthy of headlines.

7. St. Mary's Hospital and
Neighborhood Health Care

Another case illustrating the complexity of the interorganizational relationships and the difficulty of applying the Planning Council guidelines on the proper coordination of health care facilities in an area is provided by the application of St. Mary's Hospital to establish a neighborhood health care center in the Bedford-Stuyvesant area of Brooklyn. An evaluation of the grant application was made by Beatrice Kresky, M.D., who at that time was Planning Associate of the Health and Hospitals Planning Council; dated 5 April 1967, the report said that the hospital,

one of the units in the Catholic Medical Center of Brooklyn and Queens, is applying for both a Title II grant and an OEO grant.... The applicant agency for the OEO grant is the C.D.A. [Community Development Agency]. The applicant agency for the Title II project is the New York City Department of Health, the project director is Dr. Mindlin, Chief of the Bureau of Maternal and Child Welfare. ... The two projects are interdigitated [a new word coined by Dr. Kresky to represent an extremely complex interorganizational relationship] in the neighborhood health center and plan to provide comprehensive care for the population in Bedford-Stuyvesant.

The report went on to summarize the rest of the OEO grant application. and pointed out that "approximately half of the population is medically indigent by the criteria of Title XIX" (Medicaid).

A number of references in the report considered the problem of coordination with other health care facilities.

Existing medical resources in the community are as follows: the Bedford Health Center staffed by St. Mary's Hospital, Unity Hospital, and St. John's Episcopal Hospital. The Brooklyn Jewish Hospital is located just west of the area and undoubtedly serves some of the population of the Bedford-Stuyvesant section. The number of private practitioners is minimal. In addition to clinics in the district health center, the New York City Health Department staff provides school health care and two child health stations. The majority of these services are preventive and screening rather than diagnostic and therapeutical. The Health Department provides dental care in the district health center and in several of the schools.

In considering possible sites, since the location of the center had not yet been determined, it was noted that "St. John's Episcopal Hospital staffs the Bedford Health Center and is contemplating applying for an OEO grant for establishment of a comprehensive care unit in the Bedford Health Center." Four sites had been suggested for the St. Mary's project, "none of them satisfactory." Two were near St. Mary's but were also "close to the Brooklyn Jewish Hospital which has just received a Title II grant for $7,000,000 for institution of a comprehensive care program for children from birth to age 21." The other two sites were "approximately four to five blocks from St. Mary's but also five and nine blocks respectively from St. John's Episcopal Hospital."

It is clear that concern existed in the Council about the proximity of St. Mary's proposed center to others which were either proposed or already in existence, but no indication of any criteria for change of site or justification for any particular location were given. More interesting, there was no discussion of whether or not the existing district health centers could be modified, renovated, expanded, or otherwise made into comprehensive neighborhood ambulatory care facilities, why they did not serve that role, or what it would take to add the additional capacity to them. A number of criticisms of the plan referred to a lack of coordination between various existing or new facilities.

A mental health unit staffed by a psychiatrist, psychologist and psychiatric social worker will be based at the neighborhood health center. The range and type of service and the method of incorporation within the family care clinic is not delineated, although the projected mental health center at St. Mary's Hospital is mentioned as the back-up service.... The integration of the various units, the amount and frequency of consultation services are not explained. Many of these specialized services should be provided at the hospital of auspices.

In discussing the facilities of the back-up hospital, the report notes, "No assessment of the potential need for or availability of beds is given and, apparently, arrangements have not been made with an additional back-up hospital for the provision of outpatient and in-patient care which cannot be obtained at St. Mary's."

Despite these criticisms and others not summarized here, the report concludes, "The project should be approved as the need for medical care in the Bedford-Stuyvesant section is great, and existing facilities are inadequate. St. Mary's is making a sincere attempt to offer high quality comprehensive care and to involve the community in the project." Thus, it seems clear that the desperate need of the community for more health services was important enough to the council staff to allow them to overlook possible duplication of facilities. Only a casual mention of a possible conflict with St. John's Episcopal Hospital was mentioned in the following sentence: "The role of St. John's Episcopal Hospital in planning in addition a neighborhood health facility must be investigated."

On 14 August 1967, three members of the council staff (Dr. Leonard

Rosenfeld, Dr. Beatrice Kresky, and Mr. Robert McIntyre) met with two
representatives of the Catholic Charities staff (Dr. Gocke and Mr.
Murphy) to discuss the St. Mary's Hospital proposal. At this point both
the Title II and the OEO grant applications had been approved by OEO
and the Children's Bureau of HEW. A site had been selected at Utica
Avenue and Fulton Street in Bedford-Stuyvesant, two and a half blocks
from St. John's Episcopal and eight blocks from St. Mary's. The
summary of the meeting prepared by Dr. Kresky said that the "format of
the Council's 'Guidelines for Evaluating Proposals for Neighborhood
Clinics and Health Centers' [was] adhered to in reviewing this program."
The urgency of the program was indicated: "The community pressure
and commitments are such that the neighborhood health center must be
in operation early in January 1968. To meet this deadline plans must be
let out for bid by mid-September."

The community was doomed to disappointment, largely because of
conflict between the two hospitals. The conflict was referred to—"St.
John's Episcopal Hospital is disturbed about the proximity of St. Mary's
proposed neighborhood health center"—but no mention was made of
any alternative (at least none was recorded in the minutes), nor was there
any discussion of the criteria which could be used to justify the center. It
was noted that "the proposed facility is .... close to the sponsoring
hospital, and, with the exception of St. John's Episcopal Hospital, no
conflict exists with existing facilities in the area." But since the need
demonstrated by the "target population" was undeniable, the discussion
focused mainly on the specific facilities to be built, the space allocated
to various functions—pharmacy, conference rooms, telephone service,
appointment systems—and the like.

On August 14 a meeting was held between representatives of St.
Mary's and St. John's hospitals, the Health Department, the local community council, the Health Services Administration, and four Planning
Council staff members. The memorandum of the meeting (dated August
18) noted that "St. John's Hospital is violently opposed to the location"
of the St. Mary's-sponsored center. "No agreement was reached after a
discussion of two and a half hours," and no alternatives discussed,
including a hospital-based unit at St. Mary's or some other geographic
locations for the center, were acceptable to all of the parties.

On August 16 Dr. Rosenfeld called Dr. John Frankel of OEO in
Washington about the conflict. OEO said that they could not "furnish
additional funding and will not change the geographic boundaries of the
project." Thus the additional costs involved in erecting a "pre-engi-
neered clinic structure on the grounds adjoining" St. Mary's could not be

borne by OEO. Nor would an alternative definition of the service area be considered, according to Dr. Rosenfeld's summary of the telephone conversation. "OEO insists on well delineated areas with determination of eligibility on the basis of residence. It is not in favor of the free choice principle in providing service from OEO facilities." Dr. Frankel said that Dr. James Haughton, Health Services Administrator, had "visited Washington with representatives of the Community Development Agency, St. Mary's Hospital and the Provident Medical Society, at which time the boundaries of the Bedford-Stuyvesant area had been set."

On 17 August 1967 Dr. Haldeman, executive director of the Planning Council, was sent a letter from the Church Charity Foundation of Long Island, a foundation of the Episcopal Church of the diocese of Long Island, the agency controlling St. John's Episcopal Hospital. Signed by W. K. Allison, chairman of the executive committee of the board of managers, the letter was also sent to Hollis S. Ingraham, M.D. (commissioner of health of the Department of Health of New York State), Dr. Mary McLaughlin (at that time associate deputy commissioner, Department of Health of New York City), Mr. Joseph P. Peters of the Planning Council, and the administrator of St. John's. After some kind words about regional planning and the role of the council, the letter got down to business: the "projected establishment of a community health center by St. Mary's Hospital, in a locality which conflicts both with its own parent hospital and St. John's Episcopal Hospital." How and why the new center constituted a conflict was not made clear in the letter any more than why it did *not* constitute a conflict was clarified in the Planning Council review documents.

Mr. Allison then asserted that the council's own guidelines emphasized that duplication of facilities should be avoided and that the council had ignored them in this instance. He claimed that he had talked to several staff members of the council who had agreed with him that the "location of the proposed St. Mary's health center was an extremely poor one, if [the] guidelines as to the establishment of such a health center were to be considered," but these staff members had not stuck to that position either in the August 14 meeting with St. Mary's and representatives of the community council or in discussions with OEO.

Dr. Haldeman replied to Mr. Allison on 28 August 1967.

This is obviously a complex and difficult matter. There are substantial health needs which must be met in the area; and yet under the circumstances the proposed plan for meeting these needs is far from ideal. The Council is therefore working closely with various groups within the community, including officials of St. John's Episcopal Hospital and the Health Department, to explore other alternatives which would both meet the needs of the local community and provide a rational basis for the establishment of high quality ambulatory care services.

This letter, obviously a conciliatory one, seems clear evidence of the victory of St. John's Episcopal Hospital, in spite of the council's own staff recommendation of the clear need in the area, the apparent adequacy of the proposed facility to serve those needs, and the availability of financing from both OEO and the Children's Bureau.

In subsequent months the staff of the council helped in the search for alternative sites. Ultimately, St. Mary's sponsored a temporary storefront facility, called the Charles R. Drew Neighborhood Health Center, in the Bedford Health District, also with funding from Title II of HEW and OEO. It began operating in the summer of 1968 with Steven Jonas as the administrator. On August 22 Dr. McLaughlin, deputy commissioner of the city's Department of Health, wrote a letter to Dr. Donald Dickson, associate commissioner for New York City Affairs of the state Department of Health, recommending that the program be refunded.

According to a council staff memo of 19 September 1969, reporting on a conversation with Dr. Gocke of St. Mary's, the project was housed for the first year or so in a two-room, improvised facility in a Kingsborough housing project. An $80,000 remodelling of a storefront on the corner of Saratoga and St. Mark's Place was scheduled to be finished before the end of the fall of 1969, and a permanent location was scheduled for 251 Rochester Avenue, Brooklyn. According to the September 19 memo, however, "the plans for the permanent Drew Center on Rochester Avenue have been tabled indefinitely. An FHA mortgage will not be issued until OEO says that it is ready to guarantee it for a ten-year period. OEO is not ready to endorse this until it is convinced of St. Mary's ability to conduct a stable program."

The general comment in the same memo on the history of St. Mary's attempts to establish a neighborhood center is interesting. "To this day [September 19, 1969] the project is without a project director, most candidates having been scared away by the clangorous goings-on in the community health council. As a result of innumerable delays and snail-like progress, OEO conducted a site visit last month to determine whether St. Mary's grant should be continued.... St. Mary's OEO troubles have bogged the C & Y [Children's and Youth] program also."

In 1968, 4,000 patients, both children and adults, were seen in the two-room facility in the housing project. In 1969, now housed in the store-front facility, the center had 11,000 visits, but by February, 1970, the building project was "dormant," since no FHA money was available for construction.

The point here is not whether or not the council staff was right or even consistent in its judgments but only that (as staff members informed me subsequently) the criteria used for applying the guidelines for coordination were extremely flexible, that no hard data were required, and that informal assurances of commitment and intentions were regarded as more important than a detailed "empirical" justification of coordination. Given this modus operandi, if another health institution were to claim violation of its territory or its target population, there were no clear grounds for defense. What is significant is that the failure to reach agreement killed the project. Apparently, although the documentation is not complete, St. John's Episcopal Hospital was able to exert a veto power over the entire project, even though the grants had already been approved.

That there was in fact any duplication of facilities or overlapping of target populations is not at all clear. In a situation in which major neighborhood institutions perceive a threat to their resources, functions, or clientele, they are able to block new institutions which, by the flexible and reasonable criteria probably used by the council staff in its early reviews, would provide sorely needed additional health facilities. This case shows that the official guidelines for coordination and the rational criteria for regional planning can be appealed to by a threatened institution to block a new health service.

8. The Status of the NFCC
Program in 1970–71

In December 1970 the status of the NFCC program was summarized by Dr. James R. Posner, senior quantitative analyst for the Health Services Administration, in a report prepared for the Budget Bureau of the city in order to define priority allocations of scarce budget resources. Posner's summary of the situation is worth giving in full. As he said, "since it was first conceived, implementation of the NFCC program has been beset with several problems." These problems, as he saw them, were as follows.

(1) Cutbacks in income eligibility levels for Medicaid decreased by more than half the number of individuals who were eligible for this

program. These cutbacks, together with the limited ambulatory care coverage provided by Medicare and by other third-party payors, mean that total third-party reimbursement for ambulatory care services in projects which serve a diversified population is limited to roughly 50% of the costs of operation.

(2) The process of site selection, design, and contract bidding has required an inordinately lengthy time, with the result that, at this date, only a single NFCC has entered the construction stage, and only 7 are ready for bidding or construction.

(3) The rise in health care prices—roughly 15% and 7% per year for hospital and physician prices respectively—has led to dire predictions concerning the escalation of operating costs in NFCC's overtime.

(4) The scarcity of health manpower of all types has led to doubts as to whether 15 NFCC's, each of whose plans call for 50 physicians and 15 dentists, as well as a large number of other health workers, can be staffed. The advent of federally-funded comprehensive care centers has added to already stiff competition for available manpower.

(5) Paucity of central staff available for ambulatory care planning has meant that many issues governing the planning and implementation of the NFCC program, particularly its relationship to other health care programs and resources, have not been adequately explored.

This unemotional summary of the failure of a program reveals a number of major characteristics of the health system as presently constituted. The expansion and even maintenance of present health services for the poor depend almost entirely upon federal funds; budget restrictions are most likely to hit those services which already are the most inadequate—services aiming at those who do not have the means to pay for them. Recall that these ambulatory care facilities were an attempt to respond to desperate shortages of clinics and physicians in poverty-stricken areas of New York City.

The emphasis upon "bricks and mortar" is also clear, as was seen in the case study of the Manhattanville Health Group's abortive demands for a few, seemingly simple, medical, dental, and optical services for their neighborhood. The emphasis in federal programs upon capital funding of buildings rather than upon operating expenses for programs leads to a distortion of priorities which cannot be blamed on any local agency or officials simply trying to gain as many funds as possible within the constraints imposed by federal legislation.

The discontinuities of various parts of the health system are also clear in the description of potential manpower shortages and the competition of agencies funded from several different sources for the same health manpower, with no overall mechanism for deciding on needs and priorities for given areas. Posner's last point is particularly important for our concern here, since each agency, in desperation, must carry out its own mandate, and the "relationship to other health care programs and resources" of any one program simply cannot be controlled and planned, let alone "explored."

Various documents, such as Posner's report, prepared on ambulatory care facilities indicate clearly that they were designed for health care for the poor. No pretense was made that an "integrated" system was being designed. Rather, the assumption was that the middle class would pay for care individually. Posner assumed at the outset that "the City of New York is committed to assuring access to medical care *for all individuals below the median income for the City.* That is, we assume that the City will provide care for 50 per cent of the population, to whatever extent that those individuals are not able to obtain care through other sources such as medicaid, fee-for-service, or pre-payment by other parties" (italics in original). Thus, the whole subsequent analysis was predicated upon, or involved an analysis of, *deficits* in available health services in predominantly poor areas of the city.

Posner's report complained about the absence of systematic data on the health system.

In terms of direct evidence, it is difficult to argue about a 'deficit' in the amount of ambulatory care delivered to low-income individuals in New York City. Even to estimate the number of physician visits delivered, much more information would be required about what constitutes a 'visit'. . . by income and by geographical areas of the City. These problems notwithstanding, in certain geographical areas of the city there are so few physicians, that there is probably a deficit in the ambulatory care delivered.

This general assumption was echoed by officials of the Planning Council who felt that the need for more health care facilities in certain areas was so evident that hard data were not necessary. They were also willing in those cases to relax their criteria for adequate planning in order to speed up applications for funds and the rest of the lengthy bureaucratic series of approvals required. Posner singled out "at least nine health districts" which thus qualified: Central Harlem, Morrisania, Mott Haven, Pelham Bay, Brownsville, Bushwick, Red-Hook-Gowanus, Sunset Park, and Williamsburg-Greenpoint.

Posner's document summarized the "original intent and present problems." According to him the "NFCC program was originally designed to provide a network of ambulatory care centers each of which would deliver acute ambulatory medical care, preventive care, and psychiatric care to a population of some 55,000 persons. The centers

were visualized as part of a total community program which would
include a general hospital and a Community Mental Health Center, the
supporting hospitals being either municipal or voluntary, or in some
cases, both." It might be noted here that the original programs for
neighborhood family care centers as summarized in the 1 November
1967 documents mentioned nothing about the relationship of the centers
to a total community program. Here Posner cited as his source the
capital budget presentation by the Health Services Administration in
November 1967. According to Posner, the "locations of the originally-
planned 17 NFCC's were selected on the basis of (1) community health
indices, (2) availability of other health resources, (3) site availability, and
(4) political factors." No documents have been found which give any
substantive data assessing the need of the population, its use of other
health resources, and their availability.

Posner's report also developed six decision-rules for determining
priorities for the fifteen NFCC's still being planned: whether or not plans
were complete; whether or not the catchment area (aiming at 55,000
persons) could be expanded; the proportion of the population eligible for
Medicaid or Medicare; the lack of availability of alternative health
resources; the ratio of physicians in the area to the size of the Medicaid
population; and whether or not the proposed NFCC would serve as the
outpatient department of a hospital. That is, an NFCC whose plans were
complete, whose catchment area could be expanded later, whose area
had a high proportion of persons eligible for federal health benefits but
had few physicians, and which could potentially serve as the outpatient
department of a hospital ranked higher in priority.

Two of these decision-rules involved interorganizational relationships: the relationship of the NFCC to the back-up hospital and the
availability of alternative health resources. In regard to the first criterion, the NFCC was seen as a functional equivalent of an outpatient
department of the hospital, and as required partly (this is almost always
implicit) because of the failure by the hospitals to develop adequate
outpatient facilities. Thus new programs with glamorous new names
became necessary to mobilize political support for their funding and
construction. Three of the proposed NFCC's were in fact planned to
replace the outpatient departments at their respective hospitals (Williamsburg-Greenpoint, Morrisania, and East Tremont-Crotona), and
two others could become the OPD's (Soundview and East New York).
Posner commented that if this was the case, the cost of the NFCC should
be weighed against the cost of the departments it would replace.

The second interorganizational criterion—the availability of other
health resources—overlapped with the OPD criterion, since if the NFCC

was not to replace a hospital OPD, then it had lower priority because of the availability of similar services in the area. It might be noted that this report, alone of all those analyzed, considered the criteria for deciding whether or not a given OPD should be replaced by an NFCC. The criticism implicit in the replacement of one form of providing ambulatory care by another has seldom been expressed openly. The assumption seemed to be that keeping ambulatory care facilities in the hospital would freeze them in the old class-biased pattern, but this policy contradicts the other goal of centralization within the hospital to achieve economies of scale and rationalization.

In his section on program planning and coordination, Posner repeated once again the necessity for coordination and planning.

The NFCC program must be coordinated with other programs which deliver ambulatory care, in an attempt at comprehensive health planning for the City as a whole. The NFCC programs must mesh with other programs which deliver care in the municipal and voluntary hospitals (e.g., outpatient departments and emergency rooms), the Health Department (e.g., District Health Centers and Child Health Stations), other government agencies (e.g., Neighborhood Health Centers and family planning clinics funded by OEO or PHS), and with the private sector (solo practitioners and group practices). Toward this end, a working committee must be established composed of representatives from the Health Services Administration, the Health and Hospitals Corporation, the Mayor's Organizational Task Force on Comprehensive Health Planning, and other agencies. Such a committee should be responsible for developing a comprehensive plan for ambulatory care for the City.

Just to list again the varied agencies offering some form of ambulatory services indicates the complexity of the job of coordination. Posner noted that merely to recommend an interagency committee to be made "responsible for developing a more comprehensive plan of ambulatory care" seems clearly inadequate. How the "meshing" of the programs might conceivably be accomplished seems quite beyond the powers of any committee which might be named. The sources of funding and control are so diverse and the constituencies and pressures to which authoritative agencies respond are so complex and contradictory that such a recommendation seems mainly the required reflex of a person caught up in the rhetoric of bureaucratic rationality. Such a statement makes the assumption, perhaps shared by many Americans, that any committee, composed of representatives of all the interests involved, which sits down and communicates with itself honestly will thrash out its differences, arrive at a consensus, and develop a program which will solve all of the issues presented to the committee.

The HSA (Health Services Administration of the city) *News* under a headline HEALTH SPACE AGENCY REPORTS STEADY PROGRESS ON FACILITIES, noted that "the City is planning fifteen Neighborhood Family Care Centers (NFCC) at a cost of about $112 million. Virtually all of these funds will be provided by the City, with no federal participation and very little State funds." According to new Health Services Administrator Gordon Chase, "Real progress is being made in the form of site acquisition, design and state of construction in the Neighborhood Family Care Center Program" (vol. 1, no. 1 [Dec. 1970]). The article also summarized the goals of the NFCC:

[To] provide high quality health care on a continuing basis, to permit each patient or family to see the same physician each time, to offer visits on an appointment basis to minimize waiting, to safeguard personal dignity, privacy and convenience, to seek maximum community participation at all levels of planning and operations, to integrate ambulatory care with hospital and home care services, to foster the practice of preventive medicine to forestall serious illness, hospital admissions, and protracted hospital stays, to meet approximately eighty per cent of a family's or individual's total medical needs.

Achievement of these laudable goals—which are essentially identical with the goals of the best medical practice and the visions of those developing plans for the best possible health delivery system for at least the past forty years—has unfortunately been undermined by the lack of financing, coordination, and sheer generation of enough social power to implement them. As of March 1971, the city was reexamining all of its priorities in the light of the budget crisis. A Planning Council in-house memo dated March 16 said that "it seems certain at this stage that the City Council and the City Budget Director will not commit themselves to building all of the Neighborhood Family Care Centers." It was noted that the Planning Council had approved eight of the eleven NFCC's. "This. . . . was done under-the-gun. At no time did we have a proper program specifically related to the community being served or to the resources of the back-up hospital. We were never certain of how staffing would be achieved, or whether the City would be able to produce enough operational funds to carry these giant ambulatory enterprises." The difficulty of coordination was emphasized: "We also expected that we would be dealing with one responsible City official, whether from HSA, the Health Department or the Health and Hospitals Corporation [which came into existence July 1, 1970] in developing these programs. At this stage it has been impossible to find out which of these agencies will in fact be the responsible party for planning."

On 20 April 1971 the deputy administrator of HSA, Mr. Robert Harris, in a letter to Dr. Matthew Vassallo, Assistant Commissioner of the New York State Health Department, announced HSA's desire to delay the state's review process on three of the NFCC's (Bushwick, East Tremont-Crotona, Mt. Morris), plus the renovation of the East Harlem District Health Center. The current budgetary crisis in the city and the state had once again, quite aside from any other organizational or policy considerations, had its effect on the provision of adequate ambulatory care facilities for the poor.

9. Summary and Conclusions

In general, then, we have seen that the clear and comprehensive guidelines of the Planning Council concerning coordination of the proposed new ambulatory care facilities with other health services already in the same geographic area were not followed, either in the proposals themselves or in the subsequent review process, and were not regarded as of sufficient importance to warrant requiring revision and resubmission of the proposals. In no case of the reading of a proposal and the subsequent correspondence among the Planning Council, the State Department of Health, and the applying agency did the mechanisms of coordination and integration become a major or even minor bone of contention.

There seem to be several clear reasons for this lack of concern with mechanisms of coordination. First, given the sudden availability of federal funds under various programs and their accompanying pressures to act quickly, and given the danger that other agencies, cities, or even states would consume those funds, both the applying agency and the reviewing bodies—whether the Planning Council or the state—were not disposed to develop the comprehensive data necessary to document the way in which the new center would be coordinated with existing health care facilities. The best that could be done was to develop an internal program, required staff and physical facilities, and tentative financing.

Second, given the pressing needs for more ambulatory care facilities in poverty areas of the city, the latent assumption was that almost *any* additional health care services would be worth providing. Information on how the new facilities would be coordinated with old ones was not considered worth the time and resources to develop and integrate into the proposal. Almost all parties were willing to assume that mechanisms of coordination could be worked out ad hoc, or after the fact, once the funds had been obtained and the facilities were in operation.

The justification offered by the Planning Council in ultimately approving plans by the city to build "prototype 55" ambulatory care facilities without specifically tailoring each program to the needs of the community was that *any* additional health services in poverty areas were worthwhile. In the absence of any empirical specification of those needs and an evaluation of the total network of health services available to the community, it seemed utopian or excessively rigid to require the city to prepare a plan which presupposed that kind of research and policy planning. The council itself, as Dr. Leonard Rosenfeld said in the memo summarized in section 5 of this chapter, had not conducted any research which laid down criteria for community needs and had not systematically assessed the available health services in the city.

Given the complexity of the system—the diversity of origins of new services, funding sources, and controlling agencies—it would be extremely difficult to compile even a list of the capacity and services provided by health care facilities in an area, let alone assess whether or not those facilities were meeting a reasonable definition of needs of the community. Thus, requiring the city to prepare a program tailored to the community's needs would establish a standard which presupposed a level of planning capability that did not exist either in the council or anywhere else. This lack of planning capability is part of the phenomenon to be explained, not an explanation of why "coordination" did not take place or why "fragmentation" continued to exist. To assert that the fragmented system existed *because* of a lack of proper research, knowledge, or communication is merely to illustrate still another feature of a fragmented system, not to discover a cause which explains the fragmentation.

Third, in the case of the Health Services Administration, there were the political necessities of developing a new, highly visible program and of showing some results. The cost of possibly including some unnecessary facilities in one or more of the "prototypes" may have seemed, quite plausibly, justified to the city health planners, both in terms of getting something—anything—built before building costs escalated any further, and in terms of getting some additional visible services, in the form of a tangible structure labeled a Neighborhood Family Care Center, out into politically sensitive neighborhoods during the tenure of the Lindsay administration in New York City.

This last point is related to a more general one: namely, that all agencies, whether directly "political" or not, have to justify their existence by new and better programs, and the question of how these programs will be integrated with existing ones is quite low on the priority list. In fact, from the point of view of the organizational incentives involved, it may be that the *less* integrated and more autonomous, isolated, and dependent the new staff and agency are upon the adminstrative or political officials which sponsored them, the more likely the agency is to provide legitimacy for the sponsoring agency or officials and thus to become part of the resources of their political and organizational base.

Because of the absence of any coordinating mechanisms for consolidating decision making and planning, the officials of each organization went ahead on their own, trying to maintain their institutions and to solidify their position vis-a-vis relevant publics and other funding or regulating agencies. Each organization, in developing a project proposal, attempted to develop support and move ahead to the point where it would be difficult for other organizations to stop it. This may be one of the factors accounting for communication and coordination problems. If full information were available to other organizations before or at the early stages of planning, funding, designing, and so forth, they would be better able to block the project. Sometimes the interests of other organizations are well known—or at least it is known which organizations are most likely to either favor or oppose a project—so that the "friends" can be contacted and mobilized to support the project and the potential "enemies" can simply not be informed until, hopefully, it is too late. This factor seems most likely to operate where resources are either scarce or vacillating.

The history of the Neighborhood Family Care Centers illustrates the extreme dependence of local health programs upon the vicissitudes of federal legislation. The rise of a particular "hot" program such as the War on Poverty generates a flurry of activity—plans, proposals, meetings, new organizations—but this activity quickly dies down as another program appears which is advertised as solving the problems. However, the "crisis" continues, largely untouched, because no program which is politically feasible can also attack the causes of the problem and more than a few of the consequences.

The process of applications for funds for and approval of new Neighborhood Family Care Centers thus cannot be evaluated on the basis of "rational" criteria. Funding and programs, and hence priorities, constantly change, and planning organizations must take into account these persistent conditions of the organizational environment. In 1965, neighborhood health centers were funded; in 1971, family planning and abortion. The impetus behind ambulatory care has dwindled, and as of 1971 there was almost no action in that area. Only one NFCC was under construction, and the prospects for more were gloomy.

In conclusion, it can be said that despite the attention given during this period to the development of neighborhood health centers as a solution to a pressing problem, the program, "even at the height of its proliferation in New York City... never... even accounted for more than five percent of the institutional ambulatory care visits here. Today this percentage has probably shrunk. The centers are struggling to survive in the face of dwindling financing. Also, the New York City 'Prototype 55' program seems to be moribund."[8]

As was the case with other federal programs, funds were available for construction but not for operating expenses. Demonstration projects were possible in a variety of areas (such as methadone clinics), but no continuing commitment was likely, regardless of the success or failure of a project. Thus a flurry of activity occurred as separate programs rose and fell, together with their implementing organizations. This process exemplifies another aspect of a "fragmented" health system. While a proximate explanation for a particular case can be sought in failures of leadership, inadequate funding, errors of foresight or planning, mistaken decisions, or lack of public pressure for action, an ultimate explanation is probably to be found in fundamental features of the political economy of health care in the United States.

4 Health Care and New York City: Unique or Typical?

Rather than being particular manifestations of general features of the American political economy, the phenomena in New York City which I have described might conceivably be the result of the peculiar intensity and scope of New York's fiscal crisis, which produces breakdowns in the city's attempts to provide vital services in *all* areas, not just in health. This explanation is plausible enough if we take a series of studies of New York's fiscal crises at face value.[1] Significantly, these studies are of interest in their own right as a set of inquiries parallel to the health care studies which we have already scrutinized.

The 1971 City of New York Commission on State-City Relations, seeking to discover what the previous commissions had found and recommended, summarized both their analyses and their conclusions as exhibiting a "remarkable degree of consensus... concerning the causes and factors involved in the City fiscal crisis." The commission summarized that agreement on several major points: (1) there is an "inevitable" growth in the expenditure-revenue gap; (2) the city's tax structure was not responsive to economic growth and was essentially regressive; (3) the city's revenue sources were constrained by state constitution tax and debt limits; (4) although they had not caused the financial crises, managerial deficiencies in city government meant that the city was not maximizing its use of available resources; (5) New York assumed a "greater range of responsibilities than any other local government in New York State and than any other large city in the country"; and (6) New York State "assumed less responsibility for the total range of state and local government services than most states in the Union" (p. 4).

The commission report concluded that New York City, in response to these reports, had "significantly expanded its own tax effort and reformed its tax structure." New York State, in contrast, had not responded, although "time and again, with Cassandra-like regularity, previous Commissions have warned of the need for state and/or federal absorption of welfare costs, of regional funding for mass transit, for state assumption of public education financing, of state responsibility for funding the court system, and for the State assumption of the costs of the City University of New York. These basic recommendations have been talked about, debated, praised and supported—but left wholly unimplemented." The commission concluded that "the inadequate response to the works and recommendations of past Commissions should be a warning to the people of this state that the efforts of *five existing Commissions* (including this one) may only be marginally productive" (pp. 30–31; italics added).

This report, by far the most visibly self-conscious in its awareness of the political limitations of the commission-report mechanism of any I have seen, is significant here because it claims to deal with some of the underlying causes of the "crisis" in health care and thus provides an alternative explanation to the one I have offered. Essentially, the argument is that a combination of *structural* factors (constitutional limits and the division of fiscal responsibility between the city and the state) and *political* decisions (which type and level of tax the city itself chooses to impose) basically accounts for the increasing discrepancy between the revenues available to the city and its actual expenditures: the so-called "fiscal crisis." If this explanation is correct, then this is a more specific set of causes than those found in the political economy of American society—that is, in the institutions of the society as a whole, not just one city or even one state. This explanation implies that the task before us is to mobilize mass and elite support to change the constitution, to reallocate the responsibility for functions from one level of government to another, and to elect political leaders who will change the tax structure.

The problem with this line of reasoning is that it stops too soon. Further questions need to be asked: Why is it so difficult to change certain kinds of constitutional limitations or to reallocate governmental functions? Why is it so difficult to change the tax structure? Who is benefiting from the maintenance of the existing political structures and functions? These questions were not raised because, like the commissions whose reports on health I analyzed earlier, this commission was operating within fairly clear assumptions about the range of possible policy changes and the likely responses of certain elite audiences to their recommendations. Therefore, while their "intermediate" explanations in terms of the politics of New York City and New York State may be perfectly valid, it is still necessary to probe more deeply into the political economy which generates and sustains a pervasive inability to change.

My position—that although New York exhibits an unusual concentration of social and political conditions and their consequences, it is not unique—can be supported by a variety of types of evidence. First, many of the conditions discovered in New York hospitals are found in other cities, such as Boston, New Haven, San Francisco, St. Louis, Chicago, Los Angeles. Second, failures of health planning and coordination are found in cities in California, Ohio, Nebraska, and Maryland, as well as in New York. Third, commissions of investigation in other political jurisdictions make essentially the same kind of analysis and come up with the same general recommendations as have been found in New York's. Fourth, the fragmentation both of programs and of attempts at coordination are found in other areas of public policy besides health. The following sections deal briefly with each of these points.

1. Health Care in Other Cities

How far can these conditions of "crisis" and the symbolic and tangible responses to them be generalized past New York City? Such a question is difficult to answer, because, to my knowledge, no systematic comparative studies of hospitals and health care in different cities have been done. But clues are found in statements by various persons that New York City is not wildly different either in the general standards of health care provided for its citizens or in its political and administrative responses to those conditions. A recent study of the regulation of the quality of care in hospitals began by describing two suits brought by the house staff physicians of the hospitals themselves against hospitals in the District of Columbia and Los Angeles. Two large city hospitals in Boston and St. Louis lost their accreditation in 1969. The authors commented that "the quality of care alleged by these doctors to exist at two of the nation's largest hospitals can only be described as dangerously inadequate and tragically inhuman. Yet their descriptions are consistent with findings of other recent studies of hospital care in America."[2]

That the problems of coordination and of establishing comprehensive health care centers are not found only in New York is supported by the experience of Massachusetts General Hospital in Boston in its attempt to develop coordinated health services for 16,000 people in Charlestown. The project was spearheaded by an experienced and influential health leader like Dr. John Knowles, but the difficulties of working "through the multiplicity of funding arrangements from the Children's Bureau to the OEO to the other departments of the HEW" delayed the funding even of the children's portion of the program for nearly six years, "even though the authorization for federal funding of components of the project was already available and even though special arrangements were made by the assistant secretary for health... in developing and coordinating the application."[3] Nor are the problems of obsolescent hospitals or the inadequacy of federal aid peculiar to New York: "By 1967, hospital services in the major cities were reaching a point of breakdown. A study by the Department of Health, Education, and Welfare estimated that the cost of modernizing New York City hospitals was $1.25 billion; the city had received only $17.5 million from the Hill-Burton program. Similar concern was being expressed in other major cities" (ibid., p. 511).

The details set forth concerning New York City can thus probably be generalized to other large American cities, at the very least. A recent survey of Chicago concluded that

the health services system in the Chicago metropolitan area shares with the rest of the country, and certainly other large cities, generic problems.... The current private health system is inherently incapable of serving the poverty areas given its traditional incentives of physicians practicing where they can make a living and in pleasant surroundings.... [The Chicago] area faces the universal problem of rising unit costs and overall expenditures, and increasing pressures of demand on the system.... The area has problems in filling out its extended care facilities, home care, rehabilitation, and preventive medicine. There are problems of quality determinations and controls.[4]

A study of a university hospital in New Haven showed that many of the same problems which exist in the New York City hospitals are found in even a leading hospital in a small city.[5] In addition, the former first deputy commissioner of hospitals in New York, who became director of hospitals and clinics at the University of San Francisco, said in 1972 that in San Francisco "the size of the operation is smaller [than New York's], but many of the issues are identical and seemingly as intractable."[6]

Although few systematic comparative studies of health services in many communities are available, those that do exist suggest that the problems characteristic of New York City are found in smaller communities in other regions also and that certain problems may be more intense outside the major metropolitan centers. A study, sponsored by the National Commission on Community Health Services, of twenty-one communities in all regions of the country, only three of which were over 500,000 population (and six of which were under 100,000), interviewed professional, political, and business leaders and found that the issue identified as their chief health concern was

the coordination of facilities to provide care for a variety of illnesses. Nearly all the communities exhibit capacity, or potential capacity, to provide a level of population-wide medical care higher than that now prevailing. Yet the application of service to those populations most in need of it often seems haphazard and irrational against a pattern of overlapping functions and less than optimal use of extant capacities, and the proliferation of agencies for preventive and therapeutic efforts. Study after study reveals the necessity of tying the network of local services together more logically and planning in concert to meet the health imperatives of the next several decades.[7]

Related to this problem of coordination, continues the author, "is the developing cluster of problems associated with a growing, urbanizing population. These include especially the provision of care to the medically indigent, chronically ill, and aged, including the mentally ill, and the environmental health problems exemplified by sewage and water pollution in rapidly expanding communities" (p. 39). Also, the health manpower situation is, if anything, probably worse in small cities and towns than in New York since, as the author points out, "communities face severe difficulty in finding money to pay for specialists in a fiercely competitive 'seller's market'... especially in cities and towns outside the great metropolitan complexes" (p. 40).

Thus, although precise comparisons of New York City with other cities are not possible, the available evidence does not indicate a qualitative difference.

2. Planning to Plan

Since it may seem that the outcomes of some attempts at health planning in New York City recounted earlier may be entirely due to the high level of politicization and polarization in New York, resulting in nearly continuous stalemate, it may be useful to summarize the results of a field study of five of the "most successful" cases of local, regional, and state health planning efforts in 1967-68. The cases chosen were located all across the country: San Mateo, California; Rochester, New York; Cincinnati, Ohio; Lincoln, Nebraska; and the state of Maryland.[8] Cases were first recommended by panels of "nationally known leaders in the health field" (p. 14). It was agreed that success would be judged in terms of "concrete action on specified goals; evidence of a viable relationship between health planning and other public planning efforts such as city, regional or state planning; and the breadth of participation of relevant interest groups such as health agency leaders, school officials, hospital administrators and the like" (p. 15). Note that two of these are *procedural* goals for planning, not substantive ones. A "relationship" between different planners and the "participation" of different groups both counted as concrete successes. Later, Conant defined—much more appropriately in my opinion—community health planning as the "effort to bring together and make rational use of private and public resources... in such a way as to meet all important health problems in the community" (p. 99).

The five chosen cases were diverse, ranging from large metropolitan areas to relatively small communities, from local county agencies to interstate ones. The conclusions were striking: "even in communities where health planning resulted in impressive studies, precious few concrete goals were implemented" (p. 17). Remember that these are the *successful* attempts at planning. San Mateo was called a "success story," exhibiting "strong government-based leadership in community health planning" (p.31). In Rochester, former HEW secretary Marion Folsom nearly single-handedly brought about "major improvements in county-wide health services between 1961 and 1966" (p. 50). Cincinnati's community health planning "was probably as far advanced as it was in most other urban communities across the country in the 1960's" (p. 70). The Hospital and Health Council of Lincoln, Nebraska, has "moved modestly but assuredly towards tackling the problems of community health planning" (p. 83). Neither Cincinnati's nor Lincoln's planning effort had "any adequate or sustained authority or sanctions," however (p. 103). The state of Maryland's progress toward its goals was "modest" (p. 94). The author summarized the results of the studies by saying that the " 'success stories' were not very impressive successes (on their own terms) once the whole story was laid out" (p. 14).

The author had a number of possible explanations for these findings. First, "civic leaders believe health problems are being adequately met by existing services" (p. 17). Second, their "ignorance and apathy . . . leaves the field to self-interested professionals who are often more concerned about protecting their own jurisdictions than in coordinating functions with fellow agencies." Third, "comprehensive planning is considered radical in many influential quarters" (p. 17). Thus the conservatism, ignorance, and apathy of civic leadership allowed the health professionals more autonomy than they would otherwise have had. As the author's second point indicates, this was not a positive indication, because in

local health circles the professionals who run agencies constitute interests that are entrenched and frequently uncommunicative and self-protective. Civic leaders who serve on agency boards become identified with the professional interest and reinforce them. Certain other local interests are well served by inadequate or loosely enforced health regulations and also resist disturbing the status quo. Hence, we have found, the most effective blocks to inter-community or metropolitan health planning are the very persons who comprise the cadre of local health services—the same ones whose agencies would be and should be the principal participants in area-wide health planning. Realistically, they are also the ones whose position and status are most threatened by changes that planning recommendations might generate. (pp. 17–18)

From Conant's study we can thus infer that there was *no* commitment to comprehensive health planning at the community, state, inter-community, or inter-regional level in the United States if these cases are a fair sample of the *best* that has been achieved. Conant himself said that there "is in fact no firm or widespread commitment to (or understanding of) community health planning . . . anywhere in the United States except among a relatively small number of professional health planners" (pp. 99–100). (Conant places his hopes in the federal government, without indicating why he thinks its programs contribute to positive health planning.)

The reasons for the lack of comprehensive health planning lie in the conservatism of local leadership, combined with the vested interests of local health professionals in maintaining the existing division of responsibilities, services, and resources. Clearly we are dealing here with an interdependent *system*. The scaling down of Conant's criteria for judging "successful" planning—from the "rational use of public and private resources . . . in such a way as to meet all important health problems in the community" to the achievement of "relationships" among planners and the "participation" of different groups—is a mark of the extent to which students of policy-making in America are imprisoned by what they regard as pragmatic political realities. But there is a more important trap. Despite Conant's analysis of the health professionals as being a vested interest, he regards their participation as illustration or evidence of the *effectiveness* of planning, simply because they are an important interest group. This underlying pluralist assumption runs through most of this literature but gives evidence more of a political judgment than an analytic position. It may be precisely the existence of a pluralist system—in which all existing groups have the right to be heard and represented and to have a veto power over all programs which they define as challenging their basic jurisdictions and resources—which *prevents* any effective action from being taken to establish comprehensive health planning. Pluralism has become identified with democracy, so that any challenge of the legitimacy of the participation of a group which already has established its power and resources can be ruled out.

The problem is to discover just how the pluralist system works, how it manages to *throttle* effective action and *reduce* coordination to manipulation in order to secure greater resources for existing component units (whether from local, state, or federal sources). This is politically analogous to the procedures adopted by members of an oligopolistic industry in which all members are protected, even the weaker ones, once they have become members of the club.

The prevailing norm of optimism—that problems can be solved and that there can be progress, given devoted leadership—is illustrated by Conant's report, the tone and mood of which contradicts the substance of his conclusions. However, he finds some hope in the examples of "strong" leadership set by Dr. Chope in San Mateo and Mr. Folsom in Rochester. In the midst of the failure of institutions, one looks for a charismatic leader somehow to rescue us.

At least Conant gives a brief and clear description of the failure of planning. But the foreword to the study, written by the chairman of the Community Action Studies Project Committee, would give the casual reader an entirely different picture. Dr. George James (M.D., M.P.H.), a New York health professional, summarized Conant's study as follows: "Clearly discernible under Dr. Conant's microscope were the thrust and driving power of qualities of leadership—unquestioned, number one reason why the five communities enjoy national acclaim for their vigorous action against health problems" (p. 3). The five communities not only have "long records of achievement in health," but also are among those United States communities which "have enjoyed outstanding success in providing acceptable health services for their citizens" (p. 3).

Contrast this picture of Dr. Conant's study with his own conclusions, which have already been given in detail. These alleged successes are "not very impressive successes (on their own terms). . . . Precious few concrete goals were implemented." Civic leaders exhibit "ignorance and apathy" about local health problems. Local health professionals are "the most effective blocks to inter-community or metropolitan health planning." One begins to suspect that the groups which sponsor such studies as Dr. Conant's are part of that cadre of health professionals which resists any fundamental changes in the structure of the American medical system. The report is another one of a long series of investigations, commission reports, and studies, a number of which have already been summarized, which begin with an assumption of crisis and end with soothing words about progress toward leadership, planning, and coordination. Still another level of coordination and supervision will be recommended, or yet more studies. None of these grapples with substantive issues. More "participation" will occur, more meetings, conferences, and reports will take place or be written.

In one 1972 study which Clark Havighurst cited, only twenty percent of 128 health planning agencies surveyed could "project . . . a matter so elementary as the facility needs in their area" and fewer than fifty percent "knew the bed needs in their area for the current year." As Havighurst noted, many planners rationalize the absence of basic data by viewing planning as a "dynamic, political process."[9] "Planning" becomes holding meetings, consulting, and communicating, not hard analysis of empirical data on the consequences of alternative policy decisions.

The very mechanisms which are intended to insure planning guarantee that no planning takes place. The mechanisms of coordination become instruments of the status quo. And this is by no means accidental. The major parties to these investigations, councils, and commissions do not intend to "change the system." They wish to reinforce it, or at the most to allow only a little change—a few more hospitals will be built, new laundries will be constructed, affiliation of a clinic or hospital with a medical school will be achieved, a nursing program will begin. (These are the achievements of Marion Folsom, the well-known health leader of Rochester, who, incidentally, wrote the preface to Conant's study.)

Note that none of these achievements constitutes community planning in Conant's sense of the "rational use of private and public resources." They are analogous to the expansion of production by some commercial firms—it may be progress that another shoemaking plant is built or a new suburban development begun. People need shoes and houses just as they need medical care, but the building of a shoe factory or fifty new suburban homes is not necessarily a rational use of private and public resources. Quite the contrary. The shoes made in the factory may merely add another style to the seventy-five available, using up valuable natural resources not only in the factory, but also in the land it occupies and in the leather it uses. The suburban homes may use resources of labor and raw materials which might better be used in low-income apartments, given a rational assessment of the needs of the local population, and they may destroy farm land or open countryside.

Similarly, the mere citation of expansion of facilities—programs, buildings—is not evidence at all that there has been any advance toward meeting the "important health problems in the community," to use Conant's words. The assumption is that physical capacity, growth, expansion, and new programs are prima facie evidence of, first, effective coordination and the exercise of leadership—when they may actually indicate a failure of properly coordinated action to stop the expansion and also indicate the disorganization of opposition leadership; and, second, better medical services to the community—when they may actually indicate over-elaborate and expensive medical technology which is duplicative and unnecessary or simply an addition to the prestige of the hospital. In short, health "planning," like much if not most of other attempts at health reform, is more rhetoric than substance, reinforcing rather than undermining control by either dominant or challenging interest groups.[10]

Even plans for existing and new health facilities in other cities which did not, apparently, stem from the discovery of a health care "crisis" are apparently no more thorough or any less fragmented than the ones from New York City that we have analyzed. A survey[11] of thirty-three "areawide health plans" in as many communities, conducted in 1970 by a wide variety of local, state, private, and public agencies, found that: (1) the plans "devote scant attention to formulation and selection of alternative long-range goals and short-range objectives" (p. 86); (2) the plans "publish health information [on the prevalence of health or disease conditions, on utilization, and on health resources) but virtually neglect to examine its implications or to relate it to specific policy issues bearing on future health service systems" (p. 87); (3) the plans "assume that a health service area exists—that is, an area for which coordinated facilities and service should be planned. But only a few reports discuss the criteria for defining a service area, indicate the importance of defined standards, or state the basic assumptions" (p. 89); (4) "only a few plans considered specific issues related to implementation of their recommendations" (p. 91); and (5) "only a few of the plans emphasize long-range improvements or specify a target date for the implementation of recommendations" (p. 92). Although the authors of this review assert that "the crisis in medical care has led to many proposals for change in the health service system and to a variety of health planning structures" (p. 82), most of these areawide health plans "do not describe or evaluate alternative approaches or consider the interrelationships of various elements of health service systems. Too often the plans give the impression that there are no hard choices or major decisions to be made, either openly or by default, and limit their goals to patching weak spots in existing services" (p. 92).

It is interesting that the authors reach this conclusion for almost all the studies, regardless of their sponsorship. The authors agree that there has been a clear and nearly unanimous call by health reformers of whatever stripe for expanded outpatient services which would minimize expensive hospital stays, for "deliberate integration of hospitals into a network of health facilities and services" (p. 83), and for more efficient utilization of medical and nursing staffs. The failure of these areawide health plans to consider these broad alternatives leads the authors to suggest that rather than taking the "systematic approach of comprehensive planning," one should consider that "the most effective pathway to major changes in the health system may consist of a series of individual innovative programs." The authors note that "recent innovations have occurred in the planning of specific projects—such as neighborhood health centers or new hospital-based community programs—but they are hard to find in the plans covered in our survey" (p. 93). From the point of view of a health planner, this is a counsel of despair, because it is precisely the addition of one "innovative" program after another which has created many of the chaotic conditions about which these authors were and are concerned.

An academic public health planner, basing his evaluation on interviews, personal participation, and reviews of reports of Comprehensive Health Planning agencies in thirteen states and forty agencies, came to conclusions essentially the same as those stated here. There was a "lack of an organized information base upon which to do health planning," a concern with the "politics of representation, not leadership," the "disease of 'planning for planning,' " a failure to define problems, let alone programs, and "grossly inadequate funding to provide plans for comprehensive health care delivery."[12]

The Health Planning Councils established under the Comprehensive Health Planning Act of 1966 (P.L. 89-749) are nonprofit *private* agencies, although they are financed with public funds and are created for no other purpose than to apply for federal grants. One analysis of the legal framework for health planning says that "the root problem with Wisconsin's [the focus of their case study] form of voluntarism in health planning is that the regional planning agencies are private corporations performing what amounts to a public function."[13]

These private agencies are still another example of the way in which power is delegated from public authorities to private bodies in a successful attempt to combine apparent action with actual inaction, and thus prevent tangible "planning." Because these agencies are generated by federal funds, obviously their characteristics are found not only in New York City but also elsewhere. Health Planning Councils are symbolic agencies cut loose without enough direction, funds, or power to accomplish anything related to the tasks the legislation charges them with.

3. State and National
   Investigations and Plans for
   Reform

Both state and national commissions of investigations into health care employ practically the same rhetoric and come to the same conclusions as those reports previously described for New York City.[14] It seems likely that within a given society, where there is a struggle between interest groups for control of valued resources, the ideological strategies followed will be similar regardless of the "level" of the political system in which the struggle occurs.

The technique of appointing commissions of inquiry is not peculiar to New York, to health, or to the period from 1950 to the present. In the area of health, the Committee on the Costs of Medical Care is perhaps the most important national predecessor to those examined here. This committee operated from 1927 to 1932, produced twenty-eight "basic publications," an "impressive, comprehensive sweep of existing conditions and of the problems of providing, organizing, and financing medical services of good quality whose scale has not yet been duplicated." This group, interlocked with the Commission on Medical Education (three persons served jointly), was the "product of public and professional concern designed to reconcile the accelerating progress of scientific medicine in the major centers with the delivery of care to the population"[15]

The committee majority "recommended that medical personnel

should be organized in group medical practices, each including physicians, dentists, nurses, and technical personnel, and each preferably focused on a hospital. Group practice would be supported by an extension and reinforcement of public health services, governmental and private, thus spreading the costs of disease prevention" (p. 183). It also "deliberately suggested an integrated scheme whereby the providers as well as the consumers of health services would be brought into cooperative relationships. The two outstanding problems of contemporary medicine—rapidly increasing costs and steadily increasing specialization in equipment and personnel—would be dealt with together" (p. 184). Contrary to the minority (which included the AMA representatives) and the urgings of subsequent AMA attacks, the majority did *not* recommend compulsory health insurance or "government competition" with the private practitioners. The minority opposed "both voluntary and compulsory health insurance. It was only too happy, however, to recognize the duty of the state to give complete and adequate care to the indigent, thus freeing private physicians from responsibility for an unprofitable part of their practice" (p. 186).[16]

Their modest recommendations were "left unimplemented by either the private or the public sector" (p. 187). The Social Security Act of 1935, a logical place to include health insurance, was passed without any (p. 188). Needless to say, almost the same prediction can be made for most of the recommendations made by the New York City investigations we have surveyed.

The analyses of the health "crisis" in more recent state and national reports contain themes similar to those of the city investigations. An example is Governor Rockefeller's 1971 Steering Committee on Social Problems. Its report emphasized that the health "crisis" is a result *not* of shortages per se of anything—whether beds, physicians, dollars, or physician assistants (allied health manpower)—but rather maldistribution. Although the report does not generalize in this way, we might term this overabundance an "anarchy of production," almost in the classic image of a capitalist economy.

Consider its manifestations. With respect to manpower, for example, Boston "has one of the nation's greatest complexes of medical institutions [but] a severe shortage of general care practitioners" (p. 12). Two percent of medical school graduates in 1970 became general practitioners (p. 14). There are also "too many ancillary personnel—but... they are not adequately trained and not effectively deployed" (p. 22). With respect to beds, "we estimate that we need 450,000 short-term hospital beds—we now have 800,000 such beds" (p. 21). And duplication of facilities: "Needless competition [by hospitals for costly but underused equipment] results in tremendous waste of scarce resources and funds" (p. 13). And mortality rates were sharply higher in hospitals where surgeons performed few operations such as open-heart surgery. With respect to funds, increasing costs and subsidies act as an incentive to expand facilities and add to the inflation. Total expenditures on health rose from $26 billion in 1960 to $67 billion in 1970, from 5.3 percent of the gross national product to 7 percent. Two-thirds of the 1970 total was personal health expenditures, with half of this due to price increases, not to more use of services or more advanced technology. This "overproduction" of health manpower and facilities is distributed in such a way as to maintain a "two-class health system—one for the poor and a better one for those able to pay their own way. . . . The nation's poor people have been receiving inadequate and, at times, inexcusable care and treatment" (pp. 8, 15).

Using the words of the 1967 report of the National Advisory Commission on Health Manpower, the Rockefeller committee report summarized the state of affairs: "medical care in the United States is more a collection of bits and pieces (with overlapping, duplication, great gaps, high costs and wasted effort) than an integrated system in which needs and efforts are closely related." But, according to the Rockefeller committee, "the situation is more acute than four years ago, and deteriorating rapidly" (p. 41).

This picture is restated in every diagnosis of the "crisis" of the health system. The figures portray dynamics without change: a rapid increase in almost every index of growth—dollars, manpower, programs— except those pertaining to quality, distribution, accessibility, and reasonable cost to the consumer.

It should be noted that the empirical criteria and basis for the judgments of quality and the adequacy of quantity and distribution were not given in this report, nor are the basic data available which would be necessary to evaluate either a specific health service or the character of coordination of diverse health institutions. The reasons for this absence of information will be discussed later in a more theoretical context; the point here is that the many critiques of the health system are neither cumulative nor based on solid research and thus have an ideological character, rooted in images and theories about the proper way to reorganize and coordinate the system.

The Rockefeller committee, without quite saying so, attributed many of the defects of health care to the interests of the physicians, the "dominant profession."[17] The physicians have defined "health and medical care in very restricted terms," leaving out preventive medicine (pp. 18, 64). "Most clinics serving poor people are structured for the convenience of the doctor, not the patient" (p. 38). "Much care now given by a physician does not require a physician's level of training and education" (p. 64). The physicians, and especially those allied occupations which have not yet achieved similar professional controls over their incomes and work, exhibit a "great deal of sensitivity about professionalism and status" (p. 65). The committee noted the resulting situation: "We are impressed with the number of meritorious proposals for change which have been ignored, and with the tendency of the health care establishment to resist such change" (p. 23).

In a barely concealed attack on the interests of the professional monopolists in maintaining their power and privileges, the Rockefeller committee recommended coordinating all health services around hospitals into Health Center Complexes, employing "modern management approaches" (p. 57), utilizing machinery for "internal planning and systems development," and, perhaps most important, establishing "utilization controls." The recommended system would, ideally, cover the entire population for 75 percent of their medical bills (100 percent for the poor) (p. 76).

While not expressly advocating salaries for physicians, the utilization controls would exclude any public funds being used for health care services "found to be unnecessary in accordance with generally accepted practice"; furthermore, no charge would be honored which "exceeds the prevailing level of charges in the community" (pp. 57-58).

The committee accepted the hospital as the central health provider in our society. The hospital, with some qualifications, was seen as the "core of a broader health care corporation responsible for assuring comprehensive health care to a defined service area" (p. 52). Such a corporation should be franchised or licensed by a state and should participate meaningfully in "area, state and regional health care planning and regulation" (p. 54). The result should be a network of community preventive services and ambulatory and home care, integrated with in-hospital care and linked to nursing homes and extended care facilities.

Such a system would invade several traditional professional prerogatives. The proposals by the committee to end restrictive licensing of health professionals, to open up medical schools, and to reduce the length of time for training a physician challenge professional control over their own supply and over their market (p. 68). The proposals to establish physician assistants would challenge the monopoly of physicians over important areas of primary health care. As the report says, a Washington pilot program indicates that physician assistants "can perform a series of jobs with even greater skill than most physicians" (p. 70). The proposals to expand prepaid group practice and to review utilization and fees challenge the sole control by physicians over their incomes and conditions of work and thus directly undercut their professional monopoly (p. 82). Finally, the proposal to allocate health professionals, after their first training, to areas short of health manpower in return for a waiver of loans constitutes, in effect, an invasion by the government of the right of the new physician to choose his own area of practice (p. 72).

These major proposals by a New York state commission to reorganize and coordinate the health delivery system are clearly parallel to those already analyzed for New York City. They go much further, in fact, in explicitly challenging existing professional monopolies and presenting an alternative image of rational corporate organization of health care production.

Federal commissions of investigation also use the same rhetoric and come to the same kinds of conclusions. The federal role in health will be considered in more detail later in the context of the effect of vacillating federal programs and funds on urban health programs, but the assumptions which rationalize policy making at the national level seem to be similar to those at the state and city levels. One recent panel seems typical of national study groups. It was composed of ten university professors or administrators concerned with the health sciences, an executive of a systems analysis firm, two foundation executives, and one banker, a typical array of institutions and organizations representing the structural interest of corporate rationalization. The rhetoric of the recommendations reflects this perspective perfectly. The descriptive classification of recommended health services research and development areas is replete with terms suggesting the possibility of rational "systems" organization of health care: integration, coordination, regionalization, model, planning, strategies, information systems, effectiveness, evaluation, manpower, technology, automation, and measurement.[18]

Nor is the mentality of corporate rationalization confined to government-appointed commissions. It is also—appropriately—expressed by those key interest groups such as the American Hospital Association representing a challenging structural interest. While it is beyond our scope to discuss the proposals presented by such organizations in detail, one example may show that the logic and assumptions of this particular type of health reform are found elsewhere than in New York or in other government agencies.

AMERIPLAN was proposed by the American Hospital Association in 1970 as their contribution to the solutions of the health crisis.[19] It doesn't diagnose the situation, but it does present a cure. The report is an excellent example of a model of corporate rationalization of health services. It was prepared by a committee and staff appointed by the American Hospital Association: the chairman, Earl Perloff, was chairman of the board of Albert Einstein Medical Center and also chairman of the board of Philadelphia General Hospital; the other fourteen members of the committee included only three physicians, and none of these was in private practice (one was chairman of the Department of Medicine at Northwestern, and the other two were administrators of group practices); ten of the remaining eleven members held administrative posts of various kinds (including two in health organizations with the word "systems" in the title).

The core of AMERIPLAN was the establishment of Health Service Corporations chartered by State Health Commissions brought into being in turn by a National Health Commission established by federal legislation. These corporations would actually be health care providers and would "synthesize management, personnel, and facilities into a corporate structure with the capacity and responsibility to deliver the five components of comprehensive health care to the community: health maintenance, primary care, specialty care, restorative care, and health-related custodial care" (p. 7). A corporation "would ordinarily be formed by existing health care provider organizations; it could result from merger; it could be a local government authority or a private corporation." And, "many types of organizations could participate with health care providers in the formation of a . . . Corporation" (p. 16). The corporation could either provide care itself or contract for services with other providers, but regardless of its mode of provision, it would "cooperate directly with professional organizations established to evaluate the quality and adequacy of care" (p. 17).

Naturally, relations with physicians would be crucial, and from our previously stated hypotheses we would expect that the plan would gloss over the problem of control of the corporation, minimize the possibility of conflict, or try to co-opt the physicians. Sure enough, while granting that "all medical judgments related to health care must be made by or under the supervision of physicians" and agreeing that the corporation must "provide incentives to attract physicians to practice within the Health Care Corporation," AMERIPLAN affirmed that physician staff privileges must be "established through rules and regulations in accordance with his training, experience, and professional competence as measured by peer review of his credentials and performance." But, as an added incentive, they argued for bringing the "physician into the management structure and involve him in its decision-making process" (p. 24). Later the same point was repeated and expanded: that "physicians, along with professional administrators, must have a major role in deciding how institutional services should be organized, how health personnel should be deployed, how care could be rendered economically, and how evaluation should be made of the effectiveness of health services" (p. 53). It should be amply clear by now that such a statement ignores the deep divisions of interest between the professionals—both the solo practitioners and the specialists—on the one hand and the managers, administrators, and planners on the other. The whole thrust of this plan is clearly toward subordinating the physicians within a functionally coordinated system of health practitioners allocated to geographic areas and population service groups according to some reasonably rational criteria substituted for the present criteria of physician income, convenience of location, and access to a favorite clientele.

Once again, it is beside my main point to go into great detail about AMERIPLAN, and it is not my concern to criticize it as it stands—as a plan for reorganizing and innovating in health service delivery. The authors of the plan themselves were uncomfortably aware of the difficulties and were hoping to create "acceptance of the philosophy of AMERIPLAN and its emphasis on comprehensive health care and particularly, health maintenance and ambulatory care" (p. 49) as part of the painful process of transition. They acknowledged that "without a nationwide effort to coordinate such trends what is likely to result is continued fragmentation and the development of yet another inchoate, uncoordinated system." Unfortunately, in the absence of serious consideration of the conflicting interests and their base in law, custom, and organization, that is the probable outcome.

4. "Fragmentation" in Other
Policy Areas

Health policy is analogous to many other recent social problems which have required both federal and local action. As Rosemary Stevens said:

Like air pollution control (1963), community action programs (1964), neighborhood youth corps programs (1964), neighborhood facilities programs (1965), demonstration cities (1966), and the many other federal assistance activities developed in the 1960s, effectiveness depends on local coordination, planning, and control; in short, a diffuse federal bureaucracy must be matched by strong state and community initiative. But at the same time, to encourage such initiative, coordination is required among assistance programs at the federal level so that they do in fact provide assistance and support to local groups. In administering many of the programs of the Great Society of the mid-1960s, neither effective local initiative nor effective federal assistance has been forthcoming; again, Medicaid provides a classic example. . . . In the last ten years, therefore, the concept of governmental decentralization has partly given way to that of centralization, at least in terms of effective federal analysis, monitoring, management, and coordination of domestic welfare policies.[20]

Although Stevens ended on an optimistic note, there is no evidence that such effective analysis and coordination have taken or can take place. She assumed casually that the "requirement" for effective federal action will be met, simply because of the "need" for it, and that the proper "balance" between decentralization of services and centralization of direction, standards, and control will be found. She did not present any argument or evidence for this as a realistic possibility in the near future, however. Like most liberal analysts, she assumed that the combination of need, knowledge, and resources will generate, at some point, a rational reorganization at all levels, although she predicted that a pluralism of types of services and funding will be retained.

An array of examples from still other policy areas shows both that health is not unique and that such optimism is not warranted. The same pattern is found in government housing policy, which exhibits the same proliferation of federal agencies with overlapping and sometimes conflicting requirements. One program after another has been enacted by the federal government but has not been carried out because not enough money has been authorized to enable any of them to meet their goals. Such a strategy of inaction "has nevertheless created the illusion of a full-fledged federal assault on the problem. In Washington as the 1970's began there were some four dozen housing programs with a maze of rules, regulations, and fine-print procedures."[21]

A similar situation is found for environmental health services. A recent article provides a summary statement focused on air resources, water resources, waste disposal, and noise abatement in California. The political milieu (California versus New York) and the substance of the policy area (environment versus health) differ considerably, and yet the pattern was found to be the same. In 1971 there were 500 different "environmental programs" in California, provided by 127 different types of agencies. Not agencies, but *types*. Of the 127 in California in 1968, there were 40 *types* of special districts, with *3,811* special *districts* "of which the vast majority provide service directly related to the quality of the environment."[22] Of the 127 types of agencies providing environmental health services, there were 9 *federal* departments (with 74 operating bureaus); 18 "major independent agencies, commissions and councils"; 16 *state* departments plus 16 "offices, boards and commissions," excluding purely advisory boards; 6 *regional* types; 10 *county* types; and 12 *city* types of agencies. Note, lest the numbers get confusing, that they were using Los Angeles County as a model; LA County had each of the 10 county types, so that for the state as a whole there were 10 times approximately 70 counties—or, 700 agencies in California concerned with the quality of the environment.

The authors concluded that "no rational allocation of functions exists among different levels of government"; that "the same or similar functions are performed by different agencies at the same level of government with respect to the same environmental field"; and that "at the same level of government and in the same environmental field, functions that are interdependent and should be allied are split among different agencies" (p. 431). Even when large administrative units are set up for certain purposes, they still "reflect the fragmented approach" (p. 427).

The consequences of this multiplicity of jurisdictions were serious: (1) "gaps or deficiencies in services"; (2) "inefficient use of ... manpower"; (3) "duplication in facilities"; (4) "inadequate... financial resources"; (5) "weak mechanisms for coordination"; (6) "insufficient representation of the public"; and (7) "constricted planning" (p. 433).

Unfortunately, although it summarized the present situation, the article presented no analysis of the causes of this phenomenon, and thus the recommendations essentially constituted another plea for administrative reorganization. The solution recommended was a "regional environmental quality control board," which would "provide leadership in charting environmental policy, encourage affirmative improvement in the environment and balance competing interests and use of resources" (p. 451). By contrast to previous methods and various alternatives discussed, such regional boards "would have the virtue of *tying together* the disparate efforts in environmental planning and service and of still preserving the *specialized expertise* that has been built up by operating agencies" (pp. 453-54; italics added). How all of these good things would be accomplished—how the new boards would rise above the chaos—was not argued, only asserted.

Education exhibits the same pattern, if one study of Boston can be taken as a fair sample. Boston is not "immune to change or innovation." The Boston public schools are now "fairly littered with demonstration projects and experiments, head starts, preschools, enrichments, compensatory programs, second chances, reading laboratories, summer reviews, pilot schools, team-teaching trials, and a whole host of other departures. . . . But so far, the system's long list of changes. . . has had almost no effect on educational substance for most of the children most of the time.[23]

The picture is the same for social welfare programs: "In spite of the efforts to coordinate services to assist the 'multiproblem family,' primary emphasis continues to be on the traditional caseworker approach. Services remain fragmented and uncoordinated; traditional methods provide no significant amelioration of the problems of the poor; and attempts to provide better services seem to lead primarily, as in the areas of health and education, to the hiring of more personnel, thereby creating an additional layer of bureaucracy and new jobs for the professionals."[24]

Still another example is found in manpower programs. "Coordination among the major federal agencies competing for preeminence in the manpower field was frequently discussed in the 1960s, but little was accomplished."[25] Several efforts to solve the jurisdictional conflicts were made, but various arrangements "did nothing to reduce conflict between the rival agencies and led to mind-boggling administrative complexities" (p. 6). As the author of this study put it, "program fragmentation is a product not only of agency rivalries but also, and more fundamentally, of the manner in which policies are formulated and sustained in a pluralist political system. As each new pressing need is identified and publicized, a remedy or palliative is fashioned in the form of a governmental program. Thus governmental involvement tends to be a mosaic of single-purpose efforts, with inevitable discord" (p. 7). This generalization, it should be remembered, comes from a study not of health but of adult basic education, on-the-job training, prevocational and skill training, and a variety of other manpower programs found in dozens of agencies.

The factual accuracy and detail of these descriptions of health, housing, the environment, education, social welfare, and manpower programs could of course be expanded and debated at great length, as well as the question of whether or not these examples are representative of most types of public policies and administrative programs. My point here is only to emphasize that the detailed picture of health policy and reform undoubtedly has its counterparts in other policy areas.

To summarize and conclude, there is considerable evidence indicating that with respect to both the state of health care itself and attempts to improve it via commissions of investigation and health planning leading to a coordinated health delivery system, New York shares many characteristics with other cities and with the nation. But this tentative generalization merely raises again the basic question with which I started this inquiry: How can the pluralism of interest-group competition which results in the fragmentation both of health care and of attempts to plan and reform it be explained?

5   Structural Interests and Structural Reform

The repeated criticisms and recommendations made by the numerous New York City commissions of investigation into health care and the difficulty of establishing ambulatory care facilities in the city—outpatient clinics and neighborhood health centers—are disparate symptoms of some pervasive structural diseases in American health care institutions. Yet most studies have not dealt systematically with the way in which dominant structural interests have created barriers to significant change in those institutions. Neither has this one; but in the course of this research it has become apparent that just another report of defects and patch-up jobs will add nothing to the array of such documents. Therefore, the following two chapters present some hypotheses concerning the underlying causes of the diverse phenomena described previously. It must be emphasized that, despite references to a number of studies, most of the generalizations offered in the following chapters are *not* supported by historical and empirical studies but rather are an attempt at a *theoretical* synthesis based on assumptions about the functioning of structural interests in a market economy and the way in which state power is appropriated to serve those interests. It is not claimed that the substantive studies reported in chapters 2 and 3 provide supporting data—only that they are consistent with the theory.

1. Major Structural Interests

Strategies of reform based only on the "bureaucratic" or "market" models (see chapter 1) are unlikely to work. Both types of reform stress certain core functions in the health system and regard others as secondary. But both neglect the way in which the modes of organizing these functions create groups which come to develop vital interests sustaining the present system and vitiating attempts at reform.

For the market reformers, supplying trained physicians, innovating through biomedical and technological research, and maintaining competition between diverse health care producers are the main functions to be performed. They view the hospitals, medical schools, and public health agencies as only the organizational framework which sustains the primary functions of professional health care and biomedical research. However, these types of work become buttressed through institutional mechanisms which guarantee professional control, and they come to constitute the powerful structural interest which I have called "professional monopoly." Because these interests are at present the dominant ones, with their powers and resources safely embedded in law, custom, professional legitimacy, and the practices of many public and private organizations, they do not need to be as visibly active or as cohesively organized as those groups seeking change.

For the bureaucratic reformers, the hospitals, medical schools, and public health agencies at all governmental levels perform the core functions of organizing, financing, and distributing health care. Hospitals are seen ideally as the center of networks of associated clinics and neighborhood health centers, providing comprehensive care to an entire local population. The bureaucratic reformers view physicians and medical researchers as performing crucial work but, when in their proper place, as subordinated and differentiated parts of a complex delivery system, coordinated by bureaucrats, notably hospital administrators. However, these large-scale organizations represent an increasingly powerful structural interest, which I have called "corporate rationalization." These interest groups are at present the major challengers of the power of the professional monopolists, and they constitute the bulk of the membership of the various commissions of investigation and inquiry into the health care "crisis."

A third type of reform group is relatively unimportant in the American context as yet: the "equal-health advocates," who seek free, accessible, high-quality health care which equalizes the treatment available to the well-to-do and to the poor. They stress the importance of community control over the supply and deployment of health facilities, because they base their strategies upon repressed structural interests: those of the local population or community affected by the availability and character of health personnel and facilities. A community population cannot be organized as easily as can interest groups representing dominant or challenging structural interests, but obviously it has an equally great stake in the outcomes of the operations of health institutions.

Each of these three major types of structural interests is internally heterogeneous. Professional monopoly is represented by biomedical researchers, physicians in private or group practice, salaried physicians, and those in other health occupations holding or seeking professional privileges and status, all of whom differ in their relations to each other and to hospitals, medical schools, insurance plans, and government agencies. Their interests are thus affected differently by various programs of reform. But they share an interest in maintaining autonomy and control over the conditions of their work, and professional interest groups will—when that autonomy is challenged—act together in defense of that interest.

Corporate rationalization is furthered by medical schools, public health agencies, insurance companies, hospitals, and health planning agencies. Their respective organizational interests often require that they compete with each other for powers and resources. Although they differ in the priority they attach to various reform proposals, they share an interest in maintaining and extending the control of their organizations over the work of the professionals whose activities are key to the achievement of organizational goals.

The community population constitutes a set of potential interest groups which are internally heterogeneous with respect to their health needs, ability to pay, and ability to organize their needs into effective demands, but they share an interest in maximizing the responsiveness of health professionals and organizations to their concerns for accessible high-quality health care.

My assumption in making these key distinctions is that the similarities of structural location vis-à-vis each other of these major structural interests warrant an emphasis on the common aspects of each rather than on their internal differentiation. If my concern were to explain the actions of various individuals and groups with respect to a particular piece of legislation or administrative decision, lumping diverse groups and individuals together into a single structural interest would be entirely too crude. But for the purposes of explaining the main contours of the present system, its resistance to certain kinds of change, and its readiness to adopt others, finer distinctions would entail a short-term time perspective. Differences which are extremely important for tactics may be in the long run relatively unimportant for the explanation of major conflicts and structural changes.

The danger of this mode of analysis, however, is that the internal contradictions within each structural interest and type of reformer may be the source of potential strategic alliances which may have great long-term implications. For example, the vision of an ideal health system which erases the distinction between those who pay and those who don't is held up by many bureaucratic reformers as well as by the equal-health advocates. And, in the abstract, both the goal of personalized care (defended by some as viable only through fee-for-service medicine) and the goal of coordinated, comprehensive care (defended by others as possible only through hospital-organized health care) are hard to question.

But the question of whether or not these goals of personalized service and comprehensive care are sheer ideological rationalizations of its power and privileges by one or another interest group may be irrelevant if the goals can be used as a weapon for critical attack upon the inadequacies of health care. Corporate rationalizers properly accuse professional monopolists of not providing the personalized care which justifies their claim to fee-for-service practice. Professional monopolists properly accuse corporate rationalizers of not being concerned with personalized care in their drive for efficient, high-technology health care. In both cases the contradictions between rhetoric and performance provide an opportunity to the equal-health advocates to show the deficiencies in analysis and program of both dominant and challenging interests.

Differences between dominant and challenging interests should not be overemphasized, however, because both professional monopoly and corporate rationalization are modes of organizing health care within the context of a market society. Both must avoid encroachments upon their respective positions of power and privilege which depend upon the continuation of market institutions: the ownership and control of individual labor, facilities, and organizations (even nonprofit ones) by autonomous groups and individuals, with no meaningful mechanisms of public control. (The instruments of political control allegedly available to the community population are fictitious, as will be seen later.)

Corporate rationalization may thus be furthered by certain market reforms, if that will provide more doctors for the hospitals, more researchers for the medical schools, and more potential workers for medical corporations, and if it will subject these workers to market pressures which in turn will make them tractable employees. Professional monopoly may thus be furthered by certain bureaucratic reforms, particularly those aspects of planning and coordination which safeguard professional interests, or administrative rules in hospitals which guarantee continued professional dominance of medical practice.

2. Professional Monopoly

Although physicians are the most important interest group representing professional monopoly, this structural interest also includes other occupations entitled to a monopoly over certain kinds of work, either an entrepreneurial position guaranteed by law and custom or an official position defined by the hierarchy of statuses within an organization. Their incomes are derived from private practice or from foundations, governments, and universities, but they are able to exploit organizational resources for their personal and professional interests. They can be called "monopolistic" because, buttressed by the traditions of their professions and/or institutions, they have nearly complete control over the conditions of their work and because usually there is no other way to show their effectiveness except through a demonstration grant or research project or by contracting with them to perform their professional services. Frequently a clinic or health center will be set up which, although providing services, is established mainly for other purposes of the persons who hold power (and these are not always or even usually the operating staff): research, training, professional aggrandizement, power within their "home" institutions, or the prestige of extending their professional empire.

Within organizations, the major consequence of the activity of professional monopolists is a continuous proliferation of programs and projects which are established in a wide variety of ways, under many auspices, and with many sources of funding, and which undoubtedly in most cases provide real services of some kind. The professional monopolists who set them up provide a symbolic screen of legitimacy while maintaining power in their own hands through various organizational devices. A continuous flow of symbols will reassure the funding or allegedly controlling publics or constituencies about the functions being performed, while the individuals or groups which have a special interest in the income, prestige, or power generated by the agency are benefitting from its allocations of resources.

Thus, the symbolic screen will put off attempts at control or supervision by making them difficult as well as less likely (because the nominally superior agency will be reassured). The activities of the myriad projects and programs are almost impossible to plan or integrate because the interests of the individuals and groups which establish them contradict the interests of those who wish to control the functions suggested by the master symbols of the project: its title, the funding agency's contract with it, its annual report.

The professional monopolists, by and large, are satisfied with the status quo and do not form part of the market reformers, who regard them as performing the core health functions. The physicians and biomedical researchers are not in the vanguard proposing reforms, except when their powers and prerogatives are threatened by others. That physicians are not heavily represented on the various reformist committees and that the American Medical Association is losing membership and is continuously criticized for its political stance does not mean that physicians are losing power. The physicians in private practice and the voluntary hospitals still constitute the core of the health system. All of the federal, state, and local programs and projects which occupy so much time and energy of both types of reformers are still on the periphery of the health system. Almost none of the reports from numerous commissions of investigation and task forces defining the crisis and recommending solutions ever mention invading the territory of the private physicians and the voluntary hospitals.

The continuous control of the medical profession over the provision of medical services is a basic element of the American health system. As one author put it in 1932, "The legal ownership and ultimate control of the great bulk of capital invested in the practice of medicine in hospitals lies with the lay public, but the medical profession exercises a pervasive and in most instances a determining influence over the utilization of this capital and over the kinds of service which, through the use of this capital investment, are furnished to the community."[1] Twenty-three years later, the same author asserted that "the predominance of social capital has continued. Proprietary hospitals have diminished in absolute and relative importance.... More capital per physician is required than formerly."[2]

Physicians have extracted an arbitrary subset from the array of skills and knowledge relevant to the maintenance of health in a population, have successfully defined these as their property to be sold for a price, and have managed to create legal mechanisms which enforce that monopoly and the social beliefs which have mystified the population about the appropriateness and desirability of that monopoly.[3] The result of this professional monopoly by physicians has been the definition of most health problems as "illness," requiring specific and immediate diagnosis and treatment. Health care is activated by demands of persons defining themselves as "sick." Doctors, under pressure to "do" something for "sick" people, have an incentive because they are paid to do something and because patients accept the definition of the situation as one of sickness requiring medical activism: prescriptions, operations, and so forth.

The economic and professional power of physicians is not hard to document, and it is not necessary to go into great detail. A recent summary by economist Uwe Reinhardt makes the point: "physicians as a group have exercised a pervasive influence over the development of the sector and over resource allocation within that sector. . . . Current licensure laws in the health field virtually define the physician as the consumer's only legitimate, primary contact with the health-care system. . . . Through professional control over hospital accreditation and as members of individual hospital boards, physicians can, in practice, exert a powerful influence also over resource allocation within the hospital."[4]

A recent study of medical staff organization in hospitals concluded that hospitals with loosely structured medical staff organization—that is, those which make few attempts to control the behavior of physicians—are basically dominated by the medical staff who run the hospital as their "workshop." Such hospitals resist expansion of emergency room care, outpatient clinics, and other community services because of their commitment to the private practices of their attending physicians.[5] Even health reforms accommodate themselves to the existing interests and privileges of physicians. Medicare, for example, explicitly allows hospitals to provide doctors with free equipment and space.[6]

Professional power over supply also results in a distortion of training toward specialization. Responding to high status and income, too many medical students in the United States become specialists. "Although reasonable practices suggest that perhaps one-fifth of all physicians should be in the consulting specialties, approximately four-fifths of American physicians practice as specialists. Most numerous of all practitioners are the ones in the surgical specialties, and many observers believe that these practitioners are responsible for the fact that the rate of surgical operations in the United States is double the per-capita rate in England and Wales."[7] Also, contradicting the myth that internists and pediatricians substitute for the general practitioner, a survey found that the actual efforts of these specialists were "much more restricted than the replacement notion implies. The overelaboration of specialties, beyond the need for consultation or special skills, has resulted in a fragmented pattern of care and one not particularly

responsive to the human problems motivating much patient concern."[8]
Such a pattern especially contradicts the physician's claim that fee-for-service practice allows for the closest doctor-patient relationship. But these rational objections do not at all challenge the professional monopoly.

The external power of the profession also allows internal processes of increasing specialization to continue practically unchallenged. Once an occupation has gained a professional monopoly over the provision of services and the licensing of its own members, it continues to proliferate new and increasingly more specialized professions. Conflicts are endemic between specialist groups about their jurisdiction over various parts of the body and over symptoms which can be defined as belonging to particular diseases as well as about control over various medical techniques or machines. As Rosemary Stevens put it, "even in the relatively halcyon phase of specialty board development during the 1930s, problems of specialty stratification were becoming evident as each of fourteen independent specialty groups attempted to carve out the boundaries of its field, to define its content, to describe the function of certification, to establish recommended patterns of training, and—since the boards were professional organizations—to decide on acceptable modes of practice and behavior. Such issues emphasized that the definition of specialties was, at root, a political process, arising from the relative successes of interest groups."[9] In particular historical periods, these conflicts among specialty groups or between specialists and the general practitioners may be the most visible and important ones, but this does not contradict the general interest which all segments of the professional monopolists share in maintaining an institutional framework which guarantees the continuation of the *principle* of professional autonomy and control, regardless of internal conflict over the distribution of the powers and privileges involved.[10]

The success or failure of various groups in the practice of medicine to define their specialty as a professional monopoly probably has no relationship to the best scientific knowledge of disease or treatment. The rejection by the Council on Medical Education of the appeals by the abdominal surgeons for a separate specialty board has, as Stevens shows (pp. 336–39), no basis in any consistent principle. "There is something remarkably odd in a system which, in delineating in the name of the public what is a useful and proper area for specified graduate training and specialty regulation of physicians, relies on the number of partisans each side can muster" and on their success in placing their partisans on decision-making bodies (p. 339).

Within medicine itself there have been continuous battles not only between various types of specialists but also between the general practitioners and the specialists and between all of those already in the AMA and those without (the chiropractors, osteopaths, and optometrists being the main examples). According to economist Elton Rayack, "fundamentally, what is involved here is exactly the same kind of social conflict generated by the internal contradiction inherent in the concept of professionalism. . . . Organized medicine has frequently used that [professional] power as a restrictionist device, with socially undesirable results, in order to increase the incomes, power, and prestige of its members."[11] However, the general practitioners are caught in the trap of their own justification for their professional monopoly: the quality of care. The specialists can argue in their turn that only board-certified specialists should perform certain kinds of operations or procedures.

The limits to this spiral of ever-increasing specialization are probably not internal to the health care professions, but external—the degree to which the society will support the additional training and cost necessary for specialist care.

The professions face the political dilemma of maintaining a united front vis-à-vis outside threats and at the same time finding some viable method of dividing up the body and the spoils among themselves. The more they squabble—for example, over whether orthopedic or general surgeons have jurisdiction over fractures—the more they expose to the general public the mundane origins of the allegedly scientific basis for specialties. However, the more they maintain a united front, the more the technical and administrative basis for specialty dominance becomes reinforced. Thus, the potential specialties which are out in the professional cold, or losing ground, are forced in their own self-interest to fight back, regardless of the possible cost to the legitimacy of a professional united front facing such threats as group practice, universal insurance, or even socialized medicine. The progress of the medical division of labor further fragments the unity of the profession in confronting what might rationally seem to be a common enemy.

A recent book by medical sociologist Eliot Freidson summarizes the literature on the sources and nature of professional control of health care in the United States.[12] Freidson argues that organized medicine has "brought us to the present state of crisis in health services. It asserts its control over the performance of medical work at the same time its practitioners are too few to perform the work. It refuses to allow members of other occupations to perform such work except in a position of subordination from which they can gain little satisfaction. It insists on its jurisdiction over everything related to that vague word 'health,' including that vast, undifferentiated problem called 'mental illness' for which neither medicine nor any other discipline has demonstrated any consistently effective therapeutic solution" (p. 235). He shows that the monopoly of health services by individual practitioners is typical of a consumer-oriented industry dependent upon sales and volume. Professionalism provides a way of preserving monopolistic control over services without the risks of competition. Further, he asserts that "the present organization of medical practice systematically encourages the *average* physician to give indifferent medical care" (p. 70). While the average doctor in private practice is subject to the whims of patients who want something done for their pain, this is less likely in group or hospital practice. Also, the private doctor learns less from colleagues. "It is difficult to think of a worse way of organizing the practice of medicine than the traditional method I have described. The major pressures of the system are directed toward increasing the number of services and decreasing the professional quality of those services" (p. 73).

Freidson argues that "many of the rigid, mechanical, and authoritarian attributes, and much of the inadequate coordination said to characterize the health services, may stem more from their professional organization than from their bureaucratic characteristics" (pp. 132–33). In fact, he pleads for *more* bureaucratization, not less. The withholding of information from patients, for example, stems from the professional need to maintain the mystique of expertise. A bureaucratic solution to this could easily be devised and carried out—as, for example, in the case of brochures describing hospital routines (p. 140). Thus, there may actually be a contradiction between the potential for humane treatment possible through *bureaucratic* organization of medical care and the potential which is possible through *professional* dominance of the health system.

However, it must not be thought that government financing and bureaucratic control—even to the point of socialized medicine—will inevitably eliminate the special power of the professions. A recent review of the literature on the factors affecting the method of payment of physicians in ten countries concluded that "the economic power of physicians is an overriding political resource which washes away the effects of both the bargaining styles employed by physician organizations and the attributes of the political culture such as mass and elite conceptions of the nature and legitimacy of physician demands."[13]

This observation is telling evidence of the consequences of the professional monopoly of physicians for their control over the method of their payment, *even* in countries which have nearly completely socialized health care delivery.

3. Corporate Rationalization

The legal basis for private ownership of the right to practice medicine by professionals is being eroded. Legal changes in the responsibility for the quality of health care give some indication that the principle is being established that patients can be best protected by legal responsibility imposed by the hospital. As health economist Anne Somers has put it, there is "growing evidence that neither oath nor professional penalties are adequate to protect the public against improper medical care and the responsibility for such quality controls can be imposed most effectively on the hospital."[14]

According to Somers, recent changes in state laws have moved toward the fixing of responsibility for quality controls on the hospital itself, both the governing board and the medical staff (p. 114). Government action may increasingly be an agency for corporate rationalization, embedding the responsibility for health care in the hospital. This is a significant shift, if true, because one common assumption by those defending a market concept of health care organization has been that individual physicians are ultimately responsible and that legal action can most effectively be taken against individuals. The new principle asserts that organizational measures to guarantee performance are more likely to be effective than legal penalties against individual physicians activated by individual complaints through such devices as malpractice suits.

Another example of the way in which hospitals have become carriers of the social, rather than individual, practice of health care is the pressure upon hospitals to be "flexible" in the assignment of tasks. Whereas most organizational innovations in health care are hampered by guild-like restrictions on who can provide "medical" care—with even criminal liability for violations—hospitals have gone so far as actually to create new specialties, such as intravenous or operating room technicians, to meet requirements of modern health care. Technically, according to Somers, hospitals have even broken the law by doing so (p. 92).

A number of objective economic and organizational changes underlie the shift toward corporate rationalization of health care. There has been not only a striking increase in the proportion of physicians working on full-time salaries, but also an increasing importance of the equipment and facilities available only in the hospital. The very advance of specialization makes it more important that a physician be able to consult other specialists in an organizational context which makes their contribution to a given treatment feasible.

One empirical indication of this trend toward a focus upon hospitals as the core institution in the provision of care is the trend toward more rigorous medical staff organization in hospitals. According to a recent study, a higher proportion of physicians each year is becoming salaried, and there are more full-time chiefs of departments, more control committees, and many other indications of intensification of control over the individual physician's behavior.[15] The authors cite many recent developments which point toward the hospital increasingly becoming a "community health center" rather than a "doctors' workshop": Medicare and Medicaid, Regional Medical Programs, expanding government support for health manpower training, national mental health legislation, and comprehensive health planning.

As a result of these forces, "it is quite evident that the trend in recent decades has been toward the highly structured end" of the range of medical staff organization. "Almost all hospitals have taken steps to tighten the organization of their medical staffs" (p. 3). This trend is not just toward bureaucratization. Although extremely cautious in their generalizations, the authors do argue that their data support the "hypothesis that higher levels of medical staff organization are probably associated with higher quality of hospital performance," using severity-adjusted death rates as the basis for their conclusion (p. 255). Also, "a firmer medical staff organization . . . was generally associated with a higher record for the great majority of specific features indicating effective hospital performance. . . over-all performance, amplitude of staffing, diagnostic procedures, surgical facilities, other significant therapies, educational functions, and preventive and community service" (p. 279). Costs as well were lower in the more highly structured hospitals. These data clearly support the rationale for corporate rationalization—at least at the micro level of controlling the organizational environment of physician behavior.

At the macro level of government regulation of hospitals, the same processes of corporate rationalization are evident. Examples are the several forms of control over hospitals: licensing (by government, intended to set a minimum floor on quality), accreditation (a non-governmental, professional process supposedly aimed at excellence), and certification (for Medicare payments). If the first two worked, presumably there would be no need for the third, but that is not the case. Accreditation "has come to imply simply an 'acceptable' hospital." Licensing in many states is "acknowledged to have little or no influence on the quality of patient care." Somers asserts that "the predictable result of the three overlapping programs is not only confusion and financial waste but—even in their totality—inadequate safeguards of the quality of care."[16] This is a perfect case of the failure of one set of regulatory agencies and processes to work and the establishment of another, and yet another, stage or process of regulation. This continuous elaboration of overlapping bureaucratic functions is the result of two factors: first, that the actual operating characteristics of hospitals are not controllable within the potential powers of the agency, and second, that there is pressure to "do something" which looks as if it is control and regulation.

Another example of attempted corporate rationalization at the macro level is the recent trend toward state requirements that expansion of health care facilities be approved by an administrative decision. This is an example of the victory of the bureaucratic reform strategy over market reform. A recent critical examination of these new requirements, passed in some form by twenty states between 1971 and 1973, indicates that this form of response to cost escalation is a typical one. Most of the states required a "certificate of need" for new hospital construction, about half for ambulatory care facilities.[17] The American Hospital Association first indicated its acceptance of certificates of need in 1968, and actually proposed a draft of a model state law in 1972 (p. 1151). The AHA either did not see such regulation as a threat to its members or believed that by joining the movement for regulation it could influence or even control the regulatory process.

The pressure for mandatory regulation of facilities probably stemmed from the failure of voluntary health planning to control growth. Studies have concluded that "nonprofit" hospitals "do not differ greatly in their behavior from professionally managed for-profit firms, both seeking growth as the primary source of managerial gratification," and their "prices seem to behave not too differently from those of for-profit firms." Even hospitals denied public financing for expansion, for example from Hill-Burton federal funds, could "often raise the needed money from other sources," and would frequently do so "whenever an opportunity for institutional aggrandizement presented itself" (pp. 1149–50).

Law professor Clark Havighurst—the author of the above observations who basically takes a "market reform" position, argues that it is
unlikely that the new planning controls will allow health maintenance
organizations (HMO's) to compete with the hospitals and reduce costs.
Hospitals will not sit still for HMO's taking away their patients who do
not really need in-hospital care, but will create their own demand for
patients. "If the substitution of ambulatory care for inpatient care
should leave hospital beds in the fee-for-service sector empty, past
performance suggests that those beds will now be occupied by patients
who do not really require hospitalization."[18]

Havighurst believes that hospitals want to "curb competitive developments which would substitute ambulatory for inpatient care" (p.
1152). Seemingly the planners agree. Both the "hospital interests and
the planners [tend] to reach out for control over exogenous influences"
(p. 1214) such as the new developments of "surgicenters" (outpatient
surgical services), abortion clinics, acupuncture centers, and other
innovations which "threaten to reduce hospital occupancy rates." He
believes that hospitals do not introduce such innovations on their own
because the "incentives to innovate in these ways are at best weak....
To the extent the hospital's bed count and gross revenues dwindle,
managers are motivated in the opposite direction" (pp. 1211–12).
Thus, Havighurst believes that generally both hospitals and planners
will discourage the potential competitive influence of HMO's upon
hospitals and will use the certificate of need provisions to prevent their
being established if they can.

Although it may perhaps be due to his bias in favor of the market,
Havighurst sees a "potential basis for a convergence of viewpoint
between the regulated hospitals and the health planners, the group
from which most [regulatory] agency staff members are recruited.
Dedicated to developing a more rational and more humanitarian health
care system, the planners are likely to contemplate a long list of
projects which they believe would contribute to this goal.... Because
many of the desired programs could easily be hospital-based, there is at
least a potential ground for agreement between the planners and the
regulated industry on the desirability of a larger hospital sector" (p.
1183). One empirical study found that there was a "strong positive
correlation between involvement of areawide health planning agencies
in facilities regulation and bed control and the extent of financial
support drawn from the hospital industry" and concluded that a
situation of "dependency" existed in which "capture" of local planners
by local hospitals could occur (p. 1182).

The general point is that both on ideological grounds and for reasons of the material interests of their agencies, health planners are likely to act in ways consonant with the interests of hospitals. The consequences of this new attempt at regulation are thus likely, Havighurst argues, to be the exact opposite of those promised. "Larger hospitals grow while new facilities are discouraged; incumbents [e.g., existing hospitals] enjoy an unwritten presumption in proposing to replace their outmoded facilities; 'satellites' of existing hospitals are favored over new entrants; and 'chains' and other proprietaries are excluded in favor of existing facilities or community-sponsored organizations." These results are likely because of the "hospital industry's political domination of the regulatory process," but in addition, even without this factor, "regulatory policies are likely to be unduly protective and to foster both inflation and an excessive allocation of resources to the hospital sector" (pp. 1187–88). Thus, the vision of planning and integration presented by new attempts at corporate rationalization through administrative regulation is contradicted by the likely consequences of domination by hospital interests of politically feasible attempts to introduce "planning." Havighurst has documented, as few others have, the pervasive pressures upon government to act in ways which exemplify corporate rationalization.

The main forces making for corporate rationalization are probably objective changes in the technology, costs, and social organization of health care. However, an ideology of planning and coordination and the self-interest of persons holding positions within health organizations also contributes to this tendency. The structural interest of corporate rationalization is represented by persons in top positions in "health" organizations: hospital administrators, medical school directors, public health officials, directors of city health agencies, heads of quasi-public insurance (Blue Cross), state and federal health officials. Their ideology stresses a rational, efficient, cost-conscious, coordinated health care delivery system. They see the medical division of labor as arbitrary and anachronistic in view of modern hospital-based technology.

The ideology of corporate rationalization has already been detailed in the context of New York City commission reports in chapter 2, but one more example from a totally different source will indicate its pervasiveness. A professor of hospital administration, focusing upon the "role" of hospital administrator, emphasized its key importance in the changing structure of health care toward more planning, coordination, administration, regionalization, and systems research—the language of corporate rationalization. Potential conflicts both with the public and with medical staffs are recognized, particularly as the maximization of "efficiency and effectiveness" brings "resistance from those whose power would be reduced as a result," that is, the physicians.[19] Typical of the ideological content of such articles, the implicit assumption is that there are really no fundamental disagreements and that all problems can be solved. Basic conflicts are smoothed over by rhetoric which says that in a pluralist, democratic society, all groups and interests have their legitimate role. "One can assume that, in a highly developed democratic society, the major elements needed are public involvement, medical expertise, and administrative know-how. . . . It is by no means certain what type of organization and combination of talents can best supply these elements" (p. 64). Note the assumption that there *is* a "best" solution, that an organizational solution is the appropriate one, and that the necessary "elements" can be combined in some way. This is typical of a technocratic, administrative, or bureaucratic mode of analysis. Conflicts are recognized but are absorbed in a higher synthesis determined by technical criteria—themselves defined by the administrators.

Finally, given these structural and ideological factors, there are also ample incentives for individuals holding elite positions in research institutes, hospitals, universities, medical schools, health planning agencies, and government to attempt to expand the size and resources of their institution or organization. Larger organizations provide higher salaries, better fringe benefits, and greater career life-chances than smaller ones. The more successful such officials are in unifying functions, powers, and resources into a single organization under their control, the greater their incomes are likely to be and the higher their community and professional prestige.

The contradiction between the seductive ideology of corporate rationalization—coordination, integration, and planning—and the inability of the carriers of that ideology to control all of the factors in health production, lead to failures of planning and coordination in practice. A study of the factors affecting the expansion of hospitals in one community led one author to conclude that "under the present rules of the hospital-support game [which in the city he studied led to a stalemate for ten years on the decision about which hospitals should be allowed to expand], it is difficult to see how the much-trumpeted notion of the hospital as a community health center can be actualized." Each hospital in that community advertised itself as serving "the whole community," but just as important were its attempts to "gain attachments to particular segments of the community and to compete with other teams in this respect."[20]

Despite the claims for the centrality of the hospital, there is little evidence that even the internal structure of the giant hospital complexes is planned, integrated, and coordinated for the effective delivery of health services to a given target population, let alone to the public as a whole. The priorities of hospitals in fact contribute to the fragmented system. According to Dr. Ray E. Brown, writing in 1964 when he was director of the Graduate Program in Hospital Administration at Duke University, "the general hospital has integrated the resources but it has not integrated the various levels of patient care required by the community." He notes the priorities in the hospital: (1) inpatients, not outpatients, a "holdover from the old concept of the hospital as a charity institution"; (2) short-term patients who repond fast (there is even institutional segregation of short-term and long-term patients); and (3) the most expensive patients—"the rationale seems to be to feature the most expensive services that will serve the least number of patients. . . . It finds it too easy to provide a costly cobalt bomb, but finds it very difficult to provide an inexpensive well-baby clinic for a much larger number of patients." Dr. Brown goes on to say that "in a hospital setting, the total resource gamut of modern medical care is focused on patients who gain admission. At the same time, however, it has greatly increased the fragmentation of the total medical services to the community at large. Each new medical advance further fragments and widens the disparity in the scope and depth of services available between those admitted to the general hospital and those not admitted."[21]

This pattern seems typical of bureaucratic organizations in a market society. They can rationally and efficiently serve those clients or customers within their defined and limited jurisdiction who possess the proper keys (money, a legal claim, membership in a status group, etc.) to open the door to their services, but have no incentives or structural imperatives which can broaden their specific means and goals. This pattern is probably typical of priorities in both the public and the private sectors. Dr. Brown blames it in this case on the psychology of professionalism. "It apparently is difficult for professionals to maintain interest in the less rewarding progress made by . . . slow-responding, longer-term patients" (p. 41). This explanation, while plausible, probably accounts only for the immediate motives of the physician, not for the structural arrangements which lead to the saliency of those motives.

"Outreach" neighborhood health centers established by a medical center are sometimes advertised as a rational step toward coordination and integration, but instead they are really needed as a source of patients and surgical material. Because of Medicare, physicians assume they will be reimbursed and thus need not send poor patients with interesting diseases on to a university hospital. The goal in establishing a neighborhood health center is thus not coordination, but patients. Other cases of supposed coordinating mechanisms—ambulance services, referrals, communication of records and patient information—are notoriously poor in operation, and there is little evidence that the extension of control by one organization, whether via formal merger or not, results in more comprehensive care.

To conclude more generally, even if the alleged goal of corporate rationalization is to coordinate and integrate a number of organizations into a cohesive whole, the successful instituting of such bureaucratic controls over several organizations means that planning and coordination of the larger health system becomes *more* difficult. Generating enough power to integrate a portion of it successfully means, almost by definition, that this part is now insulated from outside influence and can successfully resist being integrated into a still larger system.

The rhetoric of corporate rationalization conceals this consequence by suggesting that social or political mechanisms can be created to unify and integrate the entire system. But such mechanisms do not exist—in government or anywhere else. The mere passage of legislation funding comprehensive health planning, for example, does not provide planning agencies with the necessary power and resources. If this is the case, then the act of creating another agency further complicates the system. As will be discussed later in more detail, legislators historically have responded to pressures for reform by establishing a series of agencies—none of which has sufficient power to do its job. Few of these are abolished, and subsequent legislation incorporates the previous agencies into the list of those to be coordinated, thereby further complicating the system. The resources made available to these agencies charged with planning and coordinating other agencies frequently become part of the budgets controlled by the corporate rationalizers.

A major consequence of the activity of the corporate rationalizers is thus a constant expansion of the functions, powers, and resources of their organizations. One organizational device for doing that is the institution of a bureaucratic stratum designed to coordinate and integrate the component units, at either the intra- or interorganizational level. Unfortunately, this new stratum cannot carry out this function because it is a staff operation with little power and is usually the instrument of one particular elite faction within or between the affected organizations. Thus, their recommendations frequently fail to carry enough weight to be implemented. Also the planning or research staff tends to be drawn, because of lack of any other source of personnel, from the ranks of the professional monopolists, who have little stake in truly rationalizing the operation and see the planning or research functions partly as instruments for their own personal and professional ends. Where the goals of the professional monopolists within the organization and the sponsoring faction among the corporate rationalizers coincide, an effective staff function will be performed. In that case, the committed and motivated staff will usually come into conflict with a powerful element in the top officialdom of one organization or another—either another group of professional monopolists whose toes they are stepping on, or a faction among the corporate rationalizers.[22]

Thus, the net effect of the thrust toward corporate rationalization is to complicate and elaborate both private and public bureaucratic structures, although this structural interest represents the most technologically advanced form of the medical division of labor. Corporate rationalization and professional monopoly are symbiotically related in that the ever-increasing elaboration of the bureaucratic structure is justified by the need to coordinate the expansion of health-care-providing units at the bottom. No group involved has an interest in the coordination and integration of the entire system toward the major goal of easily accessible, inexpensive, and equal health care.

This argument is consistent with that advanced by Jay Forrester, who makes the interesting and relevant point that complex systems are not easily diagnosed and that "remedies" for problems and defects may be counterproductive and actually make things worse. He asserts that "choosing an ineffective or detrimental policy for coping with a complex system is not a matter of random chance. The intuitive processes will select the wrong solution much more often than not. . . . Causes are usually found, not in prior events, but in the structure and policies of the system."[23] Translated into our terms, Forrester's point could be interpreted as saying that health reformers, regardless of their institutional base or ideological orientation, are currently almost "intuitively" likely to see establishment of a coordinating and planning instrument—whether a hospital, a regional planning board, a community advisory board, a health services corporation, or a comprehensive health center—as the organizational device potentially capable of unifying all of the health resources needed to serve a given community under one agency or one man. This solution is related to the peculiar analysis of causes in terms of previous "events," to use Forrester's term: the actions of diverse persons doing myriads of unrelated things in the past—patients going to see doctors, doctors treating patients, government providing some money to the poor, hospitals expanding, medical schools doing research, specialists getting trained, cobalt bombs being purchased. If the past is seen as an unintegrated, inchoate series of events and behaviors, then it may be natural and intuituve to see the causes of escalating costs, a maldistribution of health manpower, and the inability to provide decent health care for those unable to pay for it in the failure to establish *some* kind of organizational instrument with the necessary powers and resources capable of bringing some rational ordering and priorities into the system. However, if the causes are found in the structure and policies in the system, not in events and behavior, such an intuitive analysis may in fact select the wrong solution—one which exacerbates the very problems it is allegedly designed to solve.

4. Challenge to Dominant Structural Interests

Sometimes corporate rationalizers ally themselves with professional monopolists within their own institutions as a way of gathering more financial resources and legitimacy, and also as a way of bringing more and more health care units into their domain, even if not under their control. But usually it is in the interests of the corporate rationalizers to attempt to control the conditions of work, the division of labor, and the salaries of their employees, in view of the exigencies of funding and the need to adopt technical and organizational innovations without the built-in resistances of professional (or union, for that matter) jurisdictions over tools and tasks. They therefore attempt to convert professionals, mainly physicians, into employees and in a variety of ways to circumscribe their power in the hospital.

This basis for structural conflict is a pervasive one, even if it is concealed in many forms of rhetoric to legitimate the claims of the competing interest groups. It is significant that most definitions and diagnoses of the health "crisis" do not come from the professionals. The AMA and other professional associations have largely reacted defensively, proposing alternatives and compromises only when other interest groups have raised challenges to existing practices. When institutions and laws continuously serve dominant structural interests, challenge must come from elsewhere.

From where has the challenge come? A clue lies in the composition of the numerous commissions of inquiry at all governmental levels which have investigated the health delivery system in the last twenty years and made many recommendations for public policy. The thirty-six member "Heyman Commission" (see chapter 2) which issued its report on New York health services in 1960 included five city officials, twelve hospital administrators and executives of health associations or medical research institutes, fifteen corporate or bank executives or directors, one university president, one labor representative, and two persons representing private medical practice (both presidents of county medical societies). Of the corporate group, at least five were directors of voluntary hospitals or prepaid health plans.[24]

Seven years later, the so-called Piel Commission (see chapter 2) reported its findings to Mayor Lindsay and recommended the establishing of the Health Services Administration (1967) and the Health and Hospitals Corporation (1970). Its seven members included one publisher, one university professor, and five corporate and banking representatives, all of whom happened to hold directorships of voluntary hospitals or other health associations.[25] Of the fourteen physicians comprising the medical advisory committee to the commission, four represented hospitals; six, university medical centers; two, the New York Academy of Medicine; one, a health institute; and only one, a county medical society.

Governor Rockefeller's 1971 New York State Steering Committee on Social Problems contained seventeen members, only one of whom had an M.D.[26] Of the sixteen men who took part in the study, fourteen were high executives of some of the largest corporations, banks, or brokerage firms in the United States, including U. S. Steel, Pan American World Airways, DuPont, Equitable Life, AT&T, Xerox, and General Foods. The one physician was on the Yale medical school faculty; the other noncorporate executive was the president of the Committee for Economic Development.

At the federal level, such commissions are similar in composition. To take only one example, the Task Force on Medicaid and Related Programs was composed of twenty-seven persons, five of whom held

M.D.'s. Only one of these (according to the list of the affiliations in the report) was a physician in private practice. Four other physicians were associated with city or state health agencies or were directors of hospitals or medical schools. Of the remaining twenty-two members, seven were corporation executives (one of a proprietary hospital chain), six were connected with universities (including medical schools), three with community or state health agencies, and three with hospitals.[27] The chairman of the task force was the president of Blue Cross, a private hospital insurance association.

While I may not have accurately classified the members' multiple affiliations, the relative absence of physicians, and especially physicians in private practice, is striking. Predominant in all of these commissions are hospital administrators, hospital insurance executives, corporate executives and bankers, medical school directors, and city and state public health administrators. These organizations represent a coalition of interest groups representing the structural interest of corporate rationalization. They prefer what the AMA attacked as the "corporate practice of medicine"[28]: the control of health services by a combination of private and public health agencies, principally the hospital.

5. Conflict Between Structural Interests

In the preceding two sections, I summarized the technical and organizational bases for the structural interests labeled professional monopoly and corporate rationalization and considered a few examples of how those bases have changed. It should be noted that although these changes have intensified the recent conflict between the dominant and challenging structural interests, this conflict has deep historical roots.

A coalition in the early 1900s of private practitioners and a small group of university-hospital-based specialized teachers "represented different long-range tendencies within the AMA although at this time they were... united in pushing the reform of medical education."[29] Physicians saw their status and income being threatened by overcrowding of the profession and thus welcomed restricting the output of physicians. Even then, medical reform and the subordination of public hospitals to the medical schools were explicitly defined in terms of larger units, centralized administration, and efficiency, all seen as part of a "businesslike" system to provide health care. Reform of medical education solved several problems besides raising the income and status of the profession; it "commenced the consolidation of the components of a newly emerging university-medical school complex; restricted intraprofessional competition; organized medicine's long-term opposition to group practice and government financed hospital and clinic care, and also institutionalized a two-class medical care system" (p.85).

The result of the coalition between the rationalizing and modernizing element in the profession—the elite physicians attached to research institutions, universities, and medical schools—and the individual general practitioners was certainly change, but change which was conservative in both intent and result because it "concentrated power in the hands of a small elite, but also in the sense that for the next half-century it protected the special interests of the most outmoded segment of the profession: the private practitioner. That is to say the reforms centralized, bureaucratized, modernized and expanded medicine and medical education in the interests of physicians' own professional needs and with little regard for the needs of the public" (p. 107). However, even though the private practitioners benefited, the institutional basis was created for later challenge of their power.

The rational basis for the challenge of the professional monopolists by the corporate rationalizers is provided by the strong evidence that the professional monopoly of the provision of health services by physicians is based neither on their actual expertise nor on the necessity of sustaining the integrity of the doctor-patient relationship. Eliot Freidson has summarized the evidence as follows.[30] (1) Specialized knowledge cannot be in any one man's head any more, and thus any patient suffering from more than the most routine and simplest ailment needs referrals to more than one doctor (p. 100); therefore, a rational division of labor and referral system must be organized. (2) Physicians' performances are better under supervision. (3) Bureaucracies such as hospitals keep better records than do solo practitioners, and therefore better care is provided (p. 101). The assumption here is that patients are not likely to keep the same physician for many years because of the geographic mobility of both doctors and patients. Also, with medical specialization the "whole person" is not treated any more. (4) The settings and situation in which the doctor practices affect his behavior more than his training and background (p. 70). (5) The particular skilled behaviors which are encompassed by and controlled by the profession of medicine are historically arbitrary. There is no rational reason why certain skills in the provision of health care should be under the control of the medical profession and others not. Examples are pharmacy, dentistry, optometry, chiropractic, nursing, medical technology, and clinical psychology. These occupations, of course, are subject to controls by the organizations in which they work, their clientele, and state regulation, and they are attempting to professionalize themselves as a defense (p. 52).

These rational reasons for breaking the professional monopoly are undoubtedly less important than changes in social conditions. The gradual decline of solo practice has created one objective basis for the challenge of this monopoly by the principle of corporate rationalization. This generalization probably applies mainly to larger cities. In smaller cities the physicians still control the hospitals through the county medical societies. Administrators of the small-town hospitals are less professionalized than those in big-city hospitals and thus have a less independent view of the way their hospital should be run. A small town is also not likely to have a medical school, so that a potential coalition of corporate rationalizers comprising those from a medical school, hospital administrators, insurance companies, and public health agencies does not have the organizational or political base to challenge the control by the solo physicians of medical practice in the hospital. Potential mavericks among the doctors are controlled through the county medical board's power to refuse an appointment in the hospital. Small cities are less likely to have more than one hospital, so that a dissident physician has no place to go except to change his place of practice.

Thus, small cities are less likely to exhibit open conflict over the organization, quantity, and quality of health care than large cities. (In the pluralist sense, no "power" is being exercised.) But in small cities there may actually be more unequal allocation of health care to various segments of the community and more chance that doctors and professional associations are unchallenged than in larger cities, where different interests have reached some threshold of effective organization. Economist Elton Rayack has nicely summarized the manifold challenges of organization to the status and power of the private physician:

In attempting to retain his long-held prerogatives and power, the solo practitioner comes into conflict with hospital administrators who want to exercise control over costs and staff privileges; in trying to perpetuate the fee-for-service method of payment, he clashes with prepayment insurance programs; in rigidly adhering to the traditional principle of "free choice of physician," he is resisted by "closed panel" group practices; in battling to maintain or achieve sole control over medical service insurance plans, he is fought by labor unions and consumer cooperatives; in seeking to hold on to his traditional position as the sole arbiter of the quality of medical services, he is challenged by unions, insurance agencies and hospital administrators.[31]

Within hospitals, conflicts between the staff physicians and the hospital administration are pervasive, although varying from one type of hospital to another. According to Milton I. Roemer, "in almost every hospital today, where the leadership is dynamic and innovations are being promoted, there is a substratum of tension between the hospital administration and the medical staff."[32] In his own study of ten California hospitals, the conflicts, as one would expect, were sharpest in the hospitals with a medium level of rigorousness in medical staff organization (MSO).

> In the permissive-MSO hospitals, the behavioral values of the private medical practitioner are clearly dominant; there are few efforts at organizational innovation, and serious controversies seldom occur. In the rigorous-MSO hospitals, at the other pole, the organizational framework clearly predominates over medical individualism, but the doctors entering this arena have accepted its constraints, so that relationships are relatively peaceful. It is in the medium-MSO hospitals that numerous pressures for innovation tend to emanate from the board of directors or the hospital administrator, and the greatest resistance is encountered from the medical staff. (p. 283)

A case study of a hospital with medium-structured medical staff organization exemplifies at the micro level the conflicts between professional monopoly and corporate rationalization. "The medical staff wants [the hospital] to remain a... private doctor's workshop... [rather than] a comprehensive community medical center," the administrator's goal. The physicians perceive the administrator as allied with the board of directors: "They speak the same language, relying on the same kind of business criteria for making decisions.... The Hospital Administrator contends that the tremendous complexity of modern medical care demands the establishment and co-ordination of all the specialty services in a service-oriented institution.... It should attempt to co-ordinate its activities with those of other hospitals and agencies, in order to prevent duplication and fill gaps in community service" (p. 118).

However, the physicians are caught in a bind because some of the immediate programs they want also lead to the kind of expansion of the hospital they oppose. "They generally support the medical education program, because they recognize that the training of interns and residents brings benefits for all the doctors if only to enable them to care for more patients. But to maintain accreditation for residencies requires enlarging the full-time medical staff. Certain highly specialized services also demand the presence of full-time doctors. The more successful these programs and services, the larger the full-time staff, the larger the hospital . . . and eventually one sees the 'medical center' " (p. 119). This case illustrates the symbiotic character of the physician-hospital relationship, involving both intrinsic dependence and conflict.[33]

Rosemary Stevens sees the conflict between physician-centered and hospital-centered organization of health care manifest in other consequences as well. "At their extremes the one system assumes that medical care is a spectrum from physicians' office to hospital bed and back, with an individual physician and patient involved at each stage; from the physician's point of view, his hospital work is part of his private practice. The other system assumes a cadre of physicians whose work is predominantly or entirely in the hospital and a second cadre whose work is primarily outside the hospital; in this model the hospital is at the fringe of medical care, and the hospitalized sick are seen as requiring unusual and acute forms of diagnosis and treatment."[34]

Hospital-based group practice, advocated as far back as 1932 by the Committee on the Costs of Medical Care and opposed by the AMA, was an early attempt to rationalize the health care system around a key institution potentially capable of integrating and coordinating the specialized skills and techniques now available. A key conflict was resolved in favor of the hospitals in 1943, when the Supreme Court "found the AMA and the Medical Society of the District of Columbia guilty of restraint of trade under the Sherman Act" in attempting to exclude physician members of a health cooperative from hospital staff privileges. This decision did not establish whether or not the hospitals could control the qualifications of physicians eligible for appointment to their staffs, but it did prevent the professional associations of physicians from claiming membership in them to be a necessity. The decision opened the way for the further extension of the power of the hospital as the coordinator and controller of the health services and personnel provided within its boundaries.[35]

But the battles are not all won by the corporate rationalizers. Economist Seymour Harris described some years ago a struggle "between the hospitals and the anesthesiologists, pathologists, and radiologists on the issue of direct payments by hospitals for their services or (what is demanded by the physicians) the higher incomes obtainable through direct billing of the hospital patients."[36] This battle has apparently been won by the radiologists. According to Dr. Wallace D. Buchanan, chairman of the American College of Radiology (ACR) committee on independent practice, "for the first time in history, our judiciary committee has gone 12 months without hearing of one single ruckus between a radiologist and a hospital." He attributed this to the fact (from ACR data) that more than half of hospital-based radiologists now depend upon fees for service rather than salaries. The "realistic" *median* salary which a radiologist could expect, Dr. Buchanan estimated, was about $45,000 in 1969. "We have got to recognize that medicine generally is enjoying a pretty good gross income these days, and if radiology doesn't keep pace, it isn't very attractive."[37]

One important organizational consequence of the arbitrary division of authority between physicians and hospitals was the separate development of Blue Cross (insurance for hospital expenses) and Blue Shield (insurance for doctor bills). As Rosemary Stevens put it, "apart from their history, such a division has little logic or continuing justification. . . . In terms of administrative costs alone there is a strong case for merging Blue Cross and Blue Shield . . . but as yet . . . in almost all states Blue Cross and Blue Shield plans continue under separate administration, each with its own office to process claims for Medicare and each with its claims review mechanisms." By accepting this framework and establishing Blue Cross and Blue Shield as the private administrative agencies to handle Medicare funds in 1965, the effect of this federal action was to "freeze an outmoded form of organization."[38]

This consequence of Medicare was only one of several of its "underlying inconsistencies, which rest in turn on inconsistencies in the professional organization of medicine. In brief, these are the continuing administrative division of services given by hospitals and by physicians in private practice, and the disorganization of physicians in private practice. The continuation of private practitioners as small-scale entrepreneurs has meant that there is as yet, with few exceptions, no effective organizational focus for the development of cohesive local services" (p. 466).

The private insurance companies—designated by the government as the intermediaries between government on the one hand and the hospitals and physicians on the other—have been caught between incompatible demands for efficient, cost-effective administration of a publicly financed program and protection of the rights and privileges of two powerful structural interests. The result has been "permissive" rather than "efficient" practices by the insurance companies. Several congressional (both Senate and House) reports have criticized the administration of Medicare for alleged deficiencies, abuses, and failures to control excessive costs. It may be nearly inevitable for an organization caught between interest groups making contradictory demands upon it to behave in ways which seem vacillating and contradictory from the point of view of the efficient management of a single organization. Yet, from the point of view of the interorganizational system of which that organization is a part, there may be literally no alternative for it until the external pressures upon it change. Merely changing its personnel or its internal administrative structure or punishing it or its staff for the abuses may have no effect if functional equivalents must be found again to accommodate to the external pressures.

To conclude, the struggle between the professional monopolists and the corporate rationalizers is thus also competition between different sectors of the health industry for control of sources of profits. To quote Professor Harris again: "In the unusual market conditions since the war, there is an increasing tendency for intermediaries to intervene and absorb part of the unusual gains accruing to doctors. To some extent the spread of insurance and group practice reflects attempts to depress the income of doctors to the profit of insurance companies, their subscribers, or managers of group insurance programs. Hence the battle waged by medical societies for a generation against what they call corporate practice."[39] In effect, this is a move toward transforming the present professional monopoly into a corporate monopoly, with new health corporations taking various forms and seeking to turn individual entrepreneurs (the doctors) into employees. The slogan of "social responsibility" may be used to justify taking away some of the powers of the private physician to charge what the market will bear and to transfer these powers to the hospital, the insurance companies, or the medical corporation. The resulting health service may be better in the same way and for the same reasons that General Motors can produce more and cheaper cars than can a custom-made auto body shop or a number of craftsmen. The continuing importance of corporate profits, the focus upon a specific product, and the requirement of cost-benefit efficiency may lead to internal efficiency in the organization of health care within hospitals, but the larger issues of preventive care, neighborhood outpatient clinics, and so forth, which cannot easily be organized in a humane way by corporate structures in a market society, will be ignored.

6 Community Participation, Politics, and Bureaucracy

The major structural interests analyzed in the preceding chapter define the institutional framework within which the community population must seek health care. As we observed in chapter 1, the structural interest of the community population must be seen as "negative" or even repressed with respect to its capacity to organize into interest groups. Not only are the affected interests not represented by stable institutions, but the potential interest groups are extremely heterogeneous, and demands—even after they become defined and expressed—are easily compromised, soothed, or co-opted into bases of legitimation of the activities and role of dominant or challenging structural interests.

1. The Equal-Health Advocates

Interest groups and individual agents representing the community population's structural interest in better health care are diverse. Their spokesmen are the "equal-health advocates," comprising community-control groups in the black and white communities, full- or part-time organizers, intellectuals speaking with isolated voices, and some trade unionists. Because they are not part of the network of health institutions and agencies, they are free to demand more and better health services and also some voice in the policies which affect health care. City health bureaucracies, public health agencies, and the medical schools and universities usually contain some supporters.

The efforts of these diverse individuals and groups, whether aimed at specific or general reforms, are likely to fail. If their demands are focused upon a particular program or need, the response is likely to be the establishment of a particular kind of program or clinic—drug, alcoholism, mental health. The professional monopolists will seize upon the demand as an opportunity to legitimate their efforts to establish another project or program. While some tangible services to some people may be the outcome, the overall result is the expansion and proliferation of still more highly specialized clinics, demonstration projects, or health centers which confuse people trying to find care and are highly expensive in both staff and administrative costs and, thus, lead to a further elaboration of the overriding bureaucratic structure.

If the demands of the equal-health advocates are directed toward reorganizing the health system, the activities of the corporate rationalizers are legitimated. New planning committees and new coordinating councils will be set up with representation from the community groups and with the avowed goal of rationalizing the system. But the community representatives do not have the information necessary to play an important political role; they do not know the levers of power, the interests at stake, and the actual nature of the operating institutions, and they do not have the political resources necessary to acquire that information since they are only minority members of advisory committees. The presence of equal-health advocates on one or another committee or council is frequently a sign of legitimacy being claimed either by a set of professional monopolists or corporate rationalizers, or sometimes both, in their battle for resources and power.

Because few members of a community are self-conscious and knowledgeable about health facilities, and because food, jobs, housing, and schools have priority over doctors and hospitals—since only a few persons need health care at any given time—the equal-health advocates are likely to have a great deal of autonomy in representing community needs to official agencies. Advocates are not under much surveillance, there is little reaction to their decisions, and their victories have little collective impact. Thus, the isolation of equal-health advocates from the community increases the chances of their being co-opted into advisory boards, planning agencies, and other devices for advertising the representative character of "community participation" without much chance, let alone guarantee, that the community will be able to evaluate and control the actions of their advocates, much less of the health providers.

Thus, the major consequence of the activity of the equal-health advocates is to provide further legitimacy for both the expansion of specific research or service units controlled by professional monopolists and the expansion of the layers of bureaucratic staff controlled by the corporate rationalizers. Given the discrepancy between the inputs of manpower and funds and the outputs of health services, a continuous supply of persons from community groups will be ready to serve as equal-health advocates. However, persons who have played that role for some time are likely to become discouraged and leave, or will be co-opted into one of the established health organizations. Other persons will arise from community organizations to replace them for a wide variety of motives: prestige as a community representative, a chance to mingle with high city officials and other officials and community leaders, and possibly a chance for a better job or a political career. This chance for mobility may be good for the individuals involved, but is disastrous for the accumulation of political and organizational experience by community groups, if their leaders are constantly either being absorbed into the existing health system or dropping out of activity.

Given the personal and organizational interests at stake of the interdependent, although conflicting, network of professional monopolists and corporate rationalizers, the demands of the equal-health advocates are almost inevitably frustrated. The system as a whole, as a result of their activities, moves in a direction exactly opposite to that which they envision. Costs go up as a result of new, expensive programs. The accessibility of care goes down as a result of the proliferation of specialized, high-technology, research- or teaching-oriented health care units. Coordination and integration are reduced by the establishment of overlapping administrative bodies with no real powers.

This description of a system in equilibrium is of course only partial. The legitimacy gained for either dominant or challenging interests by the activity of the equal-health advocates is precarious because it rests upon a continuous contradiction between rhetoric and performance. Legitimacy is purchased at the escalating cost of constantly expanding provider units which duplicate each other and continuously establishing new agencies which purport to coordinate and integrate. To the extent to which equal-health advocates can create consciousness among the community population of the causes of the situation, the groundwork is laid for a more fundamental challenge to the powers of the major structural interests.

2. The Consequences of a Community "Victory"

The preceding discussion of the activities of the equal-health advocates has argued that their attempts to increase the quality and quantity of health services available to them are likely to fail. Either they will become absorbed with no real power in an advisory committee to existing agencies, or they will play a minority role in planning committees for new health facilities which take years to come to fruition. While some community participation may lead to greater political consciousness, under present conditions co-optation and stalemate are most likely."[1]

Even if community groups are represented on planning committees for new facilities, one highly likely consequence is that their activities by themselves will block new programs and projects. Once community groups are mobilized, they tend to conflict with each other and with the professionals in health organizations over funding, priorities, timing, sites, and control. Community participation is a classic instance of the "veto group" process leading to stalemate.

Such a typical pattern is no accident. The structure of participation maximizes the chances of stalemate by setting up the rules of decision making in such a way as to prevent any major interest from being seriously damaged (the requirement of "consensus"), and by failing to allocate enough power to the decision-making bodies on which community groups are represented. Because these bodies are not given enough power, there is little incentive to set up procedures and create a composition which will lead to effective decision-making processes. Just the opposite incentives exist: to make them large and unwieldy—as "representative" as possible—so that all points of view will be heard but none implemented, save those of the interests who already hold power. The net result is many meetings, speeches, and reports. Committees are set up which plan, coordinate, and communicate—and ultimately evaporate when the planning grant runs out.

One consequence of this particular scenario is that even the professionals who started the project with a sincere desire to "get the community involved" will become cynical about the competence and skills of community groups and leaders. The next time around they will join the ranks of those who try to make the mechanisms of community representation as fictitious as possible in order to preserve at least some chance of getting a health facility organized, funded, and built.

But let us assume that, as a result of sustained community organization and pressure, a neighborhood health center is, at long last, established to provide accessible, inexpensive, and high-quality care. Can it continue to do so? For several reasons—excessive *demand*, the persistence of a two-*class* health system, the likelihood of short-term funding —a community victory is likely to be short-lived.

Neighborhood health centers are selected as the example of a com-

munity victory because of their recent emergence as the focus of demand in many cities as well as New York City and their actual funding
under specific federal legislation. Parallel programs in the past and
others in the future have been or will be described by such names as
comprehensive health center, district health center, health maintenance organization, neighborhood family care center, ambulatory care
service, child health station, and mental health clinic. Such a center is
likely to be set up only in an area where few physicians are in private
practice, where there are few hospitals, and where there is a heavy
concentration of poor people. The market reformers can applaud such
an innovation because it meets demand in a flexible way, establishes
diversity in the system, and uses government resources where the
private market has no incentive to compete. The bureaucratic reformers hail such a development because it usually will be established as an
"outreach" clinic by an existing hospital, under public funding, and
therefore add to the resources of what seems to be a movement toward
integration and coordination.

Demand. Because of the inadequacy of other health facilities in poor
areas, the very success of a neighborhood health center is likely to be its
downfall. If it attempts to "deal comprehensively with patients' problems," the center becomes the "repository for all the unmet needs of
our patients." The consequence of the "lack of adequate social services
in our community will inevitably deaden staff's responsiveness to their
problems."[2] Thus, even though the staff may have begun work there in
the full flush of idealism, ready to serve the community's needs with
great energy and devotion, their very commitment will cause patients
to flood in, demanding care. The resulting overload of work will reduce
the quality of care, the enthusiasm of the staff, and the sense of
gratitude of the patients.

Establishing a facility in a poor area which provides—at its beginning
—easily accessible, inexpensive, and high-quality care will generate
enormous demand, reflecting great unmet needs, which soon reduces
both accessibility and quality. The activities of the equal-health advocates, if successfully focused upon the "realistic" end of, say, getting an
OEO grant for a neighborhood health center, are thus likely to be
fruitless from the point of view of the system as a whole. If the total
quantity of health services available to the population is increased, it
can then be argued plausibly that the community is better off than it
was before. But if the same characteristics—long waits, hurried physicians, and so forth—are reproduced after a while, the net effect may be
cynicism on the part of the previously idealistic staff and a new sense of

hopelessness in a population which had been led to expect real improvement.

Class. The same characteristics of the "old" system are reproduced not only by the demand on the facilities but also by the maintenance of a two-class system. In the case of the OEO neighborhood health centers, the requirement that service be only to the poor has meant "heavy-handed insistence"[3] by OEO on a means test, with all of the resulting downgrading of respect for the patients, lower status for the staff, and other characteristics of institutions designed for the poor.

The attempt to build health care institutions for *all*, providing free, accessible, and high-quality care, runs into an objection. Why serve the middle class? They can pay for it. Why not reserve these scarce resources for the poor who need it most? If you open up health care to all on the same basis, the argument runs, the middle class will monopolize services, since they have the information and the resources to take advantage of the available facilities. This a plausible argument, especially if one takes the position that political realism argues for a piecemeal approach to reform.

But, as we have already suggested, the consequences of a two-class institution are likely to be the extension of more of the same kind of services as before. To the extent that the sheer production of more health care facilities is better, such additions of facilities may be worthwhile; but they do not constitute structural reforms of the health system.

Funding. The argument that "more is better" assumes, for its plausibility, that these neighborhood health centers become part of the established array of health facilities available to the public, even on terms of existing costs, accessibility, and quality. This is not the case, however. The magic wand of financing moves from health area to health area and from crisis to crisis, causing one kind of facility to grow and flourish for a time, then another, leaving the first to dwindle or wither away. Community mental health centers, neighborhood health centers, and methadone clinics have each felt the impact of public concern.

Precisely because of community pressures, funding tends to flow to those kinds of facilities which can be advertised as a legitimate response to community needs. When the "old" agency or facility fails to meet those needs, community pressure builds up again after a time, and new agencies surge forward, leaving the hollow shells of under-financed, struggling agencies in their wake. The old ones are struggling partly because their failure to meet the needs has become obvious; they lose political clout, and their budgets are cut to make resources available to the new agencies, or at least they are not increased enough to enable them to do their jobs. Thus, they are further paralyzed.

The lack of permanent governmental commitment to such programs as the OEO neighborhood health centers—which by definition are peripheral and supplemental programs to the main body of the private health sector—means that they are eternally precarious and starved for funds. The consequences for their internal operations are serious. They must seek the short-term payoff, the program which will bring in the maximum number of patient visits as tangible evidence that they are playing the political role which originally generated them: cooling out the community. If they seek maximum short-term "productivity" in terms of patient visits, they run the danger of overloading their facilities, which were probably underfinanced and under-staffed in the first place. Overloading, as we have seen, in turn reduces the impact on the community and the likelihood of community pressure demanding the project's continuation. In effect, after a few years the health center becomes just another component of the two-class health system, and its theoretical goal of providing comprehensive health care is contradicted by its practice.

Another consequence of dependence on short-term financing—itself also a result of the pragmatic strategy of getting something rather than nothing for the poor—is that costs are likely to be high. In the first few years of any program, the setting-up costs—hiring, training, capital investment in buildings and facilities—are high. But in the context of demonstration projects, where an evaluation of the costs will, at least in part, be one of the bases for judging whether or not the project will continue, these high initial costs become one of the negative features in the evaluation. A common point made about demonstration projects is that they are expensive and therefore cannot be continued.

If the many sick, untreated people in a poor community ask for care once it is made available, the new, ambitious, and (let us assume) committed staff is put in a double bind. If they seek to meet all of these needs, they will quickly subject themselves to difficult work conditions, with all of the consequences mentioned earlier. If they attempt to insulate themselves against only the most pressing medical needs and try to meet those needs in a humane, careful, and thoroughly professional manner, they inevitably set up barriers to treatment for the rest. Poor patients asking for help (and also testing the new facility for its humanity) will again be subjected to "official" treatment: the appointment hassle, the inquiries (are you really sick?), and the not-so-subtle attitudes (what do you expect for nothing?). While the health care for those persons who ultimately reach a physician in the health center may be careful and competent, the cost of making it possible for their care to be of high quality may reduce the accessibility of care to many others. This consequence is a direct result of inadequate manpower and resources.

The auspices under which the neighborhood health center is organized might seem to make a difference. Linking such centers to medical schools, it is argued, will increase the chances of better care for the poor. Because of the exploitation of the poor for teaching purposes, this is not necessarily the case. The poor patients with rare diseases may, indeed, be selected for special and even superb treatment but may also be subjected to untested medicines or operations (for legitimate research and teaching purposes, of course) by inexperienced persons (medical students) who would never be allowed to practice their skills in that way on wealthy patients. The remainder of the patients—the poor with ordinary, uninteresting diseases which are useful for neither research nor training—are subjected to the normal indignities found in charity institutions of all types.

But the poor are no better off if the neighborhood health center is not connected to a medical school. In this case the medical staff, working in a facility which is of lower status precisely because it serves the poor and is not connected to a medical school, tends to be composed of foreign doctors, many of whom are not well trained; below-average medical school graduates who cannot get better jobs or practices; young idealists who get discouraged after a few years and leave; or a few good physicians who have taken the job as part of their career but intend to move on as soon as possible. The staff tends to have a high turnover and thus is relatively unable to build up continuous relationships with families in the area.[4]

What is true of one of the newest "innovations" in ambulatory care facilities—the so-called neighborhood health centers—is even more true of the older out-patient clinics of established hospitals. Here we rely upon reports by hospital administrators themselves, many of whom can be classed as bureaucratic reformers. For example, in 1964 the director of the Montefiore Hospital in New York City, Dr. Martin Cherkasky, wrote, "Outpatient facilities are a prime medical care resource and yet they often tend to be rudimentary and bypassed by the talented physician."[5] Dr. John H. Knowles, when he was general director of the Massachusetts General Hospital in Boston, wrote that:

No one would deny that the present clinic system of our urban hospitals is second-rate and that many of the current social and economic issues of medical care could be studied and remedied best in the environment of ambulatory care. The clinic is the low-status part of the urban hospital today, and the reward system for the staff is almost nonexistent. Small wonder that members of the staff do not like to work there and accordingly practice a different and poorer brand of medicine then they do with their private patients. Emotional gratification is slim, intellectual rewards are even slimmer and, of course, there are no financial rewards.[6]

Neither professional nor organizational incentives exist, therefore, to provide good health care in such facilities, even when they are sorely needed, and thus the seeming victory of a community demand may ultimately be an empty one.

To conclude, even if the equal-health advocates are victorious in their long struggle to get more health facilities in a poor area, the principles by which the rest of the health system already operates become reproduced in the new facility. The disillusionment which follows leads to either apathy or greater militance, depending on the concrete experiences of the community population, the political skills of the equal-health advocates, and the broader social and political situation at the time.

It is too soon to know whether or not these pessimistic predictions will be borne out by the history of so-called free clinics which start, at least, with the principle of patient and worker control over professional behavior. At least seventy "free clinics" were established between 1967 and 1969, and at least one hundred more in the ensuing two years, to serve "population groups that were not receiving proper nor sufficient attention: adolescents, aliented middle-class college dropouts and street people, ghetto blacks, Appalachian whites, Puerto Ricans, and Mexican-Americans."[7] It seems likely that even if the free clinics meet the needs of those groups, over a period of time they become subject to the same organizational and professional pressures as more orthodox forms of health provision, given the economic and political imperatives in the society at large. The author of a survey of free clinics concluded that free clinics "depend on established doctors and other professionals for care, established hospitals for backup, and established foundations or govern-ment for future funding and may, therefore, not actually be removed from the existing channels of care."[8]

The "free clinic" movement exhibits the dilemma of all reform movements: if they succeed, they reduce the pressures for further change; if they fail, they discourage the activists from further efforts. As a recent study of a free clinic put it, were the clinics "to become 'successful' in conventional terms, they might only succeed in further institutionalizing a two-tiered system of medical care."[9] A successful free clinic reduces the pressure upon mainstream health institutions in several ways. First, the difficult task of organizing and maintaining the clinic itself uses up the political energy of militants. Second, a difficult patient group (the poorest, sickest segment of the population) is directed toward the clinic, rather than toward established clinics and hospitals. Third, a free clinic's failure—and they are not likely to succeed, even in conventional terms—discredits alternatives to established health institutions. These factors may indeed account for the willingness of some agencies to support free clinics financially. However, there also exist internal pressures upon the clinic to abandon its treatment and participatory innovations. If the clinic becomes successful to the point that it gets past a reliance on lay staff, then the full-time professional staff will have the time and the incentives to attempt to control their own work. If the clinic still relies upon paramedics, they will want to exercise autonomy in their own use of developing skills.

3. The Federal Role in Health

Up to this point we have dealt only with the interest groups active at the local level, and the resources for which they compete have been regarded as exogenous factors. It is conceivable that the processes summarized above are due to vacillating financial support. Regular funding might solve many problems, even if health services were organized as at present. This is a plausible alternative explanation. Unfortunately, the sudden spurts of funds for new programs and then their drying up, and the continuous creation of new but under-funded and under-powered agencies, are characteristics of the political system which are not easily rectified, if they can be at all.

Most new urban health programs depend on vacillating commitments under federal and state legislation, and most analysts regard expanding and contracting state funds as exogenous factors like fate or the weather. The Ginzberg study, discussing ambulatory services and the city's plans for neighborhood family care centers, says, "In the presence of persisting financial strictures that are not likely to be loosened by the current federal administration . . . the city has nonetheless committed itself to a priority program." And the city's "ambitious program to establish neighborhood family care centers throughout the city was scarcely off the drawing board when it was undermined by Medicaid cutbacks at the state and federal levels as early as 1968."[10]

The federal government has been seen as a major force in reforming health care. Yet federal activity has intensified the problems. Government agencies are not independent forces regulating and planning in the public interest. Instead, government agencies are likely to become instruments for one or another part of the private sector. The Small Business Administration, for example, has been used on a number of occasions by one group of hospital interests to finance expansion, even while the Hill-Burton Agency has been financing the expansion of another nearby hospital.[11]

At the federal level, according to Dr. James A. Shannon, former director of the National Institutes of Health, health programs are a "broadly decentralized" and "highly fragmented" set of "patchwork" activities that make it "difficult to consider broad issues in a coherent manner." These activities touch on every problem of health care and delivery "without dealing decisively with any one," he said. Federal programs have come into being "sequentially" as "unbearable defects" are uncovered in private health care systems, rather then as "elements in a complete and unified system." During the Johnson administration alone, the Congress enacted fifty-one pieces of health legislation that provided for some 400 "discrete" authorities. The establishment of Regional Medical Programs in 1965 and Comprehensive Health Planning Programs in 1966 are additional cases in point. According to Dr. Shannon, elements of these two programs are in "direct conflict" with each other.[12]

Rosemary Stevens' 1971 study gives a brief and cogent summary of the federal role in health (pp. 500–509). "Pockets of federal action are now scattered across 221 different federal agencies and departments" (p. 502). She makes the point that even federal officials responsible for programs often do not know what programs practically identical to theirs exist in other agencies, and sometimes don't even know what programs they themselves allegedly administer. Again, this is probably not a problem of individual ignorance or incompetence, but a consequence of structural incoherence. Similarly, local or community coordination of programs is impossible because of fragmentation of funding at the federal level. Analysis of community planning thus cannot ignore the array of programs and funds available at the federal and state levels and how they have changed and are changing.

A recent analysis by Dr. Shannon of federal health expenditures was severely critical of federal activities as well as the reporting of them and the recommendations for new health activities contained in the 1971 federal budget.[13] Dr. Shannon's main point, as summarized by Senator Ribicoff, was that of the $20 billion allegedly spent by the federal government on "health," only 20 percent was actually spent on "programs whose basic

purpose is to improve and maintain the health of the general population"
(p. 1). He excluded the nearly $2 billion spent by the Department of
Defense which the federal budget includes under health expenditures but
which he says should more reasonably be charged to the "logistical
support required to satisfy the special needs of the military" (p. 12). Also,
he excluded the largest single item in the health budget—the $8 billion
Medicare program, which "is not a Federal expenditure" because it is
paid "through direct levy on employers and employees subject to social
security taxes" (p. 18). He excluded Medicaid and related programs
because, although they in fact are used to purchase health services, they
are basically income-supplement programs.

These points must be emphasized because of the common impression
that these programs represent an increase both in federal commitment
and in the quality and quantity of medical services. Rather, according to
Dr. Shannon, the

conditions under which these services are made available do not . . .
contribute to the improvement of the systems utilized. They have
not had a noticeable impact on the problems of maldistribution of
resources and services. To the contrary, the regulations governing the
operations of medicare and medicaid and some associated programs
have in many ways made these programs counter productive to the
development of more effective and more economical medical services.
The programs now provide no incentives for excellence in the services delivered or for economies in the health service system. Nor do
they provide an incentive to the development of a more equable distribution of the services to the population at large. Quite the contrary
and apart from the operational regulations, the overloading of the
health care system with no parallel provision for adequate expansion, has contributed to the present shortages in health personnel
and health service facilities. Such a circumstance tends to en-
trench more firmly the operational conventions of existing inadequate systems for health care. (pp. 19–20)

Thus, like most others these programs are tacked on to existing ones
in a complicated and irrational patchwork, subject to no consideration
of their consequences, costs, and benefits. In Dr. Shannon's terms,
federal health activities are "distributed ubiquitously within the executive agencies, lacking either central policy direction or broad program
goals as a base for program development" (p. 36).

A parallel perspective appears in the report by the Task Force on
Medicaid and Related Programs:

The existing programs that directly influence new development or
change (Partnership for Health, Regional Medical Programs, Nation-

al Center for Health Services Research and Development, Maternal and Child Health, Neighborhood Health Center, Community Mental Health Center, and Hill-Burton) have each been established by specific legislation that limits and defines eligible population, services and the roles that demonstration, experimentation, and research can play. Consequently, each program has its own grant policies, funding cycles, and requirements for review, reporting and accounting; and any group trying to develop comprehensive health care at the local level must thread its way through a maze of multiple grant applications, multiple sets of books, and inflated administrative cost— all too often to be rewarded with fragmented assistance.[14]

According to the 1971 New York State Rockefeller committee, at the federal, state, and local levels there are "68 different controlling agencies in the field."[15] The U.S. Department of Health, Education, and Welfare is "replete with overlapping and duplicating funding programs which not infrequently work in contradiction to each other. . . . 25 major programs within HEW, funded at a current cost of $12.7-billion . . . bear upon varous aspects of the health care problem and . . . operate largely independently of each other. More importantly, many of the programs have outlived their usefulness" (p. 17). Also, HEW has been

too politically defensive and not sufficiently administratively assertive. Too frequently, it reacts to individual Congressional initiative, and, in the absence of an overall health strategy of its own, fails to provide . . . leadership. . . . Many of its programs address old issues, which have been inherited from earlier days and not been re-tooled to keep abreast of contemporary needs. Overlays are put on overlays, and instead of reform and new structures, old programs are continued in their old style while new ones are added as needed—and as legislative expediency permits. (p.33)

Congress cannot be looked to for help. "Congress . . . many years ago succumbed to categorical 'disease' programs and patterns [and] has, by its actions and control over appropriations through a variety of subcommittees, contributed to many of the problems of fragmentation which now plague the present system" (p. 17).

The main consequences of Medicare and Medicaid have been the same. As a prominent medical sociologist says, "Whatever the merits of Medicare and Medicaid, they impressively illustrate that to increase investments in health care substantially without altering the framework in which services are delivered will only exacerbate the inefficiencies and absurdities of the current organization of medical care in America."[16]

The federal officials who make this kind of criticism are numerous. One more example must suffice. A former assistant secretary for health and scientific affairs of HEW cited the 1967 National Advisory Commission on Health Manpower Report to the effect that "the organization of health services has not kept pace with advances in medical science or with changes in society itself. Medical care in the United States is more a collection of bits and pieces (with overlapping, duplication, great gaps, high costs, and wasted effort), than an integrated system in which needs and efforts are closely related." The federal official, Dr. Philip R. Lee, went on to say, "That is a stern indictment, but it is a hard one to deny."[17]

These views are undoubtedly those of sincere, well-motivated men who have a vision of a well-coordinated and efficient delivery system. Unfortunately, their vision does not take into account the barriers to change. Even the data presumably necessary to administer giant federal programs have not been available because of interest group action, which illustrates again the way in which public funds and public powers are appropriated for private use without any mechanisms of accountability. Under both Medicare and Medicaid, private fiscal agents could be used to administer the programs, and "in at least one state . . . the levels of usual and customary fees for physicians as determined under Medicare were held by the carrier to be confidential information and were not released to the Medicaid administrators, and the situation is thought to have been similar in other states." In general, in both large and small states, "huge multimillion dollar programs were established without the basic mechanisms of program accountability. The tradition of inadequate statistical data was carried through from the welfare programs into Medicaid."[18] Despite the great size of federal health agencies, the staff available for long-range planning is extraordinarily small, again indicating relative priorities. "The remarkably sketchy apparatus for health policy formulation in the United States today . . . [is] understaffed, underfunded and poorly organized. . . . HEW . . . has at the secretariat level only a small handful of individuals dealing with health . . . [who] are, by necessity, preoccupied with short-term issues of importance to current legislative decisions and are heavily constrained by political exigencies." The same situation exists for the staffs of House and Senate subcommittees concerned with health legislation. They number "only some half-dozen individuals all of whom are primarily involved with practical problems related to hearings, preparation of legislation, and other pressing day-to-day matters. Only to a negligible extent can they devote their efforts to . . . policy analysis.[19]

Thus, the bodies presumably most concerned with overall policy planning in the public interest are in fact not devoting the necessary resources to that task. This too is no accident but stems from the nature of political imperatives to be discussed later.

Given the functions performed by the basic structure of the health care system for the dominant interests, legislation which allegedly establishes new principles of operation and which explicitly is designed to change the "system" is almost inevitably distorted in ways which reinforce the present system. For example, in commenting on the community mental health centers established by federal legislation in 1963, Connery et al. say, "Something appears to have been lost since the community centers program was initiated. The 'bold new approach' of 1963 shows great promise of becoming merely an expensive expansion of decentralized facilities closely resembling the outpatient clinics predating its adoption."[20]

The mechanisms through which bold new programs become timid old ones are unclear, but co-optation and direct control by interest groups play a part. The reaction by major interest groups to potential attack by federal legislation has sometimes been to create joint committees which can ward off regulation and, where possible, directly control federal activity. A good example of this is the creation of the Joint Commission on Accreditation of Hospitals in 1952 by six interest organizations, including the American Medical Association and the American Hospital Association. It established standards of accreditation for hospitals which were "grossly inadequate." Even those standards were not enforced. That 128 of the 130 state and local government hospitals registered with the AHA were accredited in 1968 "despite obvious and admitted deficiencies attests to the inadequacy of the standards applied by the JCAH and the ineffectiveness of the accreditation program in maintaining hospital quality." Despite these inadequacies, the JCAH standards have been accepted by several federal laws, notably the Social Security Act of 1965, as the basis for hospitals receiving reimbursement under Medicare. Even more important, at the administrative stage "the federal government has interpreted this section to mean that hospitals which are JCAH accredited may not be inspected or evaluated by state agencies under contract with the federal government to see if they also meet the Medicare Conditions of Participation."[21] Apparently, then, the very same laws and administrative procedures which were designed to establish a minimum standard of quality of health care in fact *guarantee* that those standards will *not* be met. Governmental acceptance of the self-regulating authority of an organization (the JCAH) representing a coalition of interest groups legally screens the private interest groups from regulation and at the same time guarantees them access to public monies and authority. Seldom has the symbiosis of public power and private interests been so clear.

However, perhaps because of these consequences of federal action, the corporate rationalizers express faith in the power of the federal government, despite their own account of its complex and fragmented structure. I intentionally omitted the optimistic rhetoric surrounding the above critiques. The Rockefeller committee softens its criticism of HEW by asserting that HEW "fails to provide the leadership it can and should be expected to give." Elsewhere it speaks of the "vital, major role" to be played by HEW in "helping to shape and rationalize the health care system" (*Preliminary Report*, p. 33). And the Task Force on Medicaid asserts, "We must focus these programs around a common Federal health-service policy, coordinate financial and administrative requirements, integrate technical services and spend what we save on new and improved services" (*Task Force*, p. 29). This brave rhetoric is nearly meaningless. Why?

4. Political Imperatives and
   Bureaucratic Autonomy

The answer is that politicians have to provide crises with solutions: a continuing series of new programs which promise to respond to the latest crisis. When one program fails, another will be offered, sometimes by the same incumbent party and politician, sometimes by the next incumbent who may have been propelled into office by his promises to provide leadership which will solve the problems his predecessor promised and failed to solve.

Thus, each impending election produces a spate of new programs designed to show either how much the incumbent has achieved or how much his challenger will achieve. Given the frequency of elections and the need to provide patronage which will solidify the support of local constituencies, each set of officials will attempt to institutionalize his programs in a new set of agencies. The liberals go along with, and even become the main proponents of, these "solutions" because of their politically realistic, pragmatic assessment of the situation.

Thus, new programs are sold; they become political commodities on the electoral market. But like other commodities their exchange value for electoral support is more important than their use value—that is, how much actual health care is provided. Once their price has been realized in the political market, new programs lose much of their value, except insofar as something tangible must be demonstrated at the time of the next election. But what is "tangible"? An agency, a building, a staff, a budget, funds being spent, but not, unfortunately, actual improvements in health services. In fact, attempts to demonstrate actual improvements are likely to show only the discrepancy between intentions (or claims) and performance and are, therefore, politically dysfunctional.

But this picture of ever-expanding programs seems to contradict the frequently made point that legislatures are losing control of state budgets as more and more programs become firmly embedded in bureaucratic agencies. Both are true. Legislatures which fund new programs are, indeed, interested in maintaining their fiscal and statutory control over as much government activity as possible. This control is steadily weakening as more agencies become securely established and remove bigger and bigger chunks of the budget (whether city, state, or federal) from legislative power.

What accounts for this apparent contradiction? The interest of the legislature as a whole in maintaining control over budgets and agencies is contradicted in specific cases by the interests of a given faction within it which wishes to turn over programs to a permanent agency, stably representing in its policies and decisions the interest of a specific constituency. As a result of logrolling between various factions within the legislature, such bills are ultimately passed in many cases. Every faction, whether liberal or conservative, wants to institutionalize its own programs—to embed them in permanently funded agencies beyond the reach of "political" decision—and prevent other factions from doing the same for their interest groups. But the consequence of continuous expansion of such bureaucratic agencies—by definition, those which are renewed or refunded with little or no debate—is to reduce the power of the legislature as a whole.

The compromise which frequently resolves this contradiction, decision by decision, is to vote to establish a new program, thus responding to constituent demands, but on a demonstration project or year-by-year basis. This solution creates additional problems for legislative operations because it means that many programs must be brought up frequently for review, thus cluttering up the legislative schedule. But at the cost of much apparently ritualistic behavior (such as passing renewal legislation or another biennial budget by a unanimous vote), the legislature maintains control over as much of the budget and agencies as possible. If a given program loses political support, or if it becomes a political liability, too expensive or obsolete, it can be cut back or eliminated. There is one sense in which it is in the interests of legislators to create public bureaucracies. Creation of an agency is a way of getting off their backs political pressure from interest groups. Depending on the cohesion, political resources, and consistency of the demands of the interest group with the dominant institutions of the society, the new agency can be a substantive rather than symbolic response to the demands.[22]

Public officials want to create bureaucracies which embody the principles to which they are committed (whether liberal or conservative). And regardless of the rhetoric about keeping the agencies under public control, it is not in the public official's interest to do so. If they are under his control, he will still be subject to the demands for performance; it is therefore to his advantage to give the agency real autonomy. Also, he wants the agency to respond to the key interests which caused it to be set up in the first place. Thus, public officials are likely to decentralize power into bureaucracies. This is a necessary form of political fragmentation in a pluralist system, for the necessary information and resources simply don't exist within the narrow confines of legitimate action for public officials. The exclusion from their legitimate jurisdiction of most decisions and policies which affect the welfare of the public means that legislatures simply do not have the power to prevent fragmentation, and in fact benefit from furthering it.

Although new agencies reduce the power of the legislature vis-à-vis the accumulating array of public bureaucracies, they also are a sign of the power of those majority coalitions within the legislature which succeed in establishing the agency and in providing it with the power to respond substantively to outside constituencies. The long-range effect of the actions of legislatures is thus to decentralize power into a wide variety of public bureaucracies. The various recommendations to create instrumentalities to coordinate and integrate agencies ignore these political functions.

The consequence of these processes at the *legislative* level is that there is continuous uncertainty among the staff at the *operating* levels of health agencies. Considerable time must be diverted from programs into preparation of the annual budget report, grant application, or whatever other document must demonstrate the need for continuation of the project or program. To some extent this continual need to justify the program would seem to maintain the priority of the original goals which established the program. This may in some cases be true. But also likely is a concern with tangible and manifest aspects of the program, those most easily measured in quantitative terms, such as adding new staff members, spending more money, adding offices and new facilities or divisions or departments which have new names. None of these has any necessary relationship to the presumed goals of the organization, but forms a visible part of the description of its recent achievements. Growth, expansion, and increased complexity can all be defined as progress toward the goals.

In addition to the pressure to develop these indicators of performance, there must be a continuing escalation of the rhetoric of claims of past performance and the promises for the next period of funding. In many situations, funds will be scarce, and different agencies will be competing against each other for them. Pressure is thereby created to exaggerate both reports and plans in order to create a favorable comparison. Because the fund-granting unit does not want to lose its own control over decisions, it is not likely to release information about how generous the available funds are in any given year, and therefore how "honest" the applying unit need be in order to compete effectively with other applying agencies. In any case, the agency which is applying (whether for funds, legislation, a new program, or any other authority being requested) has nothing to gain from being honest, because it never knows at what moment a revelation of the shortcoming of a program—even if clearly provable to be out of control of the staff—will be used against it by one or another faction higher in the organization which holds a different conception of the relative importance of one or another component department or agency.

This pluralistic competition exists because there can be no central control mechanism for making national health policy which is in the general or public interest. While legislatures have that symbolic role, they are a congeries of representatives of specific interest groups. Sometimes the bureaucratic agencies are regarded as "above politics," even if legislatures cannot be, and thus are potentially able to formulate general public policy. Many reforms aim at removing decisions from the legislature or the executive and placing them in a bureaucratic agency, for the reasons and with the consequences outlined above. These efforts assume that such agencies can become neutral instruments of general interests, but they ignore the continuous distortion of their substantive decisions in directions which fit the pervasive presence of private economic and social power. In fact, the more apparently separate the agency is from legislative representative institutions, the more vulnerable it is to influence from private organizations and groups, such as the doctors and the voluntary hospitals, in the case of the health system.

Given this sketchy outline of the structure and the processes by which it changes, one might imagine that it would quickly become both bottom- and top-heavy and collapse. That is, the multiplicity of organizational units and the differentiation of existing ones in response to the pressures summarized above would cause such a high level of overlapping, costs, complexity, and inaccessibility that a fantastically expensive chaos of organizations failing to accomplish their stated goals would result. At what point such a system would become politically and socially unbearable if difficult to say. We may be close to that point.

But there is at least one political mechanism which militates against this process and serves to maintain some equilibrium. Although this is not their intention, one consequence of the legislatures' maintaining veto power over agencies by not making them permanent is to allow the dying off (or the killing off) of a certain proportion of agencies, programs and projects.[23] Some agencies are eliminated, and some projects disappear, remarkable as it seems. There may be little or no correlation between the tangible services which an agency performs and the likelihood of its not being refunded. Certainly one should not assume from the cries of agony which are raised by the staff, its clientele, or its political sponsors when an agency is in imminent danger of being killed that, in fact, its continuation would be the best possible use of the human and material resources involved.

But from the point of view of the continuation of the existing system, the periodic elimination of some organizations may compensate for the continuous creation of new ones. Like political regimes, bureaucratic organizations may either accumulate so many liabilities that they lose political support or may become so rigid—so bureaucratic in the pejorative sense—that they are no longer able to adjust to a situation to which their political sponsors want them to respond. In that case, even if the need which generated the organization remains unfulfilled, an existing organization may be allowed to die, and a new one may be created in its place. The new one may also be, as the old one may have been, merely a symbolic response to the need. But it is a response; the organization has a fresh new name and a fresh new staff and can be advertised as the action of innovative leaders responsibly solving problems.

To conclude, seemingly inherent tendencies of bureaucracies may actually be specific features of a political economy in which autonomous, self-perpetuating organizations perform key functions in maintaining the domination of particular types of group and class interests. Once given statutory powers and a reasonably assured budget, the "natural" tendencies of bureaucracies to expand and seek autonomy take over. These independent activities conceal the continuing service to particular structured interests of the specific goals and commitments of the staff. If I am correct in this hypothesis, it further mystifies this function of "autonomous" bureaucracies to ascribe this development to inherent features of organization. Such an assertion (like the explanation of individual human behavior by intrinsic features of "personality" or "human nature") essentially stops inquiry into causes.

Constant administrative juggling is a sign of an inability to put together a functioning coalition of powers and resources which can carry out a task desired by significant elites representing dominant or challenging structural interests. Reorganizations attempt to add new elements of support or potential support or to redefine tasks in ways which cut down the resources and powers necessary to maintain a precarious balance between opposing forces.[24]

The life-history of any organization and the interests it serves thus cannot be seen in a vacuum. The organization, no matter how much it seems to be securely established by law, custom, or funding, will continue to exist only so long as the coalition of interest groups who benefit from its existence continue to support it. The more stable an organization seems—take, for example, one of the great voluntary hospitals in New York City—the more likely it is that its activities are continuously serving important structural interests. Emerging conflict over such issues as its existence, purpose, control, funding, or size indicates that the interests the organization has been serving are withdrawing their support, becoming weaker, or being challenged. Only when there is some chance of altering the balance of control over the organization are other interest groups likely to challenge its existence or character.[25] Under these circumstances, the underlying allocations of powers and privileges to different structural interests become at least partly visible in the battles of interest groups in political and legal arenas.

7 Consequences for Health Research

What may appear to be confident factual assertions in the preceding chapters do not rest upon well-confirmed and repeated studies of health institutions but rather, are hypotheses linking scattered observations. Observers and researchers agree that, unfortunately, little systematic knowledge exists about the ways in which the present system works or the alternatives that might be feasible. Not only are basic descriptive data scarce, but relevant research on the system as a whole has not been done, for reasons to be discussed.

1. The Lack of Appropriate Data

A variety of reports agree that appropriate data are not available. The 1967 report of the National Advisory Commission on Health Manpower concluded that "there is a serious lack of the consistent and comprehensive statistical information that is required for rational analysis and planning, despite a surfeit of numbers about health."[1] The research director of the Kaiser Foundation Hospitals in Portland, Oregon, commenting like others on the lack of significant change between 1933 and 1967, added that although many conferences and papers in thirty-five years have pointed out the "need for adequate medical care research," we still do not have "comprehensive, coordinated, and reliable research systematically carried on to help solve the many complex problems in the organization of health care services."[2] Medical sociologist David Mechanic has asserted that "relatively little effort has been devoted to identifying and refining criteria by which to evaluate competing programs of medical care, and few rigorous measures exist."[3] Eliot Freidson reports that "systematic and reliable information about medical practice in the United States is incredibly scanty. The extraordinary bulk of published material is composed almost entirely of special pleading or unsystematic individual impressions; the only reliable body of extensive information bears on the financing, distribution, and utilization of health services."[4]

A recent attempt to develop a comprehensive framework for the analysis of health data began by asserting that the Regional Medical Programs and Comprehensive Health Planning acts enacted by Congress in 1965 and 1966 "require the kind of data on the structure and functioning of the health services system which exist in rather fragmentary form. In fact, there is hardly even a conceptual model of the health services system by which the pertinent data can be selected and collected to reveal the chief structural and functional aspects of the system for intelligent application of the two Acts."[5] The authors go on to give a number of examples of research studies of the "system" which purport to be critical analyses but which instead consist of multitudes of isolated facts presented with no attempt to relate them or draw inferences about their causes and consequences. In a sense, the pluralism of politics and the society is thus duplicated in policy research and science. They point out that although there have been numerous complaints about the duplication of expensive facilities such as cobalt bombs, "no systematic study has been done to determine the extent of duplicating 'waste' of resources and effect of professional incentive" (p. 7). Although it is known that fewer unnecessary operations and hospital admissions occur in group practice–prepayment arrangements than in the prevailing voluntary health insurance arrangement, "there has been no systematic study of the effect on the total range of services and their costs when hospital admission and surgical rates are lowered" (p. 7). Although it is known that the use of emergency departments is increasing, it is not known whether or not "the emergency department is deliberately used by the private practitioners as an extension of their own office practices" (p. 8). These few examples illustrate the general point about the paucity of serious investigations of the interrelationships of health institutions and interest groups. Most data refer to the characteristics of patients, treatments, diseases, costs, physicians, or hospitals, seen as isolated entities about which bits of data are collected.

That study, which is essentially an inventory of the available data for Chicago, illustrates the general point perfectly, as the authors themselves are well aware. Data are given on the population of the area, mortality and morbidity rates, the numbers of hospital beds, physicians, nurses, dentists, drugstores, blood banks, medical schools, and the numbers of agencies providing for some of the health needs of the mentally ill and the poor, the numbers of admissions to hospitals, numbers of visits to physicians and dentists, the per capita expenditures for health care, room rates for hospitals, and the sources of payment for health costs. None of these data are related to each other or to a conception of the structure of institutions which generates these relationships and outcomes. The authors properly say that these bits of information *are* important, and in their absence, "the limited comprehension we now have of the structure and operation of the health services system would vanish" (p. 100). However, from these data one can, the authors plausibly argue, "in the main obtain only a static picture of the system, namely, at best the structure and at worst a simple inventory of seemingly disparate parts" (p. 100).

Unfortunately, in spelling out their conception of needed further research, the authors do not specify the kinds of *data* which would be necessary. They call for studies of the nature of physician practices, of hospital emergency departments, of health services for the poor, of long-term care facilities, and of patient flow through the health services system, and they emphasize that the linkages of "people, facilities, and personnel" should be analyzed, not as "isolated information and facts," but as illustrations of the "structure and operation of the health services system" (pp. 102-104). This goal can only be applauded, even if the means to achieve such studies of the system remain obscure.

An analysis by economist Uwe Reinhardt of the various proposals for health reform before Congress in 1973 concluded that there is a "dearth of information on the socioeconomic and medical characteristics of alternative provider systems, existing or imagined" and that "a great deal more empirical information needs to be gathered on the behavior of the participants in the health-care sector and on the technical constraints under which that sector operates before one can confidently develop and follow a coherent blueprint for a reorganization of the American health-care system."[6] This statement reflects the assumptions that the relevant data *could* be collected and that, even if appropriate data were available, their implications for policy could be followed in reorganization strategies. Both assumptions are highly questionable. If the data could be collected, why haven't they been already? Economists tend to assume that information is available to the consumer—no other assumption is compatible with a justification for a free market—or that if the information doesn't exist (for mysterious reasons), it could be gotten, and *then* the market would work.

The absence of adequate data is related to a failure to select the appropriate unit of analysis. Presumably the problem is to provide a whole range of hospital facilities within an entire region at a reasonable cost to the population within that region. Data on hospital costs do not bear on that problem, as Reinhardt says. Rather than finding direct measures of the rate of output (the rate of successful treatments per physician visit, for example), indirect measures such as the number of beds per hospital are used, which have no necessary relationship to health productivity of the institution. [7]

The lack of any system which could gain access to the basic data necessary even to *describe* the provision of health care was asserted by the president's 1972 Panel on Health Services Research and Development. Although "almost every agency within HEW involved with either health services research, development, delivery, or financing presently has its own statistical system," "the wealth of information generated by these programs is largely untapped and inaccessible." With respect to hospitals which vary "in the benefits they provide for the populations they serve, the resources they use to provide those benefits, and the charges made for their services, . . . it is impossible to compare individual hospitals with each other within a community, and similarly it is impossible to compare communities with respect to their hospital services." [8] These are astonishing revelations from a high-level panel charged with making recommendations to correct this very situation. Their inability to make any significant recommendations is just as striking, because essentially the recommendations consisted of still more *administrative* juggling. The action recommended to correct the lack of basic data was the creation of a "Bureau of Health Statistics" and still *another* task force to define that bureau's specific responsibilities, as if there were not already (as the report just pointed out) many bureaus gathering data.

2. The Lack of Relevant Research

Even the research which has been done has frequently used inappropriate measures—partly because of the inadequacy of the data. Economist Uwe Reinhardt has pointed out that there is as yet no "consensus among medical experts on an operationally meaningful definition" of an index to the quality of health care. But measures often used in practice "confuse quality with resource-intensiveness of treatment" (cost of treatment, availability of expensive and technologically sophisticated equipment, amount of physician time used), which "may result in unnecessary inflation in the cost of medical care." [9] Reinhardt's own conclusion can be extended (although perhaps he would not go this far), since in a system still dominated by fee-for-service medicine, there are enormous incentives for physicians to "overprescribe or over-supply health services to those consumers who can afford to purchase medical care" (p. 176). Under these conditions, the *more* cost, time, and equipment involved in health care, the *lower* the quality is likely to be. Research which takes the amount of money, time, and equipment used to provide service as an index of the quality of care will miss the point entirely.

Most studies of the delivery system focus on the utilization of health services by different income, occupational, and ethnic groups, on the socialization of physicians and nurses, or on the impact of the internal organization of a hospital upon patient care. Most sociological research focuses upon either the occupation or profession (doctor, nurse) as the unit, or upon the organization or institution as the unit (hospital, clinic, mental hospital). The perspective subtly shifts, depending on the problem. In the former case, the organization or institution is seen as the work setting for the occupation or profession, and problems studied are those of socialization, orientations to work, clients, knowledge, careers, mobility, and role conflicts. Characteristics of the organization or institutional environment are regarded as variables affecting one or the other dependent variable listed. In the latter case, the occupations and professions are seen as the sets of interrelated and interdependent roles which must be enacted for the goals of the institution or organization to be achieved. The research problems become the conflicts between jurisdictions of the roles, the gap or contradiction between organizational and personal or occupational goals, the conflicts between different organizational goals, and sometimes the environmental factors which affect all of the above, regarded as dependent variables.

In both cases, the larger cultural and societal framework which defines the roles and provides patients and the resources for treating them is taken as given. A few studies of cultural variations in illness behavior or variations in the financing of hospitals or state ownership are done, and the problem of the patient returning to his "environment" is pointed to, but the problem of the environment as a whole is not systematically analyzed.[10]

In response to the financial crisis, a number of studies have appeared which use econometric models—preference functions, economies of scale, demand, and so forth—to develop analyses of hospital organization and financial structure. Most of them accept the existing structure of ownership and control of medical education, and service. They accept the market environment of hospitals as given and do not attempt to counterpose another model which would alter the basic parameters of the health system. Nor do they contrast the performance of hospitals within and without the health market.

A study of four hospital "industries," for example, excludes federal hospitals because they "are typically isolated from the general market."[11] The author of this study continues:

Perhaps the most significant characteristic suggested by these data is that the short-term general and other special hospital industry, unlike the previous three hospital industries analyzed, is not dominated by public facilities. . . . somewhat more than 75 per cent of the total demand is satisfied by private institutions. The large part played by private hospitals and the pricing policy of public hospitals suggest that private benefits have usually been considered sufficient to generate a reasonably satisfactory allocation of resources in terms of the implicit social welfare function. . . . Although state and local hospitals generally treat more nonpaying welfare patients and have a higher proportion of bad receivables, their pricing policy is quite similar to those of their voluntary and proprietary counterparts in this industry. (p. 115)

The author does not raise the question of why the public hospitals' pricing policy is similar or whether demand is the same as need. As a matter of fact, elsewhere he noted that a previous study "took hospital utilization out of the ambiguous category of 'need' and placed it within a demand model."[12] From the point of view of objective analysis of data, the actual case of patients presenting themselves to hospitals is much more accurately described as that of demand rather than that of need. But whether or not an overall analysis of health care can do without an underlying category of need is doubtful. The results of such a "demand" analysis seem predetermined to accept the existing structural framework because there is no basis for criticism of failures to allocate resources to meet "needs." All one can analyze is whether or not existing health care units respond adeaquately to the demands placed upon them. This is an instance of the conceptual limitations even of those studies which have been done.

Another study—an excellent one within its own terms of reference— was a two-year demonstration project during which New York Hospital provided all medical services to welfare recipients in a certain area of New York City. The authors collected exhaustive patient and utilization data and did a survey of patient attitudes. The general conclusion was that

a voluntary teaching hospital could render a full range of medical services in a personalized and coordinated way to a population of welfare recipients in the community. The relative success of the undertaking depended on a number of innovations in customary out-patient practice[:] . . . (1) providing a clinical team within the hospital that could come to know the patients over a span of years and that would provide the continuity such care provides, (2) taking responsibility for the care of people in the community before they presented themselves for treatment. . ., (3) guaranteeing availability of services to patients so that they did not face repeated screening for eligibility.[13]

The main findings were that the experimental care cost more money than the existing system. However, even allowing for extra "start-up" costs, the estimate of all costs was less than $20 per month per patient actually served for the two years of the experiment (1961–63). Patients reported considerable satisfaction with their care. After two years, those who came to the project preferred clinic care over private care.

The project was aimed at the "fragmented" health care received by the poor in New York City. While it is undoubtedly an instance of innovative health programming within the existing institutional framework, the authors unfortunately did not place their findings within a broad enough analytic frame. They did not consider the possible economies of scale of extending this program to a wider population, nor the savings in administrative superstructure if eligibility red tape were eliminated. The basic reason is that the study was still trapped by the assumption of two health systems, one for paying and one for nonpaying patients. The authors remarked that "many factors in the medical environment of the indigent still militate against coordination of their care" (p. 215), and they proposed that several factors be taken into account by future planners. For example, "it is important to reduce the barriers to access as much as possible," and "community planning should therefore include attention to provision of facilities within easy reach."

Such recommendations have been made for generations, to no avail. The goodwill and hard work of the authors cannot be denied, but the very fact that the program disappeared after two years because of lack of funds indicates the fruitlessness of this kind of health experiment. None of their recommendations included the concept of a great voluntary teaching hospital rendering the "full range of medical services in a personalized and coordinated way to a population of welfare recipients in the community." The authors never mentioned the feasibility of establishing such a program of comprehensive, coordinated care, whether for welfare recipients or anybody else, but simply assumed that the study's findings will somehow be communicated to an audience with both the power and the motivation to act upon them. Such an audience does not exist. None of the New York City commission reports done after this experiment which ended in 1963 referred to the findings of the study.

The failures of even the best research on the health care system to draw seemingly quite modest conclusions from their own findings are striking. A good example is an important study by two Yale medical sociologists. This is a study of health care in the hospital attached to "Eastern University" [Yale University] Medical School. According to the authors, this hospital is one of the best in the nation, yet patient care is "far from what is could and should be."[14] The study compared care in wards, semiprivate rooms, and private rooms. Although the ward patients were sicker, they got less attention and poorer care than others, and of course the income and social class of the patients affected the quality of their care. The authors asserted that the problems of patients were "subordinated" to the physician's "efforts to protect the physician-patient relationship as he defined it" (p. 382). Students were trained mostly on the wards, but the authors argued that that was a poor teaching model to use, because of the poor standard of care: "the very neglect of personal and social influences upon disease, diagnosis, and care found in *all* accomodations may be viewed as extensions of the ward model" (p. 381).

The authors, commenting on their findings, rejected the possibility that "senior physicians [can be] successful private entrepreneurs or professors and at the same time effective leaders in hospital management" (p. 381). Unfortunately, they did not follow up this point to consider the internal contradictions in these roles and the way in which health care is distorted because of the ways in which institutions are organized. Individual role conflicts reflect contradictions in the goals of organizations and institutions.

After documenting the failure of this hospital—and it should be re-emphasized that the authors considered it far above average—to provide the level of health care which it could have provided, even to well-to-do private patients, the authors' recommendations seem remarkably feeble. First, they recommend that health professionals be "trained to deal systematically with the personal and social factors" affecting their patient's health. But they did not discuss the reasons why this is not possible, given the organization of health care. Second, they recommended that "continuing senior medical leadership focus on the care of patients in each patient-care division." But quite aside from ambiguity about what this means, how could it be done? Their own research identified the powerful incentives *not* to reorganize care. Third, they recommended that the nurses be responsible largely to this medical leadership. Again, their own research documented the absence of nurse-physician relationships, despite the urgent need for continuous communication between them, because of the status problems of most physicians. Fourth, they recommended that "medical auxiliaries eventually replace nurses and be given more responsibility and career opportunities in patient care" (p. 384). The structural incompatabilities of nurse-physician roles seem likely to reproduce the same problems in the new "medical auxiliaries" (or "para-professionals" as they are currently called), precisely because of the professional monopoly by the physicians. In short, the study ended with recommendations which ultimately must be seen simply as exhortations to everyone involved to be more concerned. The research focus on the sick person as the "primary actor" and upon the doctor-nurse and doctor-nurse-patient relationships may partly account for the authors' failure to analyze the structural origins of the problems they so well described.

It is striking that there is so little research on the key question of the effect of different ways of organizing health care on its cost, its quality, access to it, or anything else. Such evidence as exists—as summarized in a recent review of the literature—indicates that the prepaid form of Health Maintenance Organization (HMO) produces "lower hospital use, relatively more ambulatory and preventive service, and lower overall costs ... than conventional open-market fee-for-service patterns."[15] Clearly these measures may have little to do with the quality of care, however, since lower hospital use and costs may simply mean poorer care. With respect to the question of "how healthy [HMO's] keep their members, compared with other patterns of medical care delivery," the data are scarce. A review by Donabedian in 1969 made clear the "sparsity of data on this crucial question.... Since then, some little additional outcome data have been produced ... but not always with conclusive results" (p. 302). It is remarkable that with the continuing concern with the health care "crisis," so few studies of the consequences of alternative modes of delivering care have been done.

While all of the kinds of studies cited can be justified in their own terms, they do not touch the core problem of the structure of the *producing* institutions but focus instead either upon the *consumers* of health care or upon a specific institutional, organizational, or professional context in which a particular kind of care is provided. Such a paucity of studies is no accident; such studies would challenge structural interests of both professional monopoly and corporate rationalization in maintaining health institutions as they now exist or in directing their "orderly" expansion.

The basic information for assessing the performance of health institutions does not exist because there is no coordinated health system at the level of *delivery*: hospitals are concerned not with assessing the state of health of the patient as a total person, but only with the state of his liver at a particular time, and they therefore do not integrate various possible sources of data on persons. No organization has either the responsibility or the power to integrate and coordinate preventive care, ambulatory care, and inpatient care with regard to the efficiency of patient flows, control over duplication of facilities or the allocation of manpower in accordance with patient needs. Because of the lack of both responsibility and power, the data have not been generated which could allow policies to be made on a sound empirical foundation.

Although the community population has a real stake in accurate information on the quality and quantity of services and their costs, and also in information on a structure of controls which would be responsive to community health needs, they have no resources with which to command that information. The main information which health institutions generate is internal management information for billing and tax purposes, individual patient data, and research data useful for certain professional and scientific problems but not for assessment of outputs and the performance of the organization. But outside groups cannot easily obtain even these data to analyze for their own purposes, since the data might be used to show the ways in which the various parts of the organizations fail to achieve their ostensible goals, advertised far and wide in the efforts to obtain more funds. Even if available, information could not easily be aggregated with information from other sources to estimate the causal relationships between the inputs of money and manpower from one organization to another and the outputs of tangible health services. The professional monopolists, who tend to be strategically located in data-gathering and -processing positions, also have no incentive to release information to outside groups who might challenge their power to define their own work.

Because there is *no* "system" in the sense in which operations researchers define it, the frequently repeated solution of better information and better communication is no solution at all. Thus, while obeisance may be made to information gathering and data processing, these symbolic expressions of need screen the absence of the basic data which could be used to measure the character of services and the performance of organizations. For the same reasons, there exist no data which could allow the study of the health system as a whole, although what is really problematic is the structure of health care providing institutions—their funding, control, relationships to each other, and impact on the quality and quantity of services.

8 Crisis, Pluralism, and Perspectives on Reform

The political and economic realities of health care documented earlier in this work contrast sharply with concepts of the ideal health system. The barriers to structural change of health institutions in the class character of American society are not recognized in the optimistic pluralist image of both health care institutions and the society as a whole. Different perspectives—pluralist, bureaucratic, and class—on the possibility of health care reform are based on competing theories of the causes of the "crisis" in health care, and thus alternative paths to reform.

1. Crisis and Recent Reforms

As we have seen, periodic political crises in health care have been precipitated by corporate rationalizers in an attempt to create support for their goals, although media exposure which defines a crisis usually has nothing to do with any change in the basic performance of health institutions. The series of investigations in New York City by private, city, and state agencies from 1950 to 1970 stress the fragmentation and lack of coordination of the system, a sure sign of the ideology of corporate rationalization—as are the various reorganizations of the hospitals carried out in the last decade. But none of the reforms has touched the basic power of the private sector and its institutions. Instead, state power has reinforced private power.

A few crises have been precipitated by equal-health advocates moving outside the established framework of representation and influence to take disruptive, militant action. These have produced specific responses, usually in the form of new programs or still more "representation," taking the forms already described.[1]

As was seen in the case study of neighborhood health centers, New

York City saw a chance to use federal money to expand the city-controlled network of ambulatory care programs. The hospitals saw a chance to expand outpatient activities since they would now be funded. They may have feared loss of control of their territory if this function was taken over by the city, even if they didn't want it for its own sake. The city focused upon its programs of neighborhood family care centers, since it did not have enough power to coordinate the rest of the units of the system. Therefore, officials pushed as hard as they could to get them going; realizing the need and wanting to shorten the time, they devised a "prototype" plan which was to be used for all of the centers. The Planning Council objected on the valid ground that the prototype plan did not take into account the specific needs of the local community. The typical result was either total stalemate or the addition of another facility with no agency having the slightest idea—based on any systematic analysis—of the actual health needs of and facilities available to a neighborhood population. Incredible delays occurred in the provision of sorely needed primary care facilities in areas lacking physicians, hospitals, and clinics.

What is the likely course of change? Given the institutionalized power of both dominant and challenging structural interests and the ease with which equal-health advocates can be co-opted, the most likely changes are an expansion of health-care-providing units at the "bottom" of the system and the elaboration of bureaucratic and planning machinery at the "top." These compromises between the major structural interests have society-wide consequences—which the population as a whole must bear—of constantly increasing costs, inaccessible and complicated clinic and hospital structure, expanding governmental agencies, and reduced ability to influence the course of change through political participation and action.

2. The Ideal and the Actual
   Health System

The realities documented in the case studies and literature above contrasted sharply with the presentation by almost all commentators on health care of a consistent image of the ideal health system, which has remained essentially the same for many years. Such a system recognizes the need for both professional autonomy, on the one hand (guaranteed by strong professional organization, control over training, and high quality biomedical research), and a coordinated and integrated health care delivery system on the other (taking advantage of the knowledge and application of medical technology and a complex division of labor between paraprofessionals and various levels of specialized practitioners who provide both preventive and medical care). The primary care practitioner, responsible for families, is seen as the key "interface," linking the patient with a series of increasingly more specialized professional and hospital services. In the ideal system the services are presumed to be available without regard to income, through various types of subsidies, insurance programs, and the like.

As medical sociologist David Mechanic put it, as he focused on health care for the poor in the United States, "health care problems of the poor are a product of the larger socio-political system and of the more general organization of health care services in America." He continues, "the problems of health care are only one part of a more complex pattern of social, economic, and environmental difficulties. . . . These problems will require a more frontal attack on our national values, our priorities, and our system of social stratification itself.[2]

To summarize the argument in a nutshell, the "crisis" of health care is *not* a result of the necessary competition of diverse interests, groups, and providers in a pluralistic and competitive health economy, nor is it a result of bureaucratic inefficiencies to be corrected by yet more layers of administration established by government policy. Rather, the conflicts between the professional monopolists, who seek to erect barriers to protect their control over research, teaching, and care, and the corporate rationalizers, who seek to extend their control over the organization of services, account for many of the aspects of health care summarized above. These conflicts stem, in turn, from a fundamental contradiction in modern health care between the character of the technology of health care and the private appropriation of the power and resources involved. Health care, from the point of view of the most advanced technology, is a complex division of labor requiring highly specialized knowledge at some points, routine screening at others, and highly personalized individual care at still others. The integration of all aspects of health care—prevention, outpatient checkups, routine treatment for minor illnesses, specialized treatment for rare diseases or those requiring expensive machines, long-term care for chronic conditions—would require the defeat or consolidation of the social power that has been appropriated by various discrete interest groups and that preserves existing allocations of social values and resources. Government is not an independent power standing above and beyond the competing interest groups, but represents changing coalitions of elements drawn from various structural interests.

However, I cannot let the analysis rest here without some final comments on the possibilities of market versus bureaucratic reform. These widely perceived alternatives usually are stated in a way which creates a fictitious verbal solution of the basic conflict. For example, medical sociologist Odin Anderson has defined these alternatives as follows:

Diametrically opposite answers can be made... to the question of whether or not use and price of health services... should be subjected to a form of regulation or control: (1) allow the medical economy to follow its trends until an equilibrium is reached, without controls on use or price except insofar as they already exist, such as optimum limits on hospital beds, negotiated and contracted fee schedules between physicians and insuring agencies, and so forth; or (2) establish use and price controls at all checkpoints in hospitals, through state regulation of hospital rates and physicians' fees, regulation and standardization of insuring agencies, and so on.[3]

These alternatives correspond to what I have called the "market" versus "bureaucratic" reform views. My argument is that these alternatives should not be seen abstractly in cost-benefit terms, but rather concretely in terms of the specific advantages and disadvantages perceived by interest groups with stakes in either preserving or changing existing health institutions. Unfortunately, Anderson blunted his own analysis by relying on the vague but appealing notion of a social consensus on when costs are too great and effectiveness too low. The final judgment about these alternatives, he asserts, must be based on the "value placed on personal health services" (p. 207). Controls will be imposed when "the country feels" that costs are too high for what it can afford (p. 208). He also relied upon a vague but shifting "consensus" about the balance between the private and public sectors (p. 198) and the need for broader benefits from voluntary health insurance (p. 200). The trouble with this kind of language is that it blurs a recognition of the political and institutional barriers to change. It assumes that there is wide agreement in the population that the major features of the organization of health care should remain essentially as they are. It fails to recognize that values, feelings, and beliefs presumably held throughout the society are based on very little information about alternatives.

My analysis assumes no such consensus; or rather, it assumes that whatever consensus might be discovered by a public opinion survey is quite dependent upon the specific alternatives for health care available in the society and is not an independent force either maintaining the existing system or pushing for change. A 1971 national survey of opinions of the health care "crisis" bears this out. Fully three-quarters of the sample agreed that "there is a crisis in health care" in the United States. But queried about specifics, satisfaction with almost every aspect of health care was relatively high. The authors' only speculation was that "the individual may tend to believe that his own personal medical care is somewhat better than what the population as a whole is getting."[4] *Both* answers may reflect true attitudes: people question health care as a whole but perceive alternatives neither for themselves nor for the system.

This apparent schizophrenia may be typical of political orientations in the United States, where general dissatisfaction and alienation can exist with few viable channels being perceived for political or social action to change existing institutions. Paradoxically, the more avenues for participation that are opened up for representation on committees, for election of community advisory boards, and for public access to hearings, the more fictitious this representation becomes. The channels of communication become overloaded and no transmission of coherent demands comes through loudly and clearly to policy-making elites. As a consequence, interests which are already controlling the major resources are increasingly insulated from effective challenge. Diversion of particvipatory demands to control over peripheral resources and policies protects the core powers and privileges of dominant interest groups from challenge. Their very definition as being outside the legitimate range of political and administrative demands becomes seen as part of the "basic values," "historical traditions," or "political consensus" of the society, and therefore nearly unchangeable and almost unanalyzable in relation to concrete political actions.

These characteristics of political action have definite functions for maintaining the existing class or stratification system. Both market and bureaucratic reformers are likely to be upper-middle-class in their social origins, incomes, and occupational prestige, and thus they share an interest in moderating conflict and blunting community demands even if they are bitterly divided among themselves over the timing and scope of reforms. Noisy debate conceals an underlying unity of commitment to working through existing political channels, which may account for the unwillingness of the bureaucratic reformers—visibly more dissatisfied with the present orgnization of health care—to mobilize potential allies with the rhetoric and political tactics which could generate an effective movement for change. The ambiguous analyses of the various investigations recommending coordination and planning—and fatal compromises which result (as in the case of the Health and Hospitals Corporation in New York City)—are the ideological corollary of a political commitment not to challenge the essential power of the professional monopolists. [5] As economist Eli Ginzberg put it, "Each of the major parties insists that its essential power remain undiminished as a result of any contemplated large-scale change. . . . Inherent in pluralism is an overwhelming presumption in favor of incremental rather than large-scale reforms. [6]

An explanation of the deep-rooted character of the dynamics without change must thus ultimately go back to the dominance of the private sector and the upper middle class. To quote Ginzberg once again: "The industry remains dominated by the private sector—consumers, private practitioners, voluntary hospitals" (ibid.). Thus, a major characteristic of the public sector is that it does not have the power to challenge the domination of the private sector. Given this domination, it seems a reasonable assumption that major characteristics of the health system are due to private control. Government policy is not fundamentally important, except insofar as the policy is that of *not* interfering with the private sector or of only coming forth with financial subsidies for the private sector.

To say this does not mean that *any* program which increases the government's role will be an advance since any specific government policy may reaffirm the dominance of the private sector, provide additional subsidies for it, or further institutionalize the dichotomy between the public and private sectors. It would be possible, for example, to separate the public sphere of subsidies for the poor, or even government-owned clinics and hospitals, even further from the private sector; and this could be advertised as a step forward in public support for health services for the poor. But if the results were to insulate further the private sector from public mechanisms of funding and control, to set up new public institutions subject to the vacillating funding already discussed, and, moreover, to perpetuate a two-class system of care, then these alleged reforms might better be regarded as a setback.

It is important to emphasize that Ginzberg, in the quotation above, includes the consumers as part of the private sector. If the upper-middle-class consumers of the health care provided by fee-for-service practitioners and hospitals are, in fact, securing most of the medical services they need, then these particular consumers have no incentive to change the system and, in fact, have compelling incentives to keep it the way it is. From their point of view, the only result of a merger of the private with the public sectors would be to *reduce* their capacity to buy care, because their access to the medical and hospital market would be restricted. And this would be most true for the richest consumers. If there were a move to open up the best hospitals and the best surgeons to the public on the basis of need rather than on the basis of the ability to purchase care, the only possible result would be to reduce their access to the market, unless the supply of manpower, beds, and machines were expanded to the point where all, regardless of income, had access to equivalent care. That, of course, would be enormously expensive.

For this reason, which is intrinsically related to the class structure of American society, the vision of merging the two systems—having only one set of offices, clinics, hospitals, beds, wards—is undoubtedly utopian. The symbiosis of upper-middle-class consumers of health care, their private physicians, and their voluntary hospitals constitutes a coalition of structural interests too strong to be defeated by hospital reorganization, Comprehensive Health Planning legislation, or new neighborhood health centers—if the goal is equality of health care.

Given the continuing "crisis" resulting from a system which cannot provide decent care for all because of the domination by the private sector, there is increasing pressure upon government to step in. But, again because of the dominance of the private sector, the government cannot act in a way which could change the system without altering the basic principle of private control over the major resources of the society. Thus the health system exhibits a continuous contradiction between the expectations of the people for decent health care, the impossibility of the private sector to provide decent and *equal* health care for all, and the impossibility of the public sector to compensate for the inadequacies of the private sector.

The most recent reform is the so-called Health Maintenance Organization (HMO) agreed upon by all health reformers and politicians (including two Presidents) because it meets all of the political and economic criteria for a symbolic reform. Market reformers believe that HMO's will restore price competition with the hospitals and will offer consumers a free choice between alternative plans. Bureaucratic reformers believe that they will integrate preventive and ambulatory care in one delivery center and, through prepayment, provide an organizational incentive to reduce costs, duplication of equipment, and so forth.[7] It is premature to evaluate actual HMO's currently being funded. My argument leads me to predict their failure as a general alternative form, although specific ones may succeed in providing more, and less costly, care to special populations.

If this theory of the barriers to structural reforms is accurate, then the optimism suggested by the vision of an impending "post-industrial society" may be premature. Daniel Bell is optimistic that professions will become more "social-minded." "Within medicine... one of the central occupations of a post-industrial society, the inevitable end of the 'fee-for-service' relationship, replaced by some kind of insurance-cum-government payment scheme, means the end of the doctor as an individual entrepreneur and the increasing centrality of the hospital and group practice."[8] This casual prediction of the end of private practice is consistent with Bell's image of the inexorable character of the organization and knowledge revolutions and his central thesis that "the decisive social change taking place in our time... is the subordination of the economic function to the political order" (p. 373). However, he gives no convincing reasons to believe that the political order is in fact dominant or likely to become so or that potential or available social knowledge is in fact used rationally to plan and carry out public policy. The "constraints" upon these changes he himself enumerates seem enormous—the problem of productivity in the service sector, inflation, competition in the world market, competing allocations of resources, and the increasing participation of multiple groups which veto each other (pp. 154–60).

The problem of weighing the relative importance of complex and contradictory social, economic, and political trends is admittedly an intractable one, but I would argue that there is no evidence—in health at the very least—that Bell's image of the possibility of rational social policy is correct.

3. Pluralism in Health:
   Description or Explanation?

The view outlined above contrasts sharply with orthodox pluralist analyses of health care. Pluralism, in my view, may be an accurate description of the diverse mechanisms and institutions providing and financing health care, but it is not an adequate explanation or prescription for change. An example is Professor Dale Hiestand's chapter in Ginzberg et al., *Urban Health Services*. Professor Hiestand defines pluralism as the "division of position, power, responsibility, or obligation among groups or institutions; it implies both sharing and competition, frequently conflict, although it does not imply hostility" (p. 10). He describes the existence of pluralism in the provision of health services, in their financing, and in the institutions which provide resources. Providers (in New York City, at least) include voluntary nonprofit hospitals, municipal hospitals, state and federal hospitals, nursing homes, city clinics, independent medical or allied health practitioners, and so on. Funding sources include any or all of several levels of government, a variety of private and quasi-public (Blue Cross, for example) insurance plans, and the client himself. Resource providers, mainly of manpower, include medical and nursing schools, community colleges, government departments, and others. Any and all of these diverse functions are linked to others through complex networks of interorganizational relationships. For example, an "extensive network of clinical relationships" links the nursing program at Queens College with one or more of six voluntary or city hospitals (p. 21).

"Characteristically," says Hiestand, "the proposals for dealing with pressing problems almost invariably include an expansion in the degree and forms of pluralism. Generally, progress is sought by changing some of the relationships among different parts of the system, but its pluralistic nature is maintained" (pp. 24–25). To put the point in other words, the existing distribution of power and privileges of the various component groups is basically maintained but may be altered slightly. The consequence of this mode of changing the system is a highly conservative equilibrium, or balance, because significant change must inevitably mean stepping on some group's toes.

The high order of pluralism which has been built into the health services complex may mean that there is a strong tendency toward the maintenance of the status quo. With many interest groups built into almost every decision system, each one tends to have a veto over any changes. These vetoes are likely to be exercised by any group which fears that a new departure may undermine or be adverse to its interests. A further implication, therefore, is that innovations must almost inevitably be tailored so as not to threaten any interest groups and at the same time to provide positive incentives for the acquiescence, indeed the active support, of each of them.

Hiestand recognizes what labor leader Walter Reuther did not when the latter denied that the health services constitute a system. According to Reuther (as quoted by Hiestand), America has a "disorganized, disjointed, antiquated, obsolete, non-system of health care." The

National Advisory System on Health Manpower, in a similar conclusion said, "The word 'system' is... inaccurate if it implies the existence of an organized, coordinated, planned undertaking."⁹ Hiestand properly notes that this difference is one of evaluation, not description. "The health services complex is a system, however, but with goals beyond that of simply delivering health services. One basic goal... is to protect the *interests* of the various groups involved in the *production* of these services. This goal, perhaps more than any other factor, accounts for the complexity of the pluralism in the health services sector" (p. 28; italics added).

Part of the job of analyzing the functioning of such a pluralistic system is to ask how the interests of its segments—the health care-producing institutions—prevent any significant improvement in the quality and quantity of health services available to the entire population. From Hiestand's and other analyses, it would seem to be important to answer such questions as the following in analyzing the so-called health delivery system: What are the interests of the doctors in their professional monopoly? Of the hospitals? Of the medical schools? Of the drug and medical supply industries? How do they all draw support from various funding sources without being subjected to public control and planning? Almost no research studies whose subjects fall under the rubric of "health care delivery organization" deal with the question of the interrelated and mutually supportive operations of the pluralistic system which Hiestand has described, nor do they deal with the ways in which such a system effectively prevents significant structural change.

One reason why few such studies exist is hinted at by Hiestand's own extension of his description into normative judgment. Pluralism becomes the *necessary* mode of organization because it exists and because of a failure of organizational imagination to envision an alternative way of producing and delivering health services. Pluralism becomes a *desirable* mode of organization because it seems to represent the diversity of consumer choices and the freedom to compete for the consumer and government dollar by various types of producers—a mode which is identified as the essence of a democratic system by contemporary political theorists.¹⁰

It is within this context that we must reevaluate the diagnoses of crisis by innumerable investigations and the failures of attempts to institute such innovations as neighborhood health centers as additions to the main body of American health care institutions. Here, of course,

I have relied upon qualitative estimates of experts in the field. As we have seen, the paucity of systematic data and analyses of the system as a whole must also be explained.

What explains the initiation of a series of investigations which respond to a health "crisis," attempt to define it, and, year after year, decade after decade, come up with similar recommendations, none of which has any significant impact on the health care system? One would think that after a few such investigations which make the same diagnoses and offer the same criteria for the ideal system, the same guidelines for change, the same recommendations of more studies, coordination, planning, integration, and so forth, the charade would not find participants. This does not seem to be the case. There are always new recruits (as well as old ones) to the game.

The metaphor of a game is a useful one but is more appropriate as a description of the process than as an explanation of it. The basic factor is the separation between the political and nonpolitical and between the public and private spheres in such a way as to reduce public power to a minimum. The most important issues and decisions cannot be dealt with effectively by any governmental agency. This primary fact means that none of the juggling of decisions, of agencies, of leadership, or of administration can decisively affect the outputs of the health system. Government can do little about the basic factors which affect health (income, jobs, housing, sanitation) and also little about the care of sickness (control of the supply and quality of physicians, the distribution and quality of hospitals and ambulatory care facilities). This lack of public power—for which prima facie evidence is that government in fact has *not* exercised such power—means that politics deals with peripheral issues and decisions and becomes nonideological in the sense that conflicts are not over fundamental differences in the allocations of powers and benefits.

An important consequence of the insulation of government—despite its enormous growth—from critically important social and economic forces, is that the political system tends to become self-sustained and autonomous. The rewards possible to individuals within this "sub-system"—career, power, office, prestige, wealth—become all-important, precisely because the incentives and rewards operate within a narrow framework of consequences for other groups, except those groups which already benefit from social institutions as they exist and therefore have no need of government action. Political reality tends to become circumscribed by the battle for election and re-election, for the spoils and patronage of office, because there is relatively little feedback from the consequences of political decisions for other groups and individuals outside the political system per se, except as mediated by political symbolism and myth around elections and "crises."

Commissions of investigation—as interorganizational linkages between the "public" and "private" sectors attempting to renegotiate existing bargains allocating resources—become part of the pragmatic political process. Commissions of investigation must assume that *both* a problem *and* a solution for that problem exist; otherwise they have no reason to issue their reports. In order to appear hardheaded and realistic, they must also take as given certain parameters—the basic health care institutions of the system. They must single out a certain part of the system and the causal factors in that subsystem for analysis and recommendation of policy changes. To the extent (and this is usually problematic) that the system is composed of highly interdependent parts, the recommendations which such a commission makes are not likely to go to the heart of the problem. The men who make up such commissions are likely to be part of the "pluralist consensus," although they may favor or represent one element of a coalition or one side of a controversy in an issue of reform or change, and thus the recommendations may favor some kind of change which alters the powers and resources of one group—doctors, nurses, hospitals, researchers, patients, or the community.

Over and over again, we see even in biting critiques a contradiction between the description of barriers to change in the past and simultaneous optimism for the future. General statements on the condition of medicine almost always start by noting the extraordinary difficulty of instituting any changes, despite general agreement on the professional and organizational model for the best health care. For example, "There has been a persistent and highly laudatory effort to relate public health centers to existing medical-care facilities, and to teaching hospitals and universities.... Yet this relationship has provoked more spoken and published platitudes—with less translation into action—than any other aspect of community medicine in the last 30 years."[11] Despite this analysis of the past, the author concludes with a Panglossian vision for the future: "Fortunately the recent policy statements of the American Public Health Association on the Organization of Medical Care and the Health of the Nation, revolving about the concept of the Community Health Services Center, at last gives a clear framework within which the health professions may program" (pp. 31-32).

This apparent contradiction is not due to stupidity, lack of good will, or even the invalidity of the "clear framework" for reform. Every reform proposal becomes trapped in the pluralist political process which safeguards all existing professional and organizational interests. Following a "crisis," new sources of funds become embroiled in the pluralistic struggle between existing health agencies which are struggling for funds and attempting to define themselves as capable of handling the new, "innovative" programs. Unfortunately, most analyses neglect these constraints upon both the initiation and the implementation of structural reforms.

The "last chapter" rhetoric of many of the general analysts of health care institutions combines optimism about the possibilities of gradual and progressive change with realism about the boundaries or parameters within which whose changes must be contained, but also with a utopian view of the analyst's own role in contributing to those changes. General studies of the health care system play the same role for the informed lay public at large as the commission reports analyzed earlier in this book play for competing elites within the health sector. Their very publication is part of a process of liberal self-criticism. Academics, specialized journalists, and liberal professionals within the health field must assume that there is a public "out there" which is waiting for an insightful analysis which combines optimism and realism.[12] The latent assumption is that insight based on facts and the use of reasonable and moderate interpretations of those insights and facts to draw policy-relevant conclusions are important forces for change of health institutions. A rhetoric combining optimism and realism about the possible changes which are feasible in the near future is best designed to create and sustain the liberal coalition which can move forward to the next stage of progress. Visions of changes which go too far past the emerging consensus on the next possible stage of development will scare off the crucial elements of the coalition—those elements of the medical profession which are themselves dissatisfied and ready for some—if not much—change. The assumption is basically that change must come from within, encouraged by incentives and persuasion from without.

If the reform of health care could in fact be viewed as an isolated instance, then this liberal strategy might well work. However, the analytic and political issue which must first be faced and answered is whether or not this is true. I have argued that the institutional and interest barriers to significant change are found in many different policy areas besides health—housing, manpower training, the environment, education. If this is true, the processes and forces I have described are endemic to the structure of the society and political system as a whole and must be understood at that level, not within the context of a particular institution or the particular interests of doctors and hospitals.

4. Reform Perspectives: Pluralist, Bureaucratic, and Class

Most generally, I believe that one or another of three different models or theories of the causes of existing arrangements in health care and the possibilities of significant change lies behind most of the current debates over health care reform. It is beyond my scope here to deal with these broader issues extensively, but the wider context of theory and debate should at least be mentioned. Since these theories are relatively undeveloped and implicit, it might be better to refer to them as perspectives or viewpoints: (1) the pluralist or market perspective; (2) the bureaucratic or planning perspective; and (3) the institutional or class perspective.[13]

The *pluralist or market perspective* essentially accepts the struggle between interest groups as inevitable and even necessary. This perspective would argue that all of these groups are created and sustained by the technical and organizational requirements of a highly differentiated society and political system. The key professional functions of biomedical research and qualified physician training require that considerable autonomy be given to professional organizations. The key organizational functions of hospital administration, health planning, and the coordination of public health services require that considerable power and resources be given to those agencies and programs seeking to integrate the various components of the health delivery system. In this view, the pluralism and seeming "fragmentation" are endemic and even healthy, because they guarantee diversity by maintaining competition between alternative modes of providing health care.

This perspective on the causes of the present system essentially accepts its main structural features as appropriate for the particular historical mixture of cultural values and economic resources found in a given society. The dilemma of this perspective is that, by basically accepting the structure of health institutions as inevitable, it may neglect possible avenues of change in institutions which would substantially improve access, quality, and costs, and may underestimate the barriers to the implementation of true competition between providers and modes of payment. This perspective leads to minor structural adjustments, mainly to bringing low-income families into the market for health services by providing either free or subsidized services through income maintenance programs or direct payments for health care. However, no major institutional changes are seen as necessary or even desirable.

The *bureaucratic or planning perspective* holds that it is possible rationally to plan and coordinate the health care delivery system in ways which both preserve the necessary professional autonomy of physicians and their personal relationships with patients and also allow for allocation of resources to different sectors of health care in a way which takes account of differences in patient needs, ability to pay, and the appropriate availability of professional care. In this view, the major obstacle to change is the professional monopoly of doctors over medical education and practice, and once their power has been reduced to its proper proportions, it will be possible to devise a coordinated and integrated system, more or less equally available to all. In this view, there are no insuperable barriers to reorganization in the structure of the society as a whole—parts of it (particular institutions) can be changed without any general transformation of the culture or economic or political institutions.

This view does not adhere to a utopian solution either but, rather, believes that a significantly increased degree of coordination and integration is possible, resulting in significantly increased quality and quantity of health services to all, but especially the poor. The dilemma of this perspective is that it may neglect for various dominant interest groups the functions of existing institutions which make it very difficult to coordinate and integrate health care and, in fact, account for the failure of all of the attempts thus far to create a more rational organization of the delivery system. Also—given the complexity and diversity of the components of the system (and thus the inherent difficulty of securing basic data which simply describe the system), let alone the consequences of introducing changes—this perspective may underestimate the potential of the market as an allocative mechanism and overestimate the possibilities of rational planning.

The *institutional or class perspective* holds that the defects in the performance of health institutions are duplicated in many other areas of American society, and that the roots of these defects lie deep in the structure of a class society and create great difficulties for the effective articulation of social needs as political demands and their translation into legislation and subsequent administrative implementation. In this view, professionals and bureaucrats and planners are differentiated

sectors of class-based and class-oriented institutions, performing necessary functions within the severe limits imposed by the political and
economic privileges held by a relatively small part of the population.
The utopian vision implicit in this perspective of equality and justice
and full participation and control by a community population over its
institutions—including those dealing with health—cannot be realized
within any conceivable reform of existing institutions. The dilemma of
this perspective is that it has the danger of leading to a passive neglect
of objective possibilities of significant change—either toward increasing the options available to more persons to choose the kind and source
of health care they want, or toward sharply focusing demands for
health care reform upon elites in specific institutions and actually
significantly reorganizing them, quite apart from changes taking place
in other institutions.

Each of these perspectives implies a different program of action
appropriate to its theory about the causes of the health care "crisis"
and the scope of possible solutions. The pluralist perspective—arguing
essentially that there is no general solution, just as there is no general
crisis in the society—suggests that health insurance is the most
appropriate step to take to patch up the health care system for those
relatively few persons still without access to the system. For the poor
and elderly—those without the income to buy care or with extremely
high needs for care—the government can step in to subsidize the
insurance. Medicaid and Medicare are the prototypical programs for
this view. These are not radical or even barely liberal programs, but
might be regarded as classically conservative types of government
programs: they are—like income maintenance programs and programs
attempting to achieve equality of educational opportunity—devices for
bringing disadvantaged and unfortunate individuals and families to
the level of health, income, and education where they can compete, in
theory, on a relatively equal basis with the other members of a society.
No reorganization of health institutions is required, only a subsidy of
those individuals and families who, through no fault of their own, are
unable to procure care.

The bureaucratic perspective suggests what might be regarded as
essentially a liberal solution: create new forms of organized health care,
in addition to fee-for-service care, for those who want and can afford it.
Comprehensive prepaid care should be available to those who want it
via a variety of governmental subsidies with some kind of rational
coordination and planning of the diverse modes of provision.

As we have argued earlier, the pluralist view emphasizes the need for the autonomy of all of the elements of the health care system—the doctors, the hospitals, the researchers, the medical schools—and opposes a general program of rationalization and subsidy by the government because it will interfere with the operations of a competitive market in health care. Such a market, it is claimed, will drive out the inefficient producers and make the remaining producers more responsive to consumer demand. The bureaucratic view, on the other hand, emphasizes the need for integration of all of the same elements, in order to overcome duplication (which the pluralists hail as diversity), lack of coordination (which the pluralists welcome as competition), and lack of planning (which the pluralists condemn as both unnecessary and impossible).

There is nothing "wrong" in the abstract with any of these programs of change—be they health insurance, coordinating agencies, or new forms of provision of health care through group practices and comprehensive prepaid care. Any or all of them may significantly improve the quality and quantity of care and reduce its cost to groups who do not now have it. These different programs obviously vary in their scope and thus in the extent to which they challenge or support interest groups possessing a stake in health care institutions as they now exist. Battling to extend in any of these ways the right to health care through political action of many kinds is obviously worthwhile.

The institutional or class perspective has the most radical view of the potential and need for change, because it regards American social institutions as in need of fundamental reconstruction. This perspective rejects the implicit assumption of both the pluralist and the bureaucratic perspectives that health care (or any other social "problem") can be isolated from other "problems" and treated all by itself. The defects in current health care are regarded in this perspective as a disease of the entire social organism which must be diagnosed and treated as a whole. No specific can cure the symptoms of illness in the health care system. The institutions and groups entrusted with the provision of health care mirror the society as a whole in the sense that health care is viewed as a commodity, a product, an item of consumption, an object for cost-benefit analysis, a subject for bargaining over (health subsidies versus transportation subsidies). Both the pluralist and the bureaucratic perspectives share this piecemeal view of reform. If one accepts the assumption that the society's institutions and values are basically healthy—that America is a wealthy, democratic, egalitarian society— then it makes sense to analyze and seek to change institutions one by one. But if, as the institutional or class perspective holds, its wealth is composed of a large fraction of useless production for conspicuous consumption, if its democratic political institutions conceal a fundamental lack of access to decision-making power by a large fraction of the population, if its egalitarian ideals are contradicted by sharp inequalities of status, power, and wealth—then perhaps the packaged, public relations presentation of the American dream conceals fundamental and increasingly obvious flaws in the basic capability of the institutions of the society to provide what its technology and productive capacity make possible for the population as a whole.

If the institutional or class analysis is even partly correct, then a much more fundamental struggle to change American social institutions is called for, and this struggle will require the emergence of a social movement and political leadership which is not yet visible. A discussion of the possibility of such a movement is beyond the scope of the present essay, but it should be mentioned that the ultimate test of this perspective is whether such a movement can emerge and, once having emerged, what its fate can become. In the absence of such a movement, either or both the pluralist and the bureaucratic analyses become true by default. The success of strategies based upon them will validate their theories of the limits and sources of change in the institutions of health care. However, successes in bringing about health insurance, health maintenance organizations, and comprehensive prepaid care—valid and valuable though they are—do not rule out a more comprehensive attempt to change health institutions in ways which will fundamentally alter the pervasive tendency to reproduce continuously the same problems and defects, year after year, despite reforms. The fate of these broader struggles is the test of the possibilities suggested by an institutional or class analysis of health care in American society.

Notes

Introduction

1. For a collation of a wide variety of health statistics, see U. S. Congress, Committee on Ways and Means, *Basic Facts on the Health Industry* (Washington, D. C.: U. S. Government Printing Office, 1971).

2. *Medical Care for the American People,* the final report of the Committee on the Costs of Medical Care, adopted 31 October 1932 (reprint ed., Washington, D. C.: U. S. Department of Health, Education and Welfare, 1970.)

3. Sumner N. Rosen, "Change and Resistance to Change," *Social Policy* 1 (January-February 1971): 4.

4. Eli Ginzberg et al., *Urban Health Services: The Case of New York* (New York: Columbia University Press, 1971), p. 224.

5. Wallace S. Sayre and Herbert Kaufman, *Governing New York City: Politics in the Metropolis* (New York: Russell Sage Foundation, 1960), pp. 256–57.

6. Two earlier and shorter versions of chapters 5 and 6 have been published, in *The Social Welfare Forum* (New York: Columbia University Press, 1971), pp. 90–106, and in *Politics and Society* 2 (Winter 1972): 127–64.

1. Health Care Reform and Structural Interests

1. Harry Schwartz, "Health Care in America: A Heretical Diagnosis," *Saturday Review,* 14 August 1971, pp. 14–17, 55; and Milton I. Roemer, "Nationalized Medicine for America," *Trans-Action* 8 (September 1971): 31–36. These articles merely provide concrete illustrations of certain points, and it cannot be assumed that either man holds any views which I summarize under the general categories except those views which are specifically quoted.

2. See Sidney R. Garfield, "The Delivery of Medical Care," *Scientific American* 222 (April 1970): 15–23, for another model along these lines, which is criticized by Schwartz in "Health Care in America."

3. Roland L. Warren, "Alternative Strategies of Inter-Agency Planning," in Paul E. White et al., *Inter-Organizational Research in Health: Proceedings*

of the Johns Hopkins University Conference on Inter-Organizational Relationships in Health, document PB 198 807 (Springfield, Va.: National Technical Information Service, 1970).

4. Barbara and John Ehrenreich, *The American Health Empire: Power, Profits and Politics* (New York: Random House, 1970).

5. Milton I. Roemer, review of *The American Health Empire,* in *International Journal of Health Services* 2 (1972): 119–21. Italics added.

6. Rosemary Stevens, *American Medicine and the Public Interest* (New Haven: Yale University Press, 1971), pp. 481–82, 500.

7. David Mechanic, *Public Expectations and Health Care: Essays on the Changing Organization of Health Services* (New York: John Wiley & Sons, 1972), p. 6.

8. Odin W. Anderson, *Health Care: Can There Be Equity? The United States, Sweden, and England* (New York: John Wiley & Sons, 1972), pp. 194, 176.

9. Dorrian Apple, ed., *Sociological Studies of Health and Sickness: A Source Book for the Health Professions* (New York: McGraw-Hill Book Co., 1960).

10. For an older but still relevant statement of this perspective, see Sol Levine, Paul E. White, and Benjamin D. Paul, "Community Interorganizational Problems in Providing Medical Care and Social Services," *American Journal of Public Health* 53 (August 1963): 1183–95. For a more recent compendium, see White et al., *Interorganizational Research in Health.*

11. Wallace S. Sayre and Herbert Kaufman, *Governing New York City: Politics in the Metropolis* (New York: Russell Sage Foundation, 1960).

12. See Herbert Kaufman, "The Political Ingredient of Public Health Services: A Neglected Area of Research," *The Milbank Memorial Fund Quarterly* 44 (October 1966), part 2, pp. 30–31.

13. See Theodore R. Marmor, *The Politics of Medicare* (Chicago: Aldine Publishing Company, 1973), pp. 9, 98, 110. An English edition of this book was published in 1970. The more recent American edition contains few bibliographic or textual references past 1969.

14. Herbert Harvey Hyman, ed., *The Politics of Health Care: Nine Case Studies of Innovative Planning in New York City* (New York: Praeger Publishers, 1973), p. 188.

15. Bert E. Swanson, "The Politics of Health," in Howard E. Freeman, Sol Levine, and Leo G. Reeder, eds., *Handbook of Medical Sociology,* 2d ed. (Englewood Cliffs, N. J.: Prentice-Hall, 1972), pp. 435–55.

16. See David B. Truman, *The Governmental Process: Political Interests and Public Opinion,* 2d ed. (New York: Alfred A. Knopf, 1971), pp. 34–35. See also Harry Eckstein, *Pressure Group Politics: The Case of the British Medical Association* (Stanford: Stanford University Press, 1960), pp. 9–12, for a discussion of interest and pressure groups. Eckstein uses the term interest group for an important aspect of what I am calling a structural interest—that is, a set of objective interests which need not be involved in politics. If the interest group does become involved, it becomes a pressure group. Eckstein criticizes other pluralist political scientists (S. E. Finer, S. H. Beer, and David Truman) for neglecting the distinction between subjective values and objective interests.

17. The fate of Medicare in 1965 is a case in point. Even after a decisive legislative victory which produced an even stronger bill than proponents had thought possible, the benefits have gradually been eroding because of the escalation of costs. See Marmor, *The Politics of Medicare.*

18. Once again, see Murray Edelman, *The Symbolic Uses of Politics* (Urbana: University of Illinois Press, 1964), for the most cogent description of this process.

19. See Kaufman, "The Political Ingredient of Public Health Services," and Malcolm G. Taylor, "The Role of the Medical Profession in the Formulation and Execution of Public Policy," *The Canadian Journal of Economics and Political Science* 26 (February 1960): 108-27.

20. See Claus Offe, "Political Authority and Class Structures—An Analysis of Late Capitalist Societies," *International Journal of Sociology* 2 (Spring 1972): 73-108.

21. See Reinhard Bendix, *Work and Authority in Industry: Ideologies of Management in the Course of Industrialization* (New York: John Wiley & Sons, 1956), p. xxii, for this view of ideology, drawn from both Max Weber and Karl Mannheim.

22. See Isaac D. Balbus, "The Concept of Interest in Pluralist and Marxian Analysis," *Politics and Society* 1 (February 1971): 151-77, for a recent discussion of this point, and also Eckstein, *Pressure Group Politics.*

2. Commission of Investigation, 1950-1971

1. Report and Staff Studies of the Commission on the Delivery of Personal Health Services, *Community Health Services for New York City* (New York: Frederick A. Praeger, 1969), p. 490. The report was released on 19 December 1967. This Praeger publication is the only publicly available report of the several to be summarized in this chapter. Others were obtained from various city agencies and libraries, but are not collected in any single location, to my knowledge. Several collections of documents on New York City's health institutions can be examined at the Health and Hospital Planning Council of Southern New York, the United Hospital Fund of New York, the Municipal Reference Library (New York City Municipal Building), and the New York Academy of Medicine.

2. New York State Commission of Investigation, "An Investigation Concerning New York City's Municipal Hospitals and the Affiliation Program," eleventh report, March 1969, p. 68.

3. Eli Ginzberg et al, *Urban Health Services: The Case of New York* (New York: Columbia University Press, 1971), p. viii.

4. Ida R. Hoos, *Systems Analysis in Public Policy: A Critique* (Berkeley: University of California Press, 1972), p. 8.

5. I am indebted to Jane Gray for doing the newspaper research and writing this section on the historical background of the various commissions of investigation.

6. All of the parenthetical dates and page numbers in this historical background section refer to the *New York Times.*

7. City of New York Department of Hospitals, Marcus D. Kogel, M.D. Commissioner, "Report of the Mayor's Committee on the Needs of the Department of Hospitals," 17 February 1950, 12 pages. The other eleven members of the Mayor's Committee were George Baehr, Edward M. Bernecker, John J. Bourke, Clarence de la Chapelle, H. A. Helle, Harry S. Mustard, John B. Pastore, Elaine P. Ralli, Willard C. Rappleye, Thomas M. Rivers, and Joseph Tenopyr. All were physicians.

8. "Report of the Commission on Health Services of the City of New York," adopted 20 July 1960, 17 pages. Dr. Ray E. Trussell was the executive director; other members, besides those listed above, were George E. Armstrong, M.D.; George Baehr, M.D. (the only member also on the 1950 Committee); Leona Baumgartner, M.D.; Abraham D. Beame; Norton S. Brown, M.D.; John S. Burke; Edward F. Butler; Martin Cherkasky, M.D.; John A. Coleman; Maurice J. Costello, M.D.; James Felt; Rev. James H. Fitzpatrick; John J. Flynn, M.D.; Henry J. Friendly; Msgr. Patrick J. Frawley; Albert J. Hettinger; Mrs. Harry G. Hill; Frank L. Horsfall, Jr., M.D.; Morris A. Jacobs, M.D.; Francis Kernan; Grayson Kirk; Mrs. Albert D. Lasker; Henry L. McCarthy; Mrs. John J. McCloy; Peter Marshall Murray, M.D.; Raymond J. Nagel, D.D.S.; Charles F. Preusse; Marian Randall; Raymond H. Reiss; Alfred L. Rose; Thomas J. Ross; Victor S. Rosenfeld; Howard C. Sheperd; Harvey J. Tompkins, M.D.; Harry Van Arsdale, Jr.; and George D. Woods.

9. It might be noted here that three of the top officers of the Hospital Council —Ross, Fitzpatrick, and Murray—were members of the Heyman Commission, and nine of the thirty-nine members (23 percent) of the Heyman Commission were on the Kogel Commission.

10. Hospital Council of Greater New York, "New York City and Its Hospitals: A Study of the Roles of the Municipal and Voluntary Hospitals Serving New York City," December 1960, 35 pages. Other members were Carroll J. Dickson; James Felt; Morris A. Jacobs, M.D.; Cloyd Laporte; Peter Marshall Murray, M.D.; Hayden C. Nicholson, M.D.; Harriet I. Pickens; Thomas J. Ross; Nathan S. Sachs; Martin R. Steinberg, M.D.; and Joseph P. Walsh; with George Bugbee, chairman of the Master Plan Committee, as consultant. A longer version with documentation was published by Herbert E. Klarman, *Hospital Care in New York City: The Roles of Voluntary and Municipal Hospitals* (New York: Columbia University Press, 1963). Professor Klarman, at that time Associate Director of the Hospital Council, was the study director.

11. "Report of the Committee on Health Care System Requirements of the Mayor's Advisory Task Force on Medical Economics," 14 February 1966, 28 pages. This small committee was composed of Jack C. Haldeman, M.D., chairman, president of the Hospital Review and Planning Council of Southern New York; George Baehr, M.D., member of the New York City Board of Hospitals, chairman of the New York State Public Health Council, and director emeritus of medicine at Mount Sinai hospital, as well as a founder of the Health Insurance Plan of Greater New York; Martin Cherkasky, M.D., director of Montefiore Hospital and Medical Center in the city; George James, M.D., former Commissioner of Health of New York City and at that time dean of the newly established Mount Sinai Medical School; and

Nora K. Piore, adjunct professor of economics at Hunter College and director of the New York City Urban Medical Economics Research Project. Leonard Schrager, planning associate of the Hospital Review and Planning Council of Southern New York, was the staff for this committee. The chairman of the entire advisory task force was Robert B. Parks, Ph.D., later to be director of the staff studies for the Piel Commission (see section 8 of this chapter).

12. "System Analysis and Planning for Public Health Care in the City of New York," 25 March 1966, 166 pages.

13. Commission on the Delivery of Personal Health Services, *Community Health Services for New York City*. All page numbers are from the Praeger edition, not from the official report issued earlier.

14. Members of the commission were Eveline M. Burns, Professor Emeritus of Social Work, Columbia University School of Social Work; Benjamin J. Buttenwieser, Limited Partner, Kuhn, Loeb and Company; William T. Golden, Corporate Director and Trustee; Leo Gottlieb, Partner, Cleary, Gottlieb, Steen and Hamilton; Francis Kernan, Partner, White Weld and Company; Thomas R. Wilcox, Vice Chairman, First National City Bank; Gerard Piel, Publisher, Scientific American; and Staff Director William Glazier, Assistant for Scientific and Academic Affairs to the President of the Salk Institute for Biological Studies. (The affiliations listed for commission members are the first ones listed in the acknowledgments.)

Members of the Medical Advisory Committee were Dr. George Baehr, Director Emeritus of Medicine, Mount Sinai Hospital; Dr. Henry L. Barnett, Professor of Pediatrics, Albert Einstein College of Medicine, Yeshiva University; Dr. Leona Baumgartner, Visiting Professor of Social Medicine, Harvard Medical School; Dr. Norton S. Brown, Chairman, Committee on Social Policy for Health Care of the New York Academy of Medicine; Dr. Howard Reid Craig, Former Director, New York Academy of Medicine; Dr. Elizabeth B. Davis, Director of Psychiatry, Harlem Hospital; Dr. C. Joseph Delaney, Past President, Medical Society of the County of New York; Dr. Louis M. Hellman, Professor and Chairman, Department of Obstetrics and Gynecology, State University of New York, Downstate Medical Center; Dr. E. Hugh Luckey, Cornell University, New York Hospital Medical Center; Dr. Edwin P. Maynard, Jr., Senior Physician, Brooklyn-Cumberland Medical Center; Dr. Eugene C. McCarthy, Jr., Assistant Professor of Administrative Medicine, School of Public Health and Administrative Medicine, Columbia University; Dr. Peter Rogatz, Director, Long Island Jewish Hospital; Dr. Howard A. Rusk, Director, Institute of Rehabilitation Medicine; and Dr. E. Richard Weinerman, Professor of Medicine and Public Health, Yale School of Medicine.

15. Robb K. Burlage, *New York City's Municipal Hospitals: A Policy Review* (Washington, D.C.: Institute for Policy Studies, 1967).

16. This appendix by Dr. Burns is reprinted as the first chapter in her collection of essays, *Health Services for Tomorrow: Trends and Issues* (New York: Dunellen, 1973), pp. 1–12.

17. E. Richard Weinerman, "Discussion of Paper by Carroll L. Witten: Public-Private Partnership: Its Impact upon Physicians and their

Professional Associates," in " 'Creative Federalism,' 'Partnership in
Health': Slogans or Solutions?" reprinted from the *Bulletin of the New
York Academy of Medicine* 45 (November 1969): 1191, italics in original.
This paper was first presented in a panel at the Health Conference of the
New York Academy of Medicine, 24–25 April 1969.
18. Robert H. Connery et al., *The Politics of Mental Health: Organizing
Community Mental Health in Metropolitan Areas* (New York: Columbia
University Press, 1968), pp. 9, 484, 501, 513.
19. For an analysis of the former, see Charles H. Goodrich, Margaret C.
Olendzki, and George G. Reader, *Welfare Medical Care: An Experiment*
(Cambridge: Harvard University Press, 1970). For descriptions of the latter,
see Howard J. Brown and Raymond S. Alexander, "The Gouverneur Am-
bulatory Care Unit: A New Approach to Ambulatory Care," *American
Journal of Public Health and the Nation's Health* 54 (October 1964):
1661–65; and Howard J. Brown, "Delivery of Personal Health Services and
Medical Services for the Poor: Concessions or Prerogatives," *The Milbank
Memorial Fund Quarterly* 46 (January 1968), part 2, pp. 203–23.
20. Frank A. Sloan, "Planning Public Expenditures on Mental Health Service
Delivery," report RM-6339-NYC (New York: The New York City RAND
Institute, 1971), 94 pages plus appendixes.
21. Murray Edelman, *The Symbolic Uses of Politics* (Urbana: University of
Illinois Press, 1964).
22. Hoos, *Systems Analysis,* pp. 109–10, italics added. She also evaluates (see
pp. 173–92) ill-fated attempts at systems analysis in such diverse policy
areas as the military, water management, education, and the supersonic
transport. For a similar analysis of urban renewal programs, see Garry D.
Brewer, *Politicians, Bureaucrats, and the Consultant: A Critique of Urban
Problem Solving* (New York: Basic Books, 1973).

**3. The Planning Council and
the Coordination of
Health Care**

1. See John D. Stoeckle and Lucy M. Candib, "The Neighborhood Health
Center—Reform Ideas of Yesterday and Today," *The New England Journal of Medicine* 280 (19 June 1969): 1385–91, for a brief history which
makes these points. See Robert M. Hollister, Bernard M. Kramer, and Seymour S. Bellin, eds., *Neighborhood Health Centers* (Lexington, Mass.: Lexington Books, 1974), for a compilation of recent articles on neighborhood
health centers.
2. Herbert Kaufman, "The New York City Health Centers," Inter-University
Case Program (University, Ala.: University of Alabama Press, 1959), 18
pp. The quote is from p. 7.
3. The quotes are Kaufman's paraphrases of the original report; see pp. 3–4.
4. The details in the case studies are drawn from interviews with staff members of the council and from the files of the council, particularly those
dealing with the Neighborhood Family Care Center program for establishing ambulatory care facilities for the poor. I am indebted to the council

for allowing access to these materials. Neither the council nor any staff member is responsible, of course, for any interpretation which I place upon their remarks or the contents of any document.

5. Leonard Schrager, ed., *Planning for Better Health Services: Guidelines and Criteria for Planning Hospital and Related Health Services in New York City* (New York: Health and Hospital Planning Council of Southern New York, 1970). The guidelines referred to are summarized on pp. 38–44; the booklet contains guidelines for other types of health services as well.

6. Personal communication from Dr. Leonard Rosenfeld, 18 September 1973.

7. This account is a summary of the file at the Health and Hospital Planning Council of Southern New York, Inc. Although the proposal was not implemented, the file is complete enough to indicate some of the steps taken by various groups and organizations and the relationships and contacts between them.

8. Personal communication from Herbert Williams, Senior Planning Associate, Health and Hospital Planning Council, 18 September 1973.

4. Health Care and New York City: Unique or Typical?

1. For a summary of eight such studies conducted from 1952 to 1967, see the City of New York Commission on State-City Relations, *A Study of the Studies: An Analysis of the Work and Recommendations of a Generation of Task Forces on New York City's Fiscal Crisis* (New York, 1971), 31 pages. This commission was established by Mayor Lindsay on 15 July 1971; its chairman was William J. vandenHeuvel, and its staff director was Dr. Jewel Bellush.

2. William Worthington and Laurens H. Silver, "Regulation of Quality of Care in Hospitals: The Need for Change," *Law and Contemporary Problems* 35 (Spring 1970): 306–7.

3. Rosemary Stevens, *American Medicine and the Public Interest* (New Haven: Yale University Press, 1971), p. 506. The first quote was from Dr. Knowles' testimony before a Senate hearing in 1968.

4. Odin W. Anderson and Joanna Kravits, *Health Services in the Chicago Area: A Framework for Use of Data,* research series no. 26 (Chicago: Center for Health Administration Studies, University of Chicago, 1968), pp. 100–101.

5. Raymond S. Duff and August B. Hollingshead, *Sickness and Society* (New York: Harper and Row, 1968). See chapter 7, below, for more details on this study.

6. Robert A. Derzon, "The Politics of Municipal Hospitals," in Douglass Cater and Philip R. Lee, eds., *Politics of Health* (New York: Medcom Press, 1972), p. 137.

7. Robert N. Wilson, *Community Structure and Health Action: A Report on Process Analysis* (Washington, D.C.: National Commission on Community Health Services, Public Affairs Press, 1968), p. 38. This study was based on interviews with business, professional, and political leaders, and this summary is based on their *perceptions* of the community's problems.

8. Ralph W. Conant, *The Politics of Community Health*, report of the Community Action Studies Project, National Commission on Community Health Services (Washington, D.C.: Public Affairs Press, 1968).

9. Clark C. Havighurst, "Regulation of Health Facilities and Services by 'Certificate of Need,' " *Virginia Law Review* 59 (October 1973): 1198.

10. For an analysis of health planning as a form of technocratic ideology, see Elliott A. Krause, "Health Planning as a Managerial Ideology," *International Journal of Health Services* 3 (Summer 1973): 445-63. Krause analyzes five federal programs: Hill-Burton, Comprehensive Mental Health Planning, OEO Neighborhood Health Centers, Regional Medical Programs, and Comprehensive Health Planning.

11. Bernard J. Frieden and James Peters, "Urban Planning and Health Services: Opportunities for Cooperation," *Journal of the American Institute of Planners* 36 (March 1970): 82-95.

12. Cyril Roseman, "Problems and Prospects for Comprehensive Health Planning," *American Journal of Public Health* 62 (January 1972): 16-18.

13. Walter J. Dickey, James L. Kestell, and Carl W. Ross, "Comprehensive Health Planning— Federal, State, Local: Concepts and Realities," *Wisconsin Law Review,* 1970, p. 874.

14. See Odin W. Anderson, *Health Care: Can There Be Equity? The United States, Sweden, and England* (New York: John Wiley & Sons, 1972), pp. 175-83, for a summary and critique of several of these: the National Advisory Commission on Health Manpower (1967), the National Commission on Community Health Services (1968), the Secretary's Advisory Committee on Hospital Effectiveness (1968), the National Advisory Committee on Health Facilities (1969), and the Task Force on Medicaid and Related Programs (1970).

15. Stevens, *American Medicine and the Public Interest,* pp. 170-71. For an extended summary and discussion of the extensive research done and recommendations produced by the Committee on the Cost of Medical Care, see Odin W. Anderson, *The Uneasy Equilibrium: Private and Public Financing of Health Services in the United States, 1875-1965* (New Haven: College and University Press, 1968), pp. 91-103.

16. For a summary of the A.M.A.'s reaction to the recommendations of the 1932 report of the Committee on the Costs of Medical Care, see Elton Rayack, *Professional Power and American Medicine: The Economics of the American Medical Association* (New York: World Publishing Company, 1967), pp. 146-55. An editorial in the *Journal of the American Medical Association* appropriately identified the "great foundations, public health officialdom, social theory" as the forces advocating what I am calling corporate rationalization of health care (p. 149).

17. See Eliot Freidson, *The Profession of Medicine: A Study of the Sociology of Applied Knowledge* (New York: Dodd, Mead, & Co., 1970).

18. *Improving Health Care through Research and Development,* report of the Panel on Health Services Research and Development of the President's Science and Advisory Committee, Office of Science and Technology, Exec-

utive Office of the President (Washington, D.C.: U. S. Government Printing Office, 1972), pp. 49-50.

19. American Hospital Association, *AMERIPLAN: A Proposal for the Delivery and Financing of Health Services in the United States,* report of a Special Committee on the Provision of Health Services (Chicago: AHA, 1970).

20. Stevens, *American Medicine and the Public Interest,* p. 502.

21. Joseph P. Fried, *Housing Crisis U.S.A.* (New York: Praeger Publishers, 1971), p. 61.

22. Ruth Roemer, Jeanne E. Frink, and C. Kramer, "Environmental Health Services: Multiplicity of Jurisdictions and Comprehensive Environmental Management," *Milbank Memorial Fund Quarterly* 49, no. 4, pt. 1 (October 1971): 419-507.

23. Peter Schrag, *Village School Downtown: Politics and Education—A Boston Report* (Boston: Beacon Press, 1967), pp. 70, 71.

24. Norman I. Fainstein and Susan S. Fainstein, "Innovation in Urban Bureaucracies: Clients and Change," *American Behavioral Scientist* 15 (March/April 1972): 513.

25. Roger H. Davidson, *The Politics of Comprehensive Manpower Legislation* (Baltimore: The Johns Hopkins University Press, 1972), p. 5.

5. Structural Interests and Structural Conflict

1. Michael Davis in Michael M. Davis and C. Rufus Rorem, *Crisis in Hospital Finance* (Chicago: University of Chicago Press, 1932), p. 76.

2. Michael M. Davis, *Medical Care for Tomorrow* (New York: Harper and Brothers, 1955), pp. 34-35.

3. For a provocative discussion of the struggles of many occupations to attain prestige and higher income and to eliminate competition through occupational licensing, see Lawrence M. Friedman, "Freedom of Contract and Occupational Licensing, 1890-1910: A Legal and Social Study," *California Law Review* 53 (May 1965): 487-534. Friedman argues that once state power has been appropriated by the occupation " 'intellectual technique' and 'training' can be invented and enforced as a 'prerequisite' at the will of the leaders of the occupational group" (p. 505). His point that "the success of licensing laws depends upon the absence of organized economic adversaries" (p. 524) suggests that the current challenge to fee-for-service medical practice by HMO's and other forms of prepaid group practice is rationally feared by solo physicians.

4. Uwe E. Reinhardt, "Proposed Changes in the Organization of Health-Care Delivery: An Overview and Critique," *Milbank Memorial Fund Quarterly* 51 (Spring 1973): 172. See also Elton Rayack, *Professional Power and American Medicine: The Economics of the American Medical Association* (New York: World Publishing Company, 1967), pp. 273-74.

5. Milton I. Roemer and Jay Friedman, *Doctors in Hospitals: Medical*

Staff Organization and Hospital Performance (Baltimore: The Johns Hopkins Press, 1971), p. 8.

6. Anne R. Somers, *Hospital Regulation: The Dilemma of Public Policy* (Princeton, New Jersey: Princeton University Industrial Relations Section, 1969), p. 46. Even the Internal Revenue Service operates on the principle of "customary" allowances of very high salaries for specialists, free equipment and space, discounts, and so forth. This is an excellent example of the way various institutions function to allow the persistence of privileges for a given structural interest.

7. David Mechanic, *Politics, Medicine, and Social Science* (New York: John Wiley & Sons, 1974), p. 38.

8. Ibid., p. 49.

9. Rosemary Stevens, *American Medicine and the Public Interest* (New Haven: Yale University Press, 1971), pp. 218–19.

10. See ibid., pp. 219–43, for a discussion of pediatrics, psychiatry and neurology, radiology and pathology, internal medicine, and the various surgical specialties. With respect to the pediatrician, Stevens comments, "Whether for most of his work he needed his long specialty training was a question both unanswered and unrecognized" (p. 222).

11. Rayack, *Professional Power and American Medicine,* p. 210.

12. Eliot Freidson, *Professional Dominance: The Social Structure of Medical Care* (New York: Atherton Press, 1970).

13. Theodore R. Marmor and David Thomas, "Doctors, Politics, and Pay Disputes in Advanced Industrial Countries: An Essay Review and A Research Note," Discussion Paper No. 125, Institute for Research on Poverty, University of Wisconsin, 1972, p. 29. For the original cross-national data, see William A. Glaser, *Paying the Doctor: Systems of Remuneration and Their Effects* (Baltimore: The Johns Hopkins Press, 1970).

14. Somers, *Hospital Regulation,* p. 35. See also Roemer and Friedman, *Doctors in Hospitals,* p. 1, for a similar statement.

15. See Roemer and Friedman, *Doctors in Hospitals,* which is an intensive case study of ten hospitals and a less intensive study of 2,400 general hospitals with more than fifty beds in the United States in the middle 1960s. They developed a "medical staff organization" (MSO) score from nineteen indicators of "rigorous" versus "permissive" staff organization, to study the ten hospitals, and a "contractual physician score" (the percent of staff physicians under contract in a hospital) for the 2,400 hospitals (pp. 11, 301).

16. Somers, *Hospital Regulation,* p. 101.

17. Clark C. Havighurst, "Regulation of Health Facilities and Services by 'Certificate of Need,' " *Virginia Law Review* 59 (October 1973): 1146.

18. Ibid., p. 1210. This is the so-called Roemer effect, that the more beds there are, the more utilization there will be—because of the capacity of physicians to create demand. See Milton I. Roemer and Max Shain, *Hospital Utilization Under Insurance,* Hospital Monograph Series No. 6 (Chicago: American Hospital Assocation, 1959), and Max Shain and Milton I.

Roemer, "Hospital Costs Relate to the Supply of Beds," *Modern Hospital* 92 (April 1959): 71-73, 168.

19. Rodney F. White, "The Hospital Administrator's Emerging Professional Role," in Mary F. Arnold, L. Vaughn Blankenship, and John M. Hess, editors, *Administering Health Systems: Issues and Perspectives* (Chicago: Aldine-Atherton, 1971), p. 66.

20. See Ray H. Elling, "The Hospital-Support Game in Urban Center," in Eliot Freidson, ed., *The Hospital in Modern Society* (New York: The Free Press of Glencoe, 1963), p. 107. Elling used the metaphor of a "game" to indicate the way hospitals played off community support and federal funds against each other in order to expand.

21. Ray E. Brown, "A Hospital View: Problems of Fragmentation," *Bulletin of the New York Academy of Medicine* 41 (January 1965): 40-41.

22. For a summary of the emerging conflicts and coalitions within and between segments of the corporate rationalizers, see "Power to the Coalitions: Experts See New Balance of Health Care Forces," *Modern Hospital* 114 (April 1970): 39-40d. This article is a candid summary of the conclusions from a meeting in March 1970 of 23 leading hospital executives, hospital consultants, and health association people. The article is written by one of the participants in the off-the-record meeting. It describes three new power centers: first, the physicians (mainly those in salaried or hospital practice), allied professionals, and medical managers; second, the third-party purchasers such as Blue Cross and Blue Shield and their group and individual members; and third, government. Consistent with the ideological stance of corporate rationalization, the article just assumes a "growing identity of interest between medical practitioners and medical care managers" (p. 40). See also Charles Perrow, "Interorganizational Research in the Field of Health," paper prepared for the Johns Hopkins Conference on Interorganizational Research in Health, sponsored by HEW, New York, 21-22 October 1971, for comments on the above article from the point of view of the *lack* of concern in the interorganizational literature for such problems, focusing instead on hospital mergers and health planning and coordinating agencies. Perrow applauds the attempt in this article to deal with the emerging power centers, but questions its (and almost every other study's) exclusion of the hospital supply companies and the drug companies as powerful elements shaping the health care system.

23. Jay W. Forrester, *Urban Dynamics* (Cambridge: The MIT Press, 1969), p. 9.

24. See the Report of the Commission on Health Services of the City of New York, 20 July 1960.

25. See the Report and Staff Studies of the Commission on the Delivery of Personal Health Services, *Community Health Services for New York City* (New York: Frederick A. Praeger, 1969).

26. See the "Preliminary Report of the Governor's Steering Committee on Social Problems on Health and Hospital Services and Costs," 15 April 1971. Page numbers in parentheses refer to this report, hereafter cited as *Preliminary Report*.

27. U.S. Department of Health, Education, and Welfare, *Report of the Task Force on Medicaid and Related Programs* (Washington, D.C.: U. S. Government Printing Office, 1970). Hereafter cited as *Task Force.*

28. Quoted in Herman Miles Somers and Anne Ramsay Somers, *Medicare and the Hospitals: Issues and Prospects* (Washington, D.C.: The Brookings Institution, 1967), p. 136.

29. Gerald E. Markowitz and David Karl Rosner, "Doctors in Crisis: A Study in the Use of Medical Education Reform to Establish Modern Professional Elitism in Medicine," *American Quarterly* 25 (March 1973): p. 84.

30. Eliot Freidson, *The Profession of Medicine: A Study of the Sociology of Applied Knowledge* (New York: Dodd, Mead, & Co., 1970).

31. Rayack, *Professional Power and American Medicine,* p. 63.

32. Roemer and Friedman, *Doctors in Hospitals,* p. 283. The authors cite several studies of New England, New York, Michigan, and California hospitals which support this generalization.

33. For a case history of one hospital which illustrates the various forms of conflict as well as accommodation between trustees, administrators, and medical staff, see Charles Perrow, "Goals and Power Structures: A Historical Case Study," in Freidson, ed., *The Hospital in Modern Society,* pp. 112–46.

34. Stevens, *American Medicine and the Public Interest,* pp. 305–6.

35. Ibid., pp. 307–8. For details on the battle by the American Medical Association to maintain the professional monopoly of physicians, see "The American Medical Association: Power, Purpose, and Politics in Organized Medicine," *Yale Law Journal* 63 (May 1954): 938–1022. It is interesting to note that two key cases lost by the association involving their challenge of prepaid group practice (a U. S. Supreme Court decision in 1943 favoring the Group Health Association in the District of Columbia and a Washington Supreme Court decision in 1951 favoring the Puget Sound Group Health Cooperative) both were based on an explicit challenge to the medical monopoly (pp. 990–92). See also Rayack, *Professional Power and American Medicine,* pp. 180–95.

36. Seymour E. Harris, *The Economics of American Medicine* (New York: Macmillan, 1964), p. 10.

37. Special report, "Radiology Official Says Separate Billing Works," *Modern Hospital* 112 (January 1969): 58.

38. Stevens, *American Medicine and the Public Interest,* p. 464.

39. Harris, *The Economics of American Medicine,* pp. 9–10.

6. Community Participation, Politics, and Bureaucracy

1. For more references in an article with a similar perspective, see Michael Lipsky and Morris Lounds, Jr., "Citizen Participation and Health Care: Problems of Government-Induced Participation," unpublished paper, Massachusetts Institute of Technology, n.d.

2. Dr. Martin Luther King, Jr., Health Center, New York City, *Annual Report,* 31 December 1969, p. 15.

3. Ibid., p. 14.

4. The same problems plague the free-clinic movement as well. Sponsorship of a neighborhood health center in a poor area with few health facilities thus has little to do with the structural causes of its failure to become a long-range solution. See, for example, Health/PAC *Bulletin*, no. 34. (October 1971).

5. Martin Cherkasky, "New Dimensions for the Hospital in Meeting Community Needs: The Relationship of Public and Voluntary Hospitals," *Bulletin of the New York Academy of Medicine* 41 (January 1965): 125-31; the quote is from p. 127.

6. John H. Knowles, "The Role of the Hospital: The Ambulatory Clinic," *Bulletin of the New York Academy of Medicine* 41 (January 1965): 71.

7. Jerome L. Schwartz, "Preliminary Observations of Free Clinics," in David E. Smith, David J. Bentel, and Jerome L. Schwartz, eds., *The Free Clinic: A Community Approach to Health Care and Drug Abuse* (Beloit, Wis.: STASH Press, 1971), p. 152.

8. Ibid., p. 199. Schwartz places his faith in "patient participation in clinic decision making" as the way free clinics can avoid "becoming part of the Establishment."

9. Rosemary C. R. Taylor, "Consumer Control and Professional Accountability in the Free Clinic," unpublished paper, 1973—part of her Ph.D. dissertation in progress (1974) in the Department of Sociology at the University of California at Santa Barbara.

10. Charles M. Brecher and Miriam Ostow, "Ambulatory Services," in Eli Ginzberg et al., *Urban Health Services: The Case of New York* (New York: Columbia University Press, 1971), pp. 155-57.

11. *Federal Role in Health,* report of the Committee on Government Operations, United States Senate, made by its Subcommittee on Executive Reorganization and Government Research, 91st Congress, 2d Session, report no. 91-809 (Washington, D.C.: U. S. Government Printing Office, 1970), pp. 25-26.

12. Ibid., pp. 18-19.

13. James A. Shannon, M.D., "Health Activities: Federal Expenditures and Public Purpose," analysis submitted by the Subcommittee on Executive Reorganization and Government Research to the Committee on Government Operations, United States Senate, June 1970 (Washington, D.C.: U.S. Government Printing Office, 1970).

14. U. S. Department of Health, Education, and Welfare, *Report of the Task Force on Medicaid and Related Programs* (Washington, D.C.: U. S. Government Printing Office, 1970), p. 29; hereafter cited as *Task Force.*

15. "Preliminary Report of the Governor's Steering Committee on Social Problems on Health and Hospital Costs," 15 April 1971, p.16; hereafter cited as *Preliminary Report.*

16. David Mechanic, review of *The American Health Empire: Power, Profits, and Politics,* by Barbara and John Ehrenreich, and *The Quality of Mercy,* by Selig Greenberg, in *Science* 172 (14 May 1971): 701.

17. Philip R. Lee, M.D., "Government and the American Hospital," in James

E. Hague, ed., *The American Hospital System* (Pensacola, Fla.: Hospital Research and Development Institute, Inc., 1968), p. 84.

18. Rosemary Stevens and Robert Stevens, "Medicaid: Anatomy of a Dilemma," *Law and Contemporary Problems* 35 (Spring 1970): 405–6.

19. William B. Schwartz, "Policy Analysis in the Health Care System," *Science* 177 (15 September 1972): 968.

20. Robert H. Connery et al., *The Politics of Mental Health: Organizing Community Mental Health in Metropolitan Areas* (New York: Columbia University Press, 1968), p. 501.

21. William Worthington and Laurens H. Silver, "Regulation of Quality of Care in Hospitals: The Need for Change," *Law and Contemporary Problems* 35 (Spring 1970): 312–14.

22. See Murray Edelman, *The Symbolic Uses of Politics* (Urbana: University of Illinois Press, 1964) and *Politics as Symbolic Action: Mass Arousal and Quiescence* (Chicago: Markham Publishing Company, 1971) for an elaboration of this point.

23. I am indebted to Jonathan Cole for suggesting this possibility to me.

24. On this point, see Arthur L. Stinchcombe, *Constructing Social Theories,* (New York: Harcourt, Brace and World, 1968), pp. 189–90, in the context of a comment upon Edward C. Banfield's analysis of city politics.

25. See Richard D. Alba, "Who Governs—The Power Elite? It's All in How You Define It," *The Human Factor* [Journal of the Graduate Sociology Student Union, Columbia University] 10 (Spring 1971): 27–39, for an elaboration of this point. Although it may be obvious, it should perhaps be made more explicit that my position here directly contradicts those who assert that power is seen or is manifest only in instances of conflict and that the assessment of who wins in such conflicts is an adequate measure of power.

7. Consequences for Health Research

1. *Report of the National Advisory Commission on Health Manpower,* 2 vols. (Washington, D.C.: U. S. Government Printing Office, 1967), 1:4.

2. Merwyn Greenlick, "Imperatives of Health Services Research," *Health Services Research* 4 (Winter 1969): 259. According to Dr. Rashi Fein, "since experimentation is such a characteristic of medicine, it is surprising that delivery of care has not been an area of serious investigation and part of the serious research activity" (Rashi Fein, *The Doctor Shortage: An Economic Diagnosis* [Washington, D. C.: The Brookings Institution, 1967], p. 118).

3. David Mechanic, *Public Expectations and Health Care: Essays on the Changing Organization of Health Services* (New York: John Wiley & Sons, 1972), p. 295.

4. Eliot Freidson, "The Organization of Medical Practice," in Howard E. Freeman, Sol Levine, and Leo G. Reeder, eds., *Handbook of Medical Sociology,* 2d ed. (Englewood Cliffs, N.J.: Prentice-Hall, 1972), pp. 355–56.

5. Odin W. Anderson and Joanna Kravits, *Health Services in the Chicago Area: A Framework for Use of Data,* research series no. 26 (Chicago: Center for Health Administration Studies, University of Chicago, 1968), p. 4.

6. Uwe E. Reinhardt, "Proposed Changes in the Organization of Health-Care Delivery: An Overview and Critique," *Milbank Memorial Fund Quarterly: Health and Society* 51 (Spring 1973): 169–70.

7. See ibid., pp. 186ff., for this critique of existing research in health economics.

8. *Improving Health Care through Research and Development,* report of the Panel on Health Services Research and Development of the President's Science Advisory Committee, Office of Science and Technology, Executive Office of the President (Washington, D.C.: U. S. Government Printing Office, 1972), pp. 3–4.

9. Reinhardt, "Proposed Changes in the Organization of Health Care Delivery," p. 178.

10. See Freeman, Levine, and Reeder, eds., *Handbook of Medical Sociology,* for the most recent overview of research in medical sociology.

11. Ralph E. Berry, Jr., "Competition and Efficiency in the Market for Hospital Services: The Structure of the American Hospital Industry," Harvard University Program on Health and Medical Care, 1965, p. 114.

12. Gerald D. Rosenthal, *The Demand for General Hospital Facilities, 1964,* Hospital Monograph Series no. 14 (Chicago: American Hospital Association, 1964).

13. Charles H. Goodrich, Margaret C. Olendzki, and George G. Reader, *Welfare Medical Care: An Experiment* (Cambridge, Mass.: Harvard University Press, 1970), pp. 214–15.

14. See Raymond S. Duff and August B. Hollingshead, *Sickness and Society* (New York: Harper and Row, 1968). The quotation is from the foreword by F. C. Redlich.

15. Milton I. Roemer and William Shonick, "HMO Performance: The Recent Evidence," *Milbank Memorial Fund Quarterly: Health and Society* 51 (Summer 1973): 271.

8. Crisis, Pluralism, and Perspectives on Reform

1. See Barbara and John Ehrenreich, *The American Health Empire: Power, Profits, and Politics* (New York: Random House, 1970), a publication of the activist New York group Health/PAC, for a similar perspective, although the authors are more optimistic about the prospects for and consequences of militant community action isolated from broader movements than my argument would lead me to be. Michael J. Halberstam, in "Liberal Thought, Radical Theory and Medical Practice," *New England Journal of Medicine* 284 (27 May 1971): 1180–85, criticizes the "radical" position on health care for essentially accepting the position I have called "bureaucratic reform." Interestingly, this criticism would apply also to the proposals advanced by Robb K. Burlage, one of the founders of Health/PAC

(see his *New York City's Municipal Hospitals: A Policy Review* [Washington, D.C.: Institute for Policy Studies, 1967]). Halberstam, himself a physician, stresses the importance of reducing alienation and depersonalization and believes that only committed individual responsibility to a patient by a health professional can provide such personalized care. In this respect the "radical" position exhibits a curious schizophrenia between a faith in the potential rationality of large-scale organization and a faith in the redeeming power of community control. Perhaps the two can be reconciled, but there have been few serious efforts to think through the problem.

2. David Mechanic, *Public Expectations and Health Care: Essays on the Changing Organization of Health Services* (New York: John Wiley & Sons, 1972), p. 99.

3. Odin W. Anderson, *The Uneasy Equilibrium: Private and Public Financing of Health Services in the United States, 1875–1965* (New Haven: College and University Press, 1968), p. 207.

4. Ronald Andersen, Joanna Kravits, and Odin W. Anderson, "The Public's View of the Crisis in Medical Care: An Impetus for Changing Delivery Systems?" *Economic and Business Bulletin* 24 (Fall 1971): 51.

5. See Edmund O. Rothschild, "The Level of Health Care in Municipal Hospitals is Shocking," *New York Times,* 27 November 1971, p. 131, for another surfacing of the same old situation in the New York City hospitals, allegedly to be cured by the bureaucratic reforms recommended by the Piel Commission, including the Health and Hospitals Corporation. At the time he wrote the article, Rothschild was an attending physician at Memorial Hospital for Cancer and a member of the board of directors of the Health and Hospitals Corporation.

6. Eli Ginzberg et al., *Urban Health Services: The Case of New York* (New York: Columbia University Press, 1971), p. 226.

7. For examples of arguments for HMO's which essentially start from these different premises, see Milton I. Roemer and William Shonick, "HMO Performance: The Recent Evidence," *Milbank Memorial Fund Quarterly: Health and Society* 51 (Summer 1973): 271–317, an article mainly concerned with health planning and public monitoring of the HMO form and critical of some economists' assumption, for example, that the number of patient visits is an output measure of efficiency. A somewhat different view is presented in James F. Blumstein and Michael Zubkoff, "Perspectives on Government Policy in the Health Sector," *Milbank Memorial Fund Quarterly: Health and Society* 51 (Summer 1973): 395–431, an article emphasizing restriction of government activity which hinders "increasing effectiveness of the market mechanism" (p. 395).

8. Daniel Bell, *The Coming of Post-Industrial Society: A Venture in Social Forecasting* (New York: Basic Books, 1973), p. 154.

9. Quoted in Dale L. Hiestand, "Pluralism in Health Services," in Ginzberg et al., *Urban Health Services,* p. 27.

10. For an example in health, consider that "competition between HMOs and fee-for-service medicine would maximize consumer choice and would determine most democratically—by consumer votes—the role of each system in

the delivery of care" (Clark C. Havighurst, "Health Maintainence Organizations and the Market for Health Services, *Law and Contemporary Problems* 35 [Autumn 1970]: 724).

11. See Norman R. Ingraham, "A Public Health View: Problems of Coordination," *Bulletin of the New York Academy of Medicine* 41 (January 1965): 28–36; the quote is from p. 31.

12. For only three of the many examples which could be cited, see the October 1973 issues of the *Atlantic Monthly* and the *Washington Monthly* and the special issue of the *New Leader,* "Where Does It Hurt?" 15 April 1974.

13. For a generalization of these perspectives into paradigms of state-society relations, see Robert R. Alford, *Political Sociology* (Englewood Cliffs, N.J.: Prentice-Hall, forthcoming.)

Selected Bibliography

The following brief bibliography includes only a few recent books, articles, and journals. Some items are included because they contain extensive bibliographies themselves on particular subjects, others because they represent a point of view analyzed in the text.

Arnold, Mary F., L. Vaughn Blankenship, and John M. Hess, eds. *Administering Health Systems: Issues and Perspectives.* Chicago: Aldine-Atherton, 1971.

Twenty-three essays on issues in administering, planning, and coordinating the health system (i.e., from the point of view of "corporate rationalization"). Bibliographies, but few items published after 1968.

Edelman, Murray. *The Symbolic Uses of Politics.* Urbana: University of Illinois Press, 1964.

Presents the basic distinction between symbolic and tangible rewards from political action which underlies this book.

Ehrenreich, Barbara, and Ehrenreich, John. *The American Health Empire: Power, Profits, and Politics.* New York: Random House, 1970.

A biting critique of the drug industry and the new medical "empires" by a group of equal-health advocates. Mainly concerned with New York City institutions.

Freeman, Howard E.; Levine, Sol; and Reeder, Leo G. editors. *Handbook of Medical Sociology,* second ed. (Englewood Cliffs, N.J.: Prentice-Hall, 1972).

Twenty-one articles on every aspect of medical sociology. Sixty-page general bibliography, up to mid-1970, plus more specialized chapter bibliographies.

Freidson, Eliot. *The Profession of Medicine: A Study of the Sociology of Applied Knowledge.* New York: Dodd, Mead & Co., 1970.

The most thorough study and evaluation of the claims of physicians to a professional monopoly.

Gilb, Corinne Lathrop. *Hidden Hierarchies: The Professions and Government.* New York: Harper & Row, 1966.

An overview of the relations between professions and the state. Comprehensive bibliography.

Ginzberg, Eli, et al. *Urban Health Services: The Case of New York.* New York: Columbia University Press, 1971.

Essays on various aspects of New York City health institutions.

Havighurst, Clark C. "Regulation of Health Facilities and Services by 'Certificate of Need.'" *Virginia Law Review* 59 (October 1973): 1143–1232.

A comprehensive review of the advantages and disadvantages of state laws requiring administrative approval of new health facilities, from the point of view of a "market reformer." Extensive bibliography.

Health/PAC *Bulletin.*
Reports on national developments by militant equal-health advocates.

Hoos, Ida R. *Systems Analysis in Public Policy: A Critique.* Berkeley: University of California Press, 1972.
An analysis and critique of the assumptions of "systems analysis," one of the ideological weapons of corporate rationalization.

International Journal of Health Services. Special issue on "The Political Economy of Health Care." Summer 1973.

Journal of Health and Social Behavior.
Sociological in orientation.

Law, Sylvia A. *Blue Cross: What Went Wrong?* New Haven: Yale University Press, 1974.
This, the first comprehensive analysis of the major hospital insurance agency in the United States, concludes that Blue Cross, although acting as a fiscal intermediary for Medicare and Medicaid, is neither responsive nor accountable to either the public or its subscribers. Extensive references to the legal literature and to court cases. Prepared by the Health Law Project, University of Pennsylvania.

Law and Contemporary Problems. "Health Care," Parts I and II. Summer and Autumn 1970.
Detailed studies of fundamental policy issues in health, mainly from a legal perspective.

Mechanic, David. *Politics, Medicine, and Social Science.* New York: John Wiley & Sons, 1974.
A collection of essays and articles on a wide variety of topics.

Milbank Memorial Fund Quarterly: Health and Society.
Edited by public health officials, academics, health economists, community and social medicine specialists, and contains a wide variety of policy-related articles.

Rayack, Elton. *Professional Power and American Medicine: The Economics of the American Medical Association.* New York: The World Publishing Company, 1967.

Reinhardt, Uwe E. "Proposed Changes in the Organization of Health-Care Delivery: An Overview and Critique." *Milbank Memorial Fund Quarterly: Health and Society* 51 (Spring 1973): 169–222.
Bibliography focusing on literature in health economics.

Rutstein, David D. *Blueprint for Medical Care.* Cambridge, Mass.: The MIT Press, 1974.
An ideal vision of rationally organized health care, complete with "guidance systems," but no indication of how the barriers might be overcome.

Somers, Anne R. *Hospital Regulation: The Dilemma of Public Policy.* Princeton, N.J.: Princeton University Industrial Relations Section, 1969.
A history and analysis of various public control of hospitals through tax law, licensure, and various types of regulation. The author regards the hospital as the central institution in the provision of health care.

Stevens, Rosemary. *American Medicine and the Public Interest.* New Haven: Yale University Press, 1971.
The most comprehensive recent study of the origins and structure of medical institutions in the United States.

Index

Note: All organizations are located in New York City unless otherwise indicated. Members of the commissions whose reports are summarized in chapter 2 are not listed in the index. Their names are given on pages 270 and 271.